A Clinical Approach to Regional Anesthesiology

A Clinical Approach to Regional Anesthesiology

Editor: Mercy Rogers

FOSTER
ACADEMICS
www.fosteracademics.com

www.fosteracademics.com

FOSTER ACADEMICS

Cataloging-in-Publication Data

A clinical approach to regional anesthesiology / edited by Mercy Rogers.
p. cm.
Includes bibliographical references and index.
ISBN 978-1-64646-582-8
1. Conduction anesthesia. 2. Anesthesiology. 3. Anesthesia. 4. Local anesthesia. I. Rogers, Mercy.
RD84 .C55 2023
617.964--dc23

Foster Academics,
118-35 Queens Blvd., Suite 400,
Forest Hills, NY 11375, USA

ISBN 978-1-64646-582-8 (Hardback)

Contents

Preface

This book aims to highlight the current researches and provides a platform to further the scope of innovations in this area. This book is a product of the combined efforts of many researchers and scientists, after going through thorough studies and analysis from different parts of the world. The objective of this book is to provide the readers with the latest information of the field.

Anesthesiology refers to a type of medical specialty that focuses on the complete perioperative care of patients before, during and after surgery. It is an integral part of critical emergency medicine, anesthesia, pain medicine and intensive care medicine. Regional anesthesia, local anesthesia, general anesthesia and sedation are the four primary types of anesthesia used during surgical procedures. Regional anesthesia is a type of pain management used during surgery that numbs a significant portion of the body typically from the waist down. The drug is administered by a tiny tube or injection known as a catheter and is used when a simple injection of local anesthetic is insufficient and it is preferable for the patient to be awake. Regional anesthesia aids in the management of postoperative pain and can help patients recover quickly and safely with fewer side effects than general anesthesia. This book elucidates the concepts and innovative models around prospective developments in research with respect to regional anesthesiology. It will help new researchers by foregrounding their knowledge in this branch of medicine. Different approaches, evaluations, and advanced studies on this topic have been included in this book.

I would like to express my sincere thanks to the authors for their dedicated efforts in the completion of this book. I acknowledge the efforts of the publisher for providing constant support. Lastly, I would like to thank my family for their support in all academic endeavors.

Editor

1

Lower rate of delayed graft function is observed when epidural analgesia for living donor nephrectomy is administered

Wolfgang Baar[1], Ulrich Goebel[1], Hartmut Buerkle[1], Bernd Jaenigen[2], Kai Kaufmann[1] and Sebastian Heinrich[1*]

Abstract

Background: The beneficial effects of epidural analgesia (EDA) in terms of pain control and postoperative convalescence are widely known and led to a frequent use for patients who underwent living donor kidney nephrectomy. The objective of this study was to determine whether general anesthesia (GA) plus EDA compared to GA only, administered for living donor nephrectomy has effects on postoperative graft function in recipients.

Methods: In this monocentric, retrospective cohort analysis we analyzed the closed files of all consecutive donor-recipient pairs who underwent living donor kidney transplantations from 2008 to 2017. The outcome variable was delayed graft function (DGF), defined as at least one hemodialysis within seven days postoperatively, once hyperacute rejection, vascular or urinary tract complications were ruled out. Statistical analyses of continuous variables were calculated using the two-tail Student's t test and Fisher exact test for categorical variables with a significance level of $p < 0.05$, respectively.

Results: The study enclosed 291 consecutive living donor kidney transplantations. 99 kidney donors received epidural analgesia whereas 192 had no epidural analgesia. The groups showed balanced pretransplantational characteristics and comparable donors´ and recipients' risk factors. 9 out of all 291 recipients needed renal replacement therapy (RRT) during the first 7 days due to delayed graft function; none of these donors received EDA. The observed rate of DGF in recipients whose kidney donors received epidural analgesia was significantly lower (0% vs. 4.6%; $p = 0.031$).

Conclusions: In our cohort we observed a significantly lower rate of DGF when epidural analgesia for donor nephrectomy was administered. Due to restrictions of the study design this observation needs further confirmation by prospective studies.

Keywords: Kidney transplantation, Delayed graft function, Epidural analgesia, Donor nephrectomy

Background

Living kidney transplantation showed superior results compared to deceased donor kidney transplantation in terms of graft survival, accessibility, waiting time and cost containment for public health services [1–3]. For patients undergoing surgical procedures for another one's benefit, it is important to minimize perioperative risks and inconvenience. Furthermore, it is the healthcare providers' duty to maximize the beneficial impact of the donation for the recipient.

In numerous studies major outcome benefits like mortality of EDA could neither be confirmed nor denied [4, 5]. However, the beneficial effects of EDA in terms of intra- and postoperative pain control, intestinal motility, early mobilization and duration of ICU- hospitalization are widely known and find broad acceptance [6–9]. Therefore it is not surprising, that continuous EDA is a mandatory part of many surgical fast track programs [10–12]. In order to provide these advantages also for kidney donors and to increase their convalescence and speed up their reintegration in daily life, we offered EDA to patients for donor

* Correspondence: sebastian.heinrich@uniklinik-freiburg.de
[1]Department of Anesthesiology and Critical Care, Medical Center, Faculty of Medicine, University of Freiburg, Hugstetter Strasse 55, 79106 Freiburg, Germany

nephrectomy, if contraindications were ruled out and patients gave their informed consent. The primary intent of providing perioperative EDA for donor nephrectomy are the beneficial effects for the donor [13–15]. These EDA effects are mostly mediated by perioperative sympathicolysis which probably has effects on the kidney intended for transplantation [16, 17]. Potential effects on graft function of kidneys explanted from donors with EDA in terms of a two day follow up of glomerular filtration rate, microalbuminuria, or creatinine clearance have shown no differences in a small cohort [17]. Potential effects on the incidence of delayed graft function have not yet been reported. Therefore, the aim of this hypothesis generating study was to determine whether GA plus EDA compared to GA only, administered for living donor nephrectomy is associated with beneficial effects on postoperative graft function after transplantation.

Methods

This retrospective cohort study was approved by the local Institutional Review Board, University of Freiburg, Germany (approval number EK 555/17). The study was conducted at the Department of Anesthesiology and Critical Care and the Department of General and Visceral Surgery, Medical Center - University of Freiburg, Faculty of Medicine - University of Freiburg Germany. The study was planned and designed in accordance with the initiative for Strengthening the Reporting of Observational Studies in Epidemiology (STROBE), using the suggested checklist for epidemiological cohort studies [18]. The study was initiated and designed in March 2018; the retrospective data collection was conducted in June 2018. The onset of data collection is analogous to the existence of an electronic patient data management system on ICU which enabled data acquisition. As we enclosed only closed files and the data collection started in June 2018, cases after December 31th 2017 were not enclosed. The study cohort consists of all consecutive living donor kidney transplantations between October 2008 and December 2017 which determines the sample size. A priori sample size calculation is not applicable in this fully retrospective and observational study design. Figure 1 shows the protocol of data collection and statistical processing.

Recipient and donor evaluation were based on a check-up examination which lead to confirmation of donor suitability. Ahead of transplantation all donor- recipient pairs were evaluated by an ethics committee of the District Medical Association Suedbaden, Germany. A positive vote of this ethics committee was mandatory for transplantation.

Surgical procedure was standardized to a maximum as only two different surgeons contributed to the transplantations in this cohort. The donor nephrectomy was

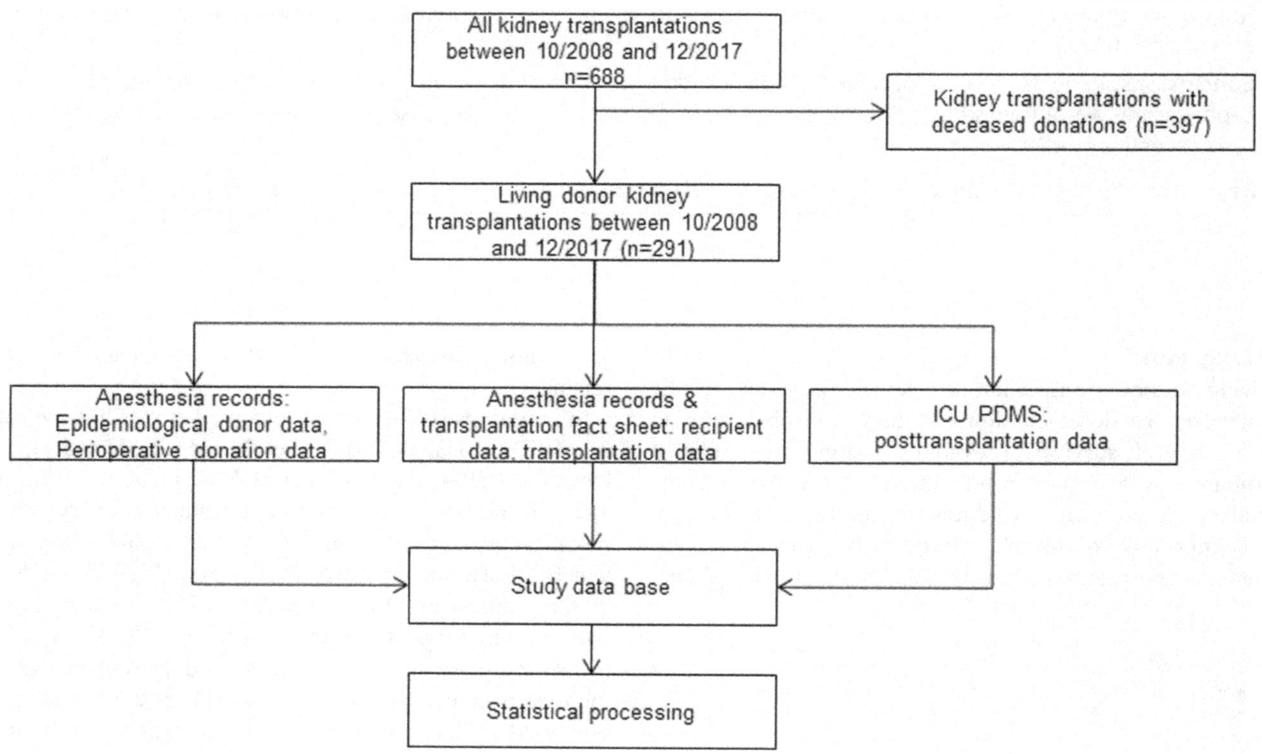

Fig. 1 Flowchart showing the data collection of the study

performed in supine position over an open anterior extraperitoneal minimal incision laparotomy. Transplantations were performed in the established technique, to the right iliac fossa of the recipient.

Decision on epidural analgesia was based on the patients´ preference. All patients that received epidural analgesia gave their informed consent on that procedure. Epidural analgesia was performed directly preoperatively according a specific departmental standard operating procedure: Epidural catheter was placed between the 7th and the 11th thoracic intervertebral space, followed by an application of 25 µg sufentanil and 10 ml ropivacaine 0.2%. After the initial dose a continuous epidural application of 45 ml ropivacaine 0.2% mixed with 25 µg sufentanil (= ropivacaine 0.18% and sufentanil 0.5 µg/ml) with an infusion rate of 8 ml/h during the surgery was established. Anesthesia procedures for donor nephrectomy with and without epidural analgesia followed a unique mandatory standard operating procedure (SOP) which differed only regarding the administration of EDA and was performed by a specialized transplantation team. Our transplantation team consists of 8 to 10 attending anesthesiologists, who underwent special training (transplant fellowship) and are used to perform anesthesiology for kidney transplantation in accordance to our mandatory in-house standard operating procedure. Over the years the attending anesthesiologists in charge changed, so that in total a number of 25 anesthesiologists took care of the patients. Postoperatively all donors were transferred to a transplantation ICU. Patients who received epidural analgesia were visited daily by the acute pain service of our department. Epidural catheters were removed between the second and the fifth postoperative day by the acute pain service.

Anesthesia for transplantation was performed without epidural analgesia for the recipient and followed a departmental SOP which was established and revised where necessary in close collaboration between the responsible surgeons and anesthetists The SOP addresses the need for 250 mg prednisolone and 10 g mannitol ahead of reperfusion. With the onset of reperfusion of the transplant kidney 125 mg furosemide were administered. Intraoperative fluid and catecholamine management was performed by the attending anesthetist referring to the SOP.

Renal replacement therapy (RRT) was initiated when patients were threatened by volume overload or increased serum potassium levels. Delayed graft function was defined as any renal replacement therapy in the first postoperative week, once hyperacute rejection, vascular or urinary tract complications were ruled out [19–21] .

Statistics

The data was collected in a MS Excel™ (Microsoft, Redmond, USA) datasheet. Further statistical processing was performed using SPSS™ (IBM, Armonk, USA). Statistical analyses of continuous variables were calculated using the two-tail Student's t test and Fisher Exact test for categorical variables with a significance level of $p < 0.05$, respectively.

Results

The study enclosed 291 consecutive living donor kidney transplantations between October 2008 and December 2017. 99 kidney donors received epidural analgesia whereas 192 had no epidural analgesia. Table 1 shows the distribution of patients, the rate of EDA and the incidence of RRT and DGF for every year. For none of the years RRT or DGF rate are significantly increased. All recipients underwent kidney transplantation due to end stage renal disease. No mortality was reported in either group. In the EDA group no epidural catheter associated complications were found.

The perioperative characteristics are shown in Table 2. The two study groups showed no significant differences in several donors´ risk factors except a significantly shorter nephrectomy time (135 vs. 144 min, $p < 0.003$). The intraoperative fluid consumption (1813 vs. 2191 ml; $p = 0.053$) and maximum dose of vasopressor (0.03 vs. 0.06 µg/kg/min; $p = 0.300$) showed no statistically significant difference. None of the recipients´ pre- and intra-transplantation data showed a significant difference (Table 2). After transplantation, 14 out of all 291 recipients needed renal replacement therapy during the first 7 days after transplantation, but only 9 cases due to delayed graft function. The other 5 recipients suffered humoral rejection, thrombosis of the iliac vessel or bleeding complications with the need of a surgical revision (Table 3). All kidney donors to these 9 recipients received GA without epidural analgesia. The incidence of DGF was significantly higher in recipients whose donors did not receive epidural analgesia (4.6% vs. 0%; $p = 0.031$) (Fig. 2). In line with this finding the serum creatinine level as well as the maximum serum potassium level within 7 days were significantly lower in the recipients whose donors received EDA (2.17 vs. 2.04 mg/dl, $p = 0.036$; 5.15 vs. 5.11 mmol/l, $p < 0.001$).

Discussion

The benefits of EDA regarding pain control, ICU stay, intestinal motility and early mobilization are frequently reported [22–27]. The beneficial effects of EDA in terms of pain control and return to normal daily activities specifically for kidney donors have also been reported in the past [28, 29]. This retrospective cohort study of 291 living donor kidney transplantations compared 99 cases whose donors received EDA with 192 cases that received GA only, with regard to DGF in the recipients. The main result is that DGF is significantly more frequent in

Table 1 Distribution of patients, rate of EDA, incidence of RRT and DGF throughout the observation period

Year	Number of patients	With EDA (n/%)	RRT within 7 days (n/%)	DGF (n/%)
2008	7	0/0%	0/0%	0/0%
2009	31	1/3%	0/0%	0/0%
2010	33	0/0%	1/3%	1/3%
2011	34	6/18%	3/9%	3/9%
2012	35	15/43%	3/9%	1/3%
2013	32	14/44%	0/0%	0/0%
2014	35	8/23%	2/6%	1/3%
2015	31	14/45%	2/6%	2/6%
2016	30	25/83%	2/7%	1/3%
2017	23	16/70%	1/4%	0/0%

Table 2 Main results of the study. Continuous variables are given as mean ± standard deviation, categorical variables are given as absolute number and percentage

	Without EDA (n = 192)	With EDA (n = 99)	Significance
Donor and nephrectomy data			
Donor male sex [n/(%)]	71 (37%)	32 (32%)	0.469
Donor BMI [kg/m^2]	25.7 ± 4.1	25.5 ± 3.5	0.165
Donor age [years]	52	52	0.416
Donor preoperative hemoglobin [g/dl]	14.1 ± 1.2	14.1 ± 1.2	0.919
Crystalloid fluid for nephrectomy [ml]	1813 ± 907	2191 ± 1113	0.053
Max. dose of noradrenaline after cut [µg/kg/min]	0.03 ± 0.04	0.06 ± 0.05	0.300
Nephrectomy time (cut – suture) [min]	135 ± 38	144 ± 48	**0.003**
Recipient and transplantation data			
Recipient BMI [kg/m^2]	24.8 ± 3.9	25.6 ± 4.2	0.168
Recipient male sex [n/(%)]	121 (62%)	61 (62%)	0.899
Recipient age [years]	44 ± 13	47 ± 13	0.853
Recipient rest diuresis [ml]	1098 ± 907	1134 ± 858	0.062
Recipient preoperative creatinine [mg/dl]	8.0 ± 2.8	7.6 ± 2.8	0.744
Duration of transplantation [min]	161 ± 55	145 ± 41	0.129
Warm ischemic period [min]	29 ± 9	26 ± 7	0.138
MAP for anastomosis [mmHg]	93 ± 11	88 ± 16	0.165
Fluid intake during transplantation [ml]	2782 ± 1366	3477 ± 1233	0.559
Posttransplantation data			
Diuresis first hour [ml]	425 ± 430	383 ± 390	0.358
Diuresis 24 h [ml]	9947 ± 5313	10,871 ± 6419	0.062
Recipient creatinine 12–24 h postoperative [mg/dl]	4.37 ± 2.2	4.09 ± 1.8	0.189
Recipient creatinine 36–48 h postoperative[mg/dl]	3.15 ± 2.1	3.04 ± 1.7	0.404
Recipient creatinine 7 days postoperative [mg/dl]	2.17 ± 1.6	2.04 ± 1.1	**0.036**
Max. recipient serum potassium level within 7d	5.15 ± 0.6	5.11 ± 0.4	**0.001**
Renal replacement therapy first postoperative week [n/(%)]	11 (6%)	3 (3%)	0.312
Delayed graft function [n/(%)]	9 (4.6%)	0 (0%)	**0.031**

statistical significance is indicated by bold numbers

Table 3 Underlying reasons for renal replacement therapy (RRT) and met definition of delayed graft function (DGF)

Case Number	Year	EDA	Underlying reason leading to RRT within 7 days	DGF
507	2010	no	graft perfusion deficit	yes
581	2011	no	insufficient graft function, later sepsis	yes
588	2011	no	critical potassium levels, good graft function later on	yes
624	2011	no	acute tubules necrosis	yes
666	2012	yes	humoral rejection	no
692	2012	no	bleeding complication, needed operative revision	no
701	2012	no	insufficient graft function	yes
829	2014	no	humoral rejection	no
859	2014	no	graft perfusion deficit	yes
888	2015	no	insufficient graft function, critical potassium levels	yes
935	2015	no	insufficient graft function	yes
1017	2016	no	insufficient graft function	yes
1023	2016	yes	humoral rejection	no
1089	2017	yes	thrombosis of recipients iliac vessel	no

patients whose kidney donors did not receive EDA. The incidence of DGF in cohorts of living kidney transplantations varies from 4 to 10% and increases morbidity, healthcare costs, hospitalization times and complicates post- transplantation care [30–33]. DGF predisposes for chronic rejection, chronic allograft nephropathy and seems to be causal for increased rates of graft failure and mortality [34, 35].

In line with the significantly lower rate of DGF in EDA group, we found that serum creatinine level, as well as the maximum serum potassium level within 7 days, were significantly lower in the EDA group. Although these

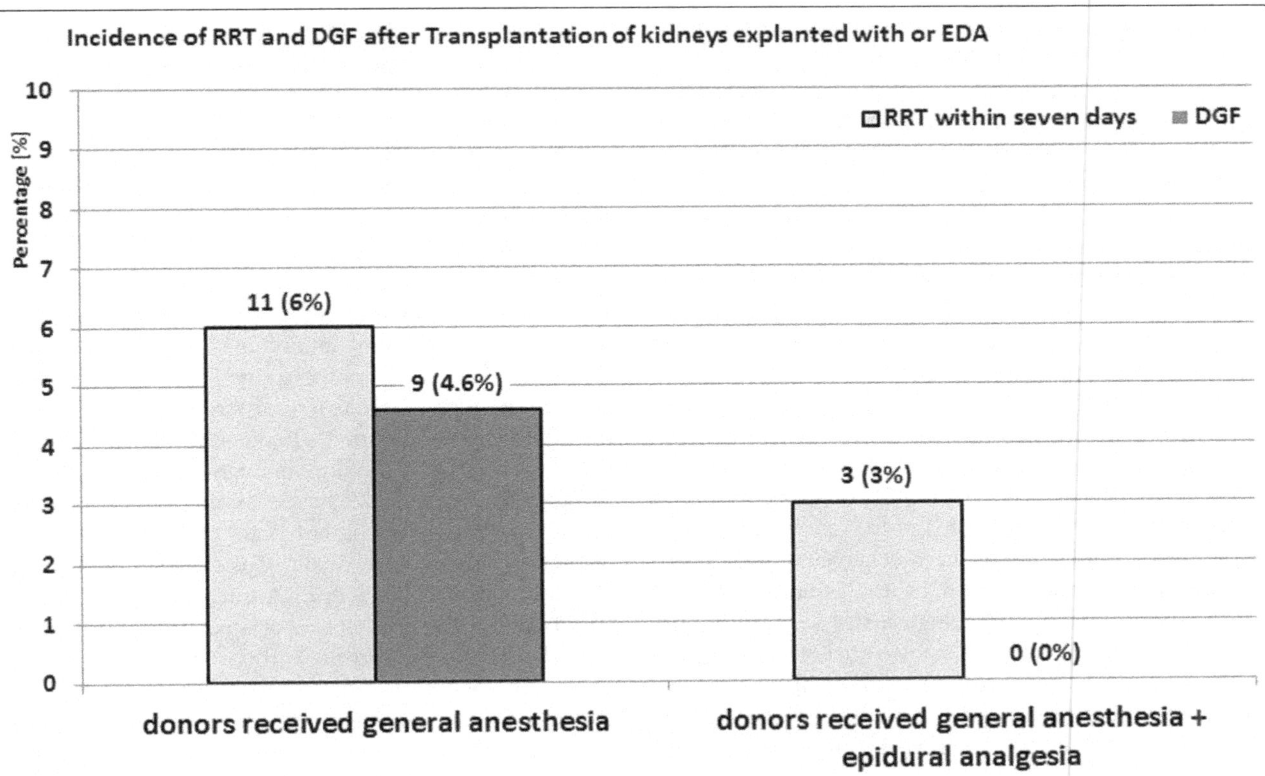

Fig. 2 The incidence of renal replacement therapy (RRT) with the first seven days and delayed graft function (DGF) depending on the anesthesia procedure for donor nephrectomy

findings are statistically significant, their measured levels and differences in numbers are clinically not of relevance. Even when looking at the decline of the serum creatinine levels over the first two days postoperatively no significant or clinically relevant difference can be found. The recipients of the no-EDA group start at a slightly higher level of serum creatinine which should be taken into account. Further baseline characteristics of donors and recipients showed no statistically significant difference or clinically relevant imbalance between the donors and recipients of both groups. An increased intraoperative fluid and vasopressor consumption in the EDA group could be associated with the EDA mediated inhibition of the sympatho- adrenal response with consecutive vasodilatation. However, neither intraoperative fluid nor vasopressor consumption showed a statistically significant difference in our study.

The standard surgical technique for donor nephrectomy in our institution is an open anterior extraperitoneal minimal incision laparotomy. Open surgical technique for donor nephrectomy is associated with inferior cosmetic result, longer hospitalization and more intra- and postoperative pain with consecutively increased need for pain medication [36, 37]. However, the open surgical approach showed superior results in terms of warm ischemia period, surgical costs, length of operation, intraperitoneal complications, recovery of graft function, recipient anastomosis difficulties and incidence of acute tubulus necrosis [38–40]. It is reported that up to 25% of living kidney donors after open surgical technique nephrectomy suffer from chronification of postoperative pain [41]. A reduction of somatic pain within the first six postoperative weeks is associated with improved mental health of kidney donors [37]. These findings underline the need for EDA from the donors' perspective. The described clinical benefits of EDA for the donor might lose their relevance and have to be reconsidered in case the surgical approach in our institution changes to laparoscopic technique.

The reasons why kidney grafts fail to function immediately after transplantation when acute rejection, urological or vascular reasons are ruled out are associated with the transplanted kidney. DGF is modulated and caused by complex mechanisms of hypoxic and ischemic injuries and insufficient repair mechanisms [42]. These cascades seem to be induced by the operative trauma and the corresponding physiological stress response during donor nephrectomy. It is known that surgical procedures and the physiological stress response are associated with intra- and postoperative hypercoagulability which results in postoperative thromboembolic and vaso-occlusive events [43, 44]. Increased levels of tissue factor, tissue plasminogen activator, plasminogen activator inhibitor-1, and von Willebrand factor which all contribute to hypercoagulability are reported to be found proximately after surgical stimulus [45]. Due to inhibition of nociceptive and non-nociceptive pathways of sympathetic innervation of the adrenal glands, EDA with local anesthetics leads to a perioperative sympathicolysis [46]. Experimental reports on rats showed a significantly improved microcirculation in the areas of EDA mediated sympathetic blockage [47]. In an ovine model with artificially administered pulmonary embolism therapeutic EDA improved macrohemodynamic parameters [48]. It is also reported that EDA modulates postoperative hypercoagulability by normalizing antithrombin III- activity and a decrease of platelet aggregation [49–51]. We hypothesize that a decreased risk of thrombotic and vasoocclusive events which is mediated by therapeutic EDA could be one of the reasons that we found a significantly increased rate of DGF in the non-EDA group.

The potential benefit of EDA performed for the transplantation could not be investigated by our study group. In our institution the transplantation itself is performed without EDA due to the mandatory immune suppressive therapy and the high incidence of platelet dysfunction in patients suffering from end stage renal disease [52, 53]. Hadimioglu and colleagues found improved clinical results and an attenuated stress response in kidney transplantations performed with EDA and general anesthesia compared to general anesthesia alone [54]. Against the background of these results and the results of our study, we will reconsider our previous approach with regard to the use of EDA in kidney transplants.

The present study has several distinct limitations

First, the retrospective and non-randomized design implies that a study protocol which addresses randomization on who receives EDA is missing. It is speculative why patients opted for or against EDA, possibly the way whether EDA was offered by the visiting anesthesiologist or rather recommended plays an important role. Perhaps patients who opted for EDA were more trustful of their physicians and therefore had less anxiety or stress levels which may have influenced DGF of their donated kidney. The way EDA was offered to the donors might have been changed throughout the years. We have seen that EDA is more frequently performed in the last years of the program compared to the very early years of the observation period. However, this imbalance of EDA rates throughout the observational period was not associated with an accumulation of RRTs or DGF in the early or the late years of the observation. RRT was initiated by visiting nephrology specialists and the request of the attending ICU physician when patients were threatened by volume overload or increased serum potassium levels. We are fully aware that living donor kidney transplantation is a highly complex procedure. The outcome quality is affected by various confounding variables for which we have not adjusted in our study due to the limited number of cases with DGF.

There are also several slightly different definitions on delayed graft function in literature. In our study DGF was defined as any renal replacement therapy in the first postoperative week, when hyperacute rejection, vascular and urinary tract complications were ruled out. More than 22 different definitions of DGF are described, the most common definition refers to any RRT within the first posttransplantational week [55, 19]. Due to the manageable size of our cohort we could screen every case of RRT for the underlying reasons. Knowing these reasons leading to RRT for every patient, we decided to choose a more specific definition of delayed graft function. Beyond the discussion about the definition we have to state, that in the EDA group none of the patients who received RRT showed graft associated reasons leading to RRT. In no case of the EDA group, graft perfusion deficits or insufficient otherwise unexplainable graft dysfunction led to RRT. Finally, we can report of an association between EDA for donor nephrectomy and a lower rate of DGF in our study. However, we are fully aware that correlation does not proof causality. Especially in a multifactorial context such as living kidney transplantations, larger numbers of prospectively randomized assigned patients are needed to provide stronger evidence.

Conclusions

In this retrospective cohort study, we found an association between epidural analgesia for living kidney donors and significantly less delayed graft function in the corresponding kidney recipients. These results favor not only the beneficial analgesic effect of epidural analgesia for donors, but also show significant beneficial effects for kidney recipients. As our analysis depends on the authors' experience, derived from a very low level of evidence with consecutive relevant shortcoming in terms of study design, number of index cases and adjustment of confounding variables, our findings have to be confirmed by prospective randomized trials.

Abbreviations

DGF: Delayed graft function; EDA: Epidural analgesia; GA: General anesthesia; RRT: Renal replacement therapy; SOP: Standard operating procedure; STROBE: Strengthening the reporting of observational studies in epidemiology

Acknowledgements

Not applicable.

Authors' contributions

SH initiated the study, performed statistically processing, contributed to the writing of the manuscript, UG developed the study design, contributed to data collection and proofread the manuscript, HB advised the study design, is responsible for the anesthesia SOPs and proof read the manuscript, BJ operated most of the patients is responsible for the postoperative care of the patients and contributed to data collection, KK contributed to data collection and writing of the manuscript, WB contributed to data collection and wrote the manuscript. All authors contributed substantially to this work and all of them revised and agreed to the final version of the manuscript with full access to all data.

Author details

[1]Department of Anesthesiology and Critical Care, Medical Center, Faculty of Medicine, University of Freiburg, Hugstetter Strasse 55, 79106 Freiburg, Germany. [2]Department of General and Visceral Surgery, Medical Center, Faculty of Medicine, University of Freiburg, Hugstetter Strasse 55, 79106 Freiburg, Germany.

References

1. Lionaki S, Kapsia H, Makropoulos I, Metsini A, Skalioti C, Gakiopoulou H, et al. Kidney transplantation outcomes from expanded criteria donors, standard criteria donors or living donors older than 60 years. Ren Fail. 2014; 36:526–33.
2. Axelrod DA, Schnitzler MA, Xiao H, Irish W, Tuttle-Newhall E, Chang S-H, et al. An economic assessment of contemporary kidney transplant practice. Am J Transplant Off J Am Soc Transplant Am Soc Transpl Surg. 2018;18: 1168–76.
3. Guimarães J, Araújo AM, Santos F, Nunes CS, Casal M. Living-donor and deceased-donor renal transplantation: differences in early outcome--a single-center experience. Transplant Proc. 2015;47:958–62.
4. Liu SS, Wu CL. Effect of postoperative analgesia on major postoperative complications: a systematic update of the evidence. Anesth Analg. 2007;104: 689–702.
5. Liu SS, Wu CL. The effect of analgesic technique on postoperative patient-reported outcomes including analgesia: a systematic review. Anesth Analg. 2007;105:789–808.
6. Guay J, Nishimori M, Kopp SL. Epidural local anesthetics versus opioid-based analgesic regimens for postoperative gastrointestinal paralysis, vomiting, and pain after abdominal surgery: a Cochrane review. Anesth Analg. 2016; 123:1591–602.
7. Feldheiser A, Aziz O, Baldini G, Cox BPBW, Fearon KCH, Feldman LS, et al. Enhanced recovery after surgery (ERAS) for gastrointestinal surgery, part 2: consensus statement for anaesthesia practice. Acta Anaesthesiol Scand. 2016;60:289–334.
8. Salicath JH, Yeoh EC, Bennett MH. Epidural analgesia versus patient-controlled intravenous analgesia for pain following intra-abdominal surgery in adults. Cochrane Database Syst Rev. 2018;8:CD010434.
9. Pöpping DM, Elia N, Van Aken HK, Marret E, Schug SA, Kranke P, et al. Impact of epidural analgesia on mortality and morbidity after surgery: systematic review and meta-analysis of randomized controlled trials. Ann Surg. 2014;259:1056–67.
10. Vukovic N, Dinic L. Enhanced recovery after surgery protocols in major urologic surgery. Front Med. 2018;5. https://doi.org/10.3389/fmed.2018.00093.
11. Bonde C, Khorasani H, Eriksen K, Wolthers M, Kehlet H, Elberg J. Introducing the fast track surgery principles can reduce length of stay after autologous breast reconstruction using free flaps: a case control study. J Plast Surg Hand Surg. 2015;49:367–71.
12. Feo CV, Lanzara S, Sortini D, Ragazzi R, De Pinto M, Pansini GC, et al. Fast track postoperative management after elective colorectal surgery: a controlled trail. Am Surg. 2009;75:1247–51.
13. Torgay A, Donmez A, Varol G, Durmaz L, Arslan G, Haberal M. Intra- and postoperative complications of donor nephrectomies. Transplant Proc. 2005; 37:2941–3.
14. Milan Z, Das S, Kocarev M, Rawari V. Is single-shot epidural analgesia more effective than morphine patient-controlled analgesia for donor nephrectomy? Transplant Proc. 2011;43:3588–92.
15. Peters TG, Repper SM, Jones KW, Walker GW, Vincent M, Hunter RD. Living kidney donation: recovery and return to activities of daily living. Clin Transpl. 2000;14(4 Pt 2):433–8.
16. Li Y, Zhu S, Yan M. Combined general/epidural anesthesia (ropivacaine 0. 375%) versus general anesthesia for upper abdominal surgery. Anesth Analg. 2008;106:1562–5 table of contents.
17. Sener M, Torgay A, Akpek E, Colak T, Karakayali H, Arslan G, et al. Regional versus general anesthesia for donor nephrectomy: effects on graft function. Transplant Proc. 2004;36:2954–8.

18. Vandenbroucke JP, von Elm E, Altman DG, Gøtzsche PC, Mulrow CD, Pocock SJ, et al. Strengthening the reporting of observational studies in epidemiology (STROBE): explanation and elaboration. Int J Surg Lond Engl. 2014;12:1500–24.
19. Yarlagadda SG, Coca SG, Garg AX, Doshi M, Poggio E, Marcus RJ, et al. Marked variation in the definition and diagnosis of delayed graft function: a systematic review. Nephrol Dial Transplant Off Publ Eur Dial Transpl Assoc - Eur Ren Assoc. 2008;23:2995–3003.
20. Avihingsanon Y, Ma N, Pavlakis M, Chon WJ, Uknis ME, Monaco AP, et al. On the intraoperative molecular status of renal allografts after vascular reperfusion and clinical outcomes. J Am Soc Nephrol JASN. 2005;16:1542–8.
21. Moreso F, Serón D, Gil-Vernet S, Riera L, Fulladosa X, Ramos R, et al. Donor age and delayed graft function as predictors of renal allograft survival in rejection-free patients. Nephrol Dial Transplant Off Publ Eur Dial Transpl Assoc - Eur Ren Assoc. 1999;14:930–5.
22. Wang L, Li X, Chen H, Liang J, Wang Y. Effect of patient-controlled epidural analgesia versus patient-controlled intravenous analgesia on postoperative pain management and short-term outcomes after gastric cancer resection: a retrospective analysis of 3,042 consecutive patients between 2010 and 2015. J Pain Res. 2018;11:1743–9.
23. Malyshev AA, Sviridov SV, Vedenina IV. Effect of prolonged epidupal analgesia on respiratory function after major laparoscopic surgery. Anesteziol Reanimatol. 2015;60:30–3.
24. Mouawad NJ, Leichtle SW, Kaoutzanis C, Welch K, Winter S, Lampman R, et al. Pain control with continuous infusion preperitoneal wound catheters versus continuous epidural analgesia in colon and rectal surgery: a randomized controlled trial. Am J Surg. 2018;215:570–6.
25. Peyton PJ, Myles PS, Silbert BS, Rigg JA, Jamrozik K, Parsons R. Perioperative epidural analgesia and outcome after major abdominal surgery in high-risk patients. Anesth Analg. 2003;96:548 table of contents.
26. Feltracco P, Bortolato A, Barbieri S, Michieletto E, Serra E, Ruol A, et al. Perioperative benefit and outcome of thoracic epidural in esophageal surgery: a clinical review. Dis Esophagus Off J Int Soc Dis Esophagus. 2018;31.
27. Gendall KA, Kennedy RR, Watson AJM, Frizelle FA. The effect of epidural analgesia on postoperative outcome after colorectal surgery. Colorectal Dis Off J Assoc Coloproctology G B Irel. 2007;9:584–98 discussion 598-600.
28. Oliveira B, Mascarenhas C, Cardoso G, Sá J, Casal M. Assessment of the degree of satisfaction among living kidney donors. Transplant Proc. 2011;43:43–7.
29. Suarez-Sanchez L, Perales-Caldera E, Pelaez-Luna MC, Bernal-Flores R. Postoperative outcome of open donor nephrectomy under epidural analgesia: a descriptive analysis. Transplant Proc. 2006;38:877–81.
30. Perico N, Cattaneo D, Sayegh MH, Remuzzi G. Delayed graft function in kidney transplantation. Lancet Lond Engl. 2004;364:1814–27.
31. Almond PS, Troppmann C, Escobar F, Frey DJ, Matas AJ. Economic impact of delayed graft function. Transplant Proc. 1991;23(1 Pt 2):1304.
32. Almond PS, Matas AJ, Canafax DM. Fixed-rate reimbursement fails to cover costs for patients with delayed graft function. Pharmacotherapy. 1991;11: 126S–9S.
33. Taber DJ, DuBay D, McGillicuddy JW, Nadig S, Bratton CF, Chavin KD, et al. Impact of the new kidney allocation system on perioperative outcomes and costs in kidney transplantation. J Am Coll Surg. 2017;224:585–92.
34. Butala NM, Reese PP, Doshi MD, Parikh CR. Is delayed graft function causally associated with long-term outcomes after kidney transplantation? Instrumental variable analysis. Transplantation. 2013;95:1008–14.
35. Giral-Classe M, Hourmant M, Cantarovich D, Dantal J, Blancho G, Daguin P, et al. Delayed graft function of more than six days strongly decreases long-term survival of transplanted kidneys. Kidney Int. 1998;54:972–8.
36. Perry KT, Freedland SJ, Hu JC, Phelan MW, Kristo B, Gritsch AH, et al. Quality of life, pain and return to normal activities following laparoscopic donor nephrectomy versus open mini-incision donor nephrectomy. J Urol. 2003; 169:2018–21.
37. Nicholson ML, Elwell R, Kaushik M, Bagul A, Hosgood SA. Health-related quality of life after living donor nephrectomy: a randomized controlled trial of laparoscopic versus open nephrectomy. Transplantation. 2011;91:457–61.
38. Jamale TE, Hase NK, Iqbal AM. Laparoscopic donor nephrectomy versus open donor nephrectomy: recipient's perspective. Saudi J Kidney Dis Transplant Off Publ Saudi Cent Organ Transplant Saudi Arab. 2012;23:1175–80.
39. Simforoosh N, Basiri A, Shakhssalim N, Gooran S, Tabibi A, Khoshdel A, et al. Long-term graft function in a randomized clinical trial comparing laparoscopic versus open donor nephrectomy. Exp Clin Transplant Off J Middle East Soc Organ Transplant. 2012;10:428–32.
40. Subramanian T, Dageforde LA, Vachharajani N, Wellen J, Doyle MBM, Lin Y, et al. Mini-incision versus hand-assisted laparoscopic donor nephrectomy in living-donor kidney transplantation: a retrospective cohort study. Int J Surg Lond Engl. 2018;53:339–44.
41. Owen M, Lorgelly P, Serpell M. Chronic pain following donor nephrectomy--a study of the incidence, nature and impact of chronic post-nephrectomy pain. Eur J Pain Lond Engl. 2010;14:732–4.
42. Schröppel B, Legendre C. Delayed kidney graft function: from mechanism to translation. Kidney Int. 2014;86:251–8.
43. Warltier DC, Pagel PS, Kersten JR. Approaches to the prevention of perioperative myocardial ischemia. Anesthesiology. 2000;92:253–9.
44. Meissner A, Rolf N, Van Aken H. Thoracic epidural anesthesia and the patient with heart disease: benefits, risks, and controversies. Anesth Analg. 1997;85:517–28.
45. Bombeli T, Spahn DR. Updates in perioperative coagulation: physiology and management of thromboembolism and haemorrhage. Br J Anaesth. 2004; 93:275–87.
46. Nygård E, Kofoed KF, Freiberg J, Holm S, Aldershvile J, Eliasen K, et al. Effects of high thoracic epidural analgesia on myocardial blood flow in patients with ischemic heart disease. Circulation. 2005;111:2165–70.
47. Daudel F, Freise H, Westphal M, Stubbe HD, Lauer S, Bone H, et al. Continuous thoracic epidural anesthesia improves gut mucosal microcirculation in rats with Sepsis. Shock. 2007;28:610–4.
48. Jahn UR, Waurick R, Van Aken H, Hinder F, Meyer J, Bone HG. Therapeutic administration of thoracic epidural anesthesia reduces cardiopulmonary deterioration in ovine pulmonary embolism. Crit Care Med. 2007;35:2582–6.
49. Fant F, Tina E, Sandblom D, Andersson S-O, Magnuson A, Hultgren-Hörnkvist E, et al. Thoracic epidural analgesia inhibits the neuro-hormonal but not the acute inflammatory stress response after radical retropubic prostatectomy. Br J Anaesth. 2013;110:747–57.
50. Grass JA. The role of epidural anesthesia and analgesia in postoperative outcome. Anesthesiol Clin N Am. 2000;18:407–28 viii.
51. Liu S, Carpenter RL, Neal JM. Epidural anesthesia and analgesia. Their role in postoperative outcome. Anesthesiology. 1995;82:1474–506.
52. Pluta J, Nicińska B, Grzeszczyk M, Kołacz M, Jureczko L, Kwiatkowski A, et al. Assessment of the hemostatic parameters and platelet function on Thromboelastometry and impedance Aggregometry in hemodialysis patients qualified for kidney transplantation: preliminary report. Transplant Proc. 2016;48:1431–4.
53. Kaw D, Malhotra D. Platelet dysfunction and end-stage renal disease. Semin Dial. 2006;19:317–22.
54. Hadimioglu N, Ulugol H, Akbas H, Coskunfirat N, Ertug Z, Dinckan A. Combination of epidural anesthesia and general anesthesia attenuates stress response to renal transplantation surgery. Transplant Proc. 2012;44: 2949–54.
55. Decruyenaere P, Decruyenaere A, Peeters P, Vermassen F. A single-center comparison of 22 competing definitions of delayed graft function after kidney transplantation. Ann Transplant. 2016;21:152–9.

2

Effects of regional anesthesia techniques on local anesthetic plasma levels and complications in carotid surgery

Thomas Rössel[1*†], Christopher Uhlig[1†], Jörg Pietsch[2], Stefan Ludwig[3], Thea Koch[1], Torsten Richter[1], Peter Markus Spieth[1] and Stephan Kersting[3,4]

Abstract

Background: The ultrasound guided intermediate cervical plexus block with perivascular infiltration of the internal carotid artery (PVB) is a new technique for regional anesthesia in carotid endarterectomy (CEA). We conducted a pilot study investigating the effects of deep cervical block (DCB), intermediate cervical block alone (ICB) and PVB on perioperative complications in patients undergoing elective CEA. We hypothesized, that the ropivacaine plasma concentration is higher in patients receiving DCB compared to PVB and ICB.

Methods: In a randomized controlled pilot study thirty patients scheduled for elective CEA were randomly assigned into three groups: DCB receiving 20 mL ropivacaine 0.5% ($n = 10$), ICB receiving 20 mL ropivacaine 0.5% ($n = 10$) and PVB receiving 20 mL ropivacaine 0.5% and 10 mL ropivacaine 0,3% ($n = 10$). As primary outcome, plasma levels of ropivacaine were measured with high performance liquid chromatography before, 5, 10, 20, 60, and 180 min after the injection of ropivacaine. Secondary outcomes were vascular and neurological complications as well as patients' and surgeons' satisfaction. All analyses were performed on an intention-to-treat basis. Statistical significance was accepted at $p < 0.05$.

Results: No conversion to general anesthesia was necessary and we observed no signs of local anesthetic intoxication or accidental vascular puncture. Plasma concentration of ropivacaine was significantly higher in the DCB group compared to PVB and ICB ($p < 0.001$) and in the PVB group compared to ICB ($p = 0.008$). Surgeons' satisfaction was higher in the PVB group compared to ICB ($p = 0.003$) and patients' satisfaction was higher in the PVB group compared to ICB ($p = 0.010$) and DCB group ($p = 0.029$). Phrenic nerve paralysis was observed frequently in the DCB group ($p < 0.05$). None of these patients with hemi-diaphragmatic paralysis showed signs of respiratory distress.

Conclusion: The ultrasound guided PVB is a safe and effective technique for CEA which is associated with lower plasma levels of local anesthetic than the standard DCB. Considering the low rate of complications in all types of regional anesthesia for CEA, larger randomized controlled trials are warranted to assess potential side effects among the blocks.

(Continued on next page)

* Correspondence: thomas.roessel@ukdd.de
†Thomas Rössel and Christopher Uhlig contributed equally to this work.
[1]Department of Anaesthesiology and Critical Care Medicine, University Hospital Carl Gustav Carus Dresden, Technische Universität Dresden, Fetscherstr. 74, 01307 Dresden, Germany

(Continued from previous page)

Keywords: Carotid endarterectomy, Cervical plexus block, Plasma concentration, Regional anesthesia, Local anesthetic, Ropivacaine

Background

In carotid endarterectomy (CEA), regional anesthesia is associated with beneficial effects regarding sensitivity and specificity of patients neurological monitoring [1, 2]. CEA in awake patients requires the blockade of cervical nerves from C2 to C4. The blockade can be performed on the nerve roots or on the terminal nerve fibers. The most frequently used regional anesthetic techniques for this purpose are superficial, intermediate and deep cervical block. The anesthetic effects of these three techniques are comparable [3, 4]. However, during dissection of the internal carotid artery (ICA) the need for local anesthetic supplementation by the surgeon ranges from 20 to 60% [5].

Over the last decade, the use of ultrasound has improved the safety and efficacy of regional anesthesia [6, 7]. The major advantages of ultrasound-guided regional anesthesia are the visualization of the target structures, the direct observation of the spread of the local anesthetic and the reduction of puncture-related complications compared to nerve stimulation or land mark technique. Furthermore, new ultrasound-guided anesthetic approaches for blockade of various nerves were developed [8–11]. Our group previously demonstrated a good clinical efficacy with a low rate of intraoperative local anesthetic supplementation by surgeons for the combination of ultrasound-guided intermediate cervical block with perivascular infiltration of the ICA, so called perivascular block (PVB) [8]. On the other hand, due to the vicinity of the vessels the PVB may result on higher plasma levels of local anesthetic compared to ultrasound-guided intermediate cervical block alone (ICB). This may cause more perioperative complications such as dizziness and seizures as described for the deep cervical block (DCB) [4]. In addition to potential toxic effects of local anesthetics, respiratory distress by phrenic nerve paralysis is possible [4].

To our knowledge, ultrasound-guided PVB, ICB and DCB have not been assessed in regard to block performance, perioperative complications and plasma levels of local anesthetics.

Therefore, we investigated the effects of PVB, ICB and DCB on ropivacaine plasma levels, anesthesia related nerve paralysis and efficacy of the block in patients undergoing elective CEA. We hypothesized that the ropivacaine plasma concentration is higher in patients receiving DCB for elective CEA compared to PVB and ICB.

Methods

We conducted a randomized controlled, single-center pilot study. The trial is reported according to the Consolidated Standards of Reporting Trials (CONSORT) statement [12]. The experimental protocol is depicted in Fig. 1. After approval by the local institutional review board of the Technische Universität Dresden, Germany (EK 130042013), thirty consecutive patients scheduled for elective CEA in the University Hospital Carl Gustav Carus, Dresden, Germany were screened for eligibility in a 6 month period. Inclusion and exclusion criteria are summarized in Table 1. The patients were randomized directly before start of ultrasound-guided regional anesthesia to three groups: DCB with 20 mL ropivacaine 0.5%, ICB alone with 20 mL ropivacaine 0.5% and combination of intermediate cervical block and perivascular infiltration, PVB, with 20 mL ropivacaine 0.5% and 10 mL ropivacaine 0.3%, respectively. The random sequence was compiled using a computer-generated random numbers table and group allocation was concealed by sequentially numbered opaque closed envelopes. Surgeons and data collectors were blinded to the study group.

Regional anesthesia

Regional anesthesia was performed by two senior anesthesiologists with substantial experience in performance of ultrasound guided deep and intermediate cervical plexus block. The regional anesthetic techniques used in this study were performed as previously described [6, 8]. Briefly, patients were placed for regional anesthesia in supine position with their heads turned 30° to the opposite side. Prior to performing the block, the anatomic conditions of the neck region were analyzed by ultrasound. During this examination, first the transverse process with the corresponding nerve roots from the second to the seventh cervical vertebrae (C2 to C7) as well as the distal part of cervical plexus were visualized and recorded using a Philips HD 11 with a 12.5 MHz linear ultrasound transducer (Philips Medicine Systems GmbH, Hamburg, Germany). Subsequently, the ICA was identified and the distance between the skin and the ICA was recorded. The cervical block was performed according to group allocation (Fig. 2). The success of the

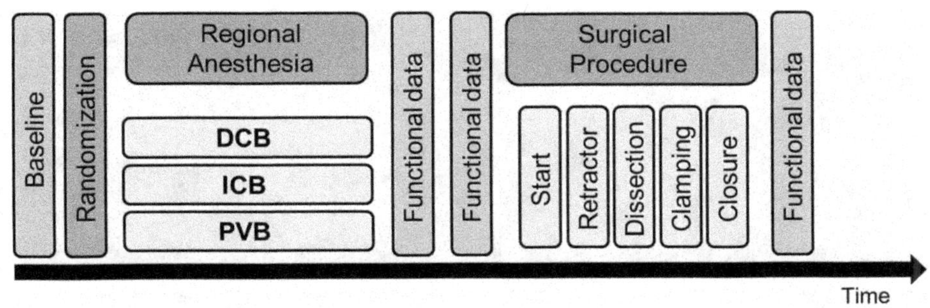

Fig. 1 Time course of intervention. DCB: deep cervical block, ICB: intermediate cervical block, PVB: intermediate cervical block with perivascular infiltration of the internal carotid artery

blockade was evaluated 5, 10, and 15 min after regional anesthesia by pin prick test in the dermatomes from C2 to C5. Additionally, 20 min after the block was performed, sensory skin testing at the hand, shoulder and motor testing at the wrist, arm and shoulder were performed. Puncture related complications, such as respiratory distress, hypoglossal and facial nerve palsy or Horner's syndrome were also assessed.

Intraoperative management and hemodynamic monitoring

The evening before surgery, patients received 25 mg of clorazepate (Aventis GmbH, Bernburg, Germany) per os by request. No premedication was administered at the day of surgery. In the operating room, peripheral venous access, a 5-lead ECG including ST-segment analysis, a pulsoxymetry and an arterial line for continuous monitoring of arterial blood pressure were placed. Hemodynamic data were continuously recorded using a Philips Intellivue MP 70 (Philips Medicine Systems GmbH, Hamburg, Germany). An arterial blood gas analysis was performed before, as well as 15 and 30 min after regional anesthesia. To improve intraoperative comfort, all patients received 0.03 μg/kg/min remifentanil (Aspen-Germany GmbH, Germany; dosage in relation to ideal body weight). After surgery, the patients were observed for 24 h under cardiovascular and neurological monitoring in the intermediate care unit, post anesthesia care unit or regular ward, as appropriate.

Surgical management

All CEAs were performed by two senior vascular surgeons. Surgery was started when the surgical site had been sufficiently anesthetized. Pain was intraoperatively evaluated by means of the Numeric Analgesia Scale (NAS) graded from 0 (no pain) to 10 (worst pain) during the performance of regional anesthesia and during skin incision, retractor placement, dissection, cross-clamping, and skin closure. If patients complained of intraoperative pain NAS > 2 an additional local infiltration of lidocaine 1% (mibe GmbH, Brehna, Germany) was administered by the surgeon in 1 ml steps until a sufficient anesthetic level was achieved. The total amount of supplemented lidocaine was recorded. At the end of surgery, the surgeons assessed the surgical conditions on a subjective scale ranging from 1 to 5 (1-very good, 2-good, 3-reasonable, 4-poor, 5-very poor). All patients underwent follow-up visits on the first post-operative day. Patients were asked to assess their satisfaction with anesthesia in five grades from 1-very good, 2-good, 3-reasonable, 4-poor to 5-very poor and if they would again undergo surgery under regional anesthesia.

Plasma level measurement

Arterial blood samples for plasma level of ropivacaine were collected before and 5, 10, 20, 60, and 180 min after the injection of ropivacaine. After immediate centrifugation, plasma samples were stored at − 20 °C. The unbound ropivacaine plasma level was measured by the Institute of Legal Medicine, Dresden Technical University. After a liquid-liquid extraction procedure for sample preparation specimens were analyzed with a high performance liquid chromatography photodiode array detection system (Agilent 1100 series, Agilent Technologies, Waldbronn, Germany). For quantification, drug-free serum was spiked at five different concentrations of ropivacaine (100, 200, 500, 1000, 2000 ng/ml). Ropivacaine concentration was calculated using linear

Table 1 Inclusion and exclusion criteria. CEA: carotid endarterectomy, ICA: internal carotid artery

Inclusion	Exclusion
-age > 18 years -elective CEA surgery for treatment of ICA stenosis -written informed consent	-history of anaphylactic reaction to local anesthetics -local infection in the lateral cervical region -presumed limitation of patients' compliance

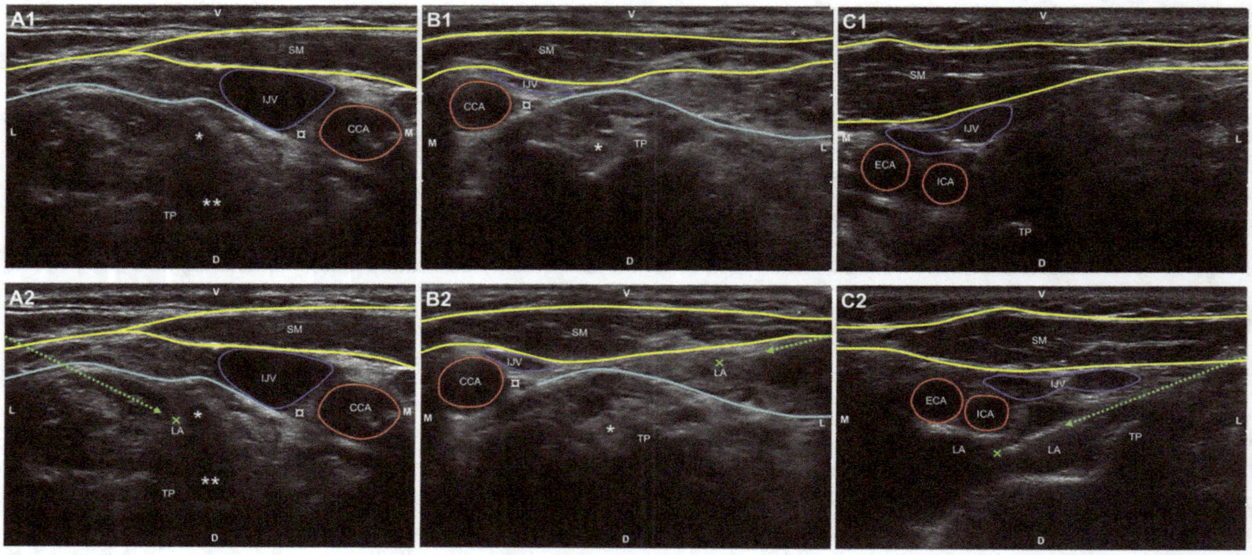

Fig. 2 Ultrasound images of cervical block. **a**: deep cervical block, **b**: intermediate cervical block, **c**: intermediate cervical block with perivascular infiltration of the internal carotid artery. Ultrasound images were acquired with Philips HD-11-XE (Philips Healthcare GmbH, Hamburg, Germany using a linear probe (12 MHz, L-12-4, Philips Healthcare GmbH, Hamburg, Germany). Direction of the ultrasound enhanced puncture needle is depicted as green dashed line and the needle tip as green cross. Yellow line: superficial cervical fascia, blue line: deep cervical fascia. LA: local anesthetic, ECA: external carotid artery, ICA: internal carotid artery, IJV: internal jugular vein, CCA: commune carotid artery, TP: Processus transversus of the respective cervical vertebra, V: ventral, D: dorsal, SM: M. steroncleidomastoideus. *: C5 nerve root, **: C6 nerve root, ¤: N. vagus, x: N. auricularis magnus and *N. transversus* colli

regression. The limit of quantification of the method was 100 ng/ml.

Assessment of phrenic nerve paresis

The quantitative analysis of phrenic nerve paresis was performed by electrical impedance tomography (EIT, PulmoVista 500, Dräger Medical, Lübeck, Germany) [13]. Images were obtained at baseline, 15, 30 and 180 min after successful establishment of the cervical block. The images containing 32 × 32 pixels were recorded at a rate of 50 frames/s during 2 min for offline analysis. Using a MATLAB (Vers. R2006b, The Mathworks Inc., Natick, MA, USA) based routine, changes in impedance (region of interest – ROI) were determined. The ROI was divided into two zones with equal size corresponding with the left and right lung. Relative changes in impedance were computed. A phrenic nerve paresis was defined as a decrease in change of impedance of more than 50% compared to baseline in one ROI. Phrenic nerve paresis was assessed qualitative and quantitatively by an investigator blinded to the group allocation.

Neurological monitoring

Neurologic function was perioperatively continuously monitored by observing the level of consciousness and the response to verbal commands. During 5 min test cross-clamping of the ICA, the patient was challenged to squeeze a squeaking rubber toy with the contralateral hand every 10–15 s and to answer simple questions for close judgment of neurological function. A shunt was placed if any signs of neurological dysfunction occurred during test cross-clamping. Additionally, the function of recurrent laryngeal nerve, hypoglossal nerve and facial nerve was monitored before and 30 min after regional anesthetic blockade, as well as before and after cross clamping and at the end of surgery.

Statistical analysis

Statistical analysis was performed with SPSS (Vers. 20, IBM Deutschland GmbH, Ehningen, Germany). Graphs were computed using Graph Pad Prism Vers. 6.01 (GraphPad Software Inc., La Jolla, CA, USA). Values are given as total numbers and percentage, mean and standard deviation or median and interquartile range as appropriate. Statistical significance was considered at two-sided $p < 0.05$. All analyses were performed on an intention-to-treat basis. Normal distribution was assessed visually using Q-Q Plot of standardized residuals. For the primary outcome, the ropivacaine plasma level, among- and within-groups differences for repeated measures were tested with a general linear model followed by adjustment according to the Sidak method. For secondary outcomes, frequency distributions were analyzed with a Chi-square test followed by a multiple regression approach using adjusted residuals and Bonferoni post hoc test, if appropriate. One-way ANOVA followed by Bonferroni adjustment or Kruskal Wallis test followed by Dunn-Bonferroni test for multiple comparison were used for independent parameters depending on the data distribution. Among- and within-groups differences for repeated measures were tested with a general linear model followed by adjustment according to the Sidak method. Since this study was planned as an explorative trial, no sample size estimation was performed. We opted for 30 patients (10 per group).

Results

Over a period of 7 months, 30 consecutive patients undergoing CEA were enrolled in the trial (Fig. 3). All patients completed the follow-up according to the trial protocol. The three groups were comparable regarding baseline characteristics (Table 2).

Block execution and performance

The identification of the nerve roots, of the intermediate cervical plexus, of the ICA and the bifurcation of carotid artery using ultrasound was successful in all patients. The distances from the skin to the ICA was 1.8 ± 0.3 cm in the DCB group, 2.1 ± 0.3 cm in the ICB group and 2.1 ± 0.5 cm in the PVB group ($p = 0.143$). The time required to perform the block was significantly higher in the DCB group compared to PVB ($p = 0.003$, Table 3). The time until full expression of regional anesthesia is depicted in Fig. 4. All three groups showed sufficient analgesia in the dermatomes C3 and C4, but PVB was the only block providing analgesia in the dermatome C2 in all patients.

During surgery, 18 patients complained about pain NAS ≥ 2 resulting in supplementation of the block with local lidocaine 1% by the surgeon (6 vs. 8 vs. 4 patients, DCB vs. ICB vs. PVB, $p = 0.189$, respectively). In the PVB group a lower dosage of supplementation was required (Table 3). No conversion to general anesthesia due to an incomplete block or any other reasons was necessary. The duration of surgery was 103 ± 33 mins in the DCB group, 103 ± 17 mins in the ICB and 107 ± 21 min in the PVB group ($p = 0.874$). The cross-clamping time was 37 ± 10 min in the DCB group, 37 ± 9 min in the ICB group and 29 ± 5 min in group with PVB ($p = 0.061$). Planned or unplanned shunt placement was not necessary in any case. Surgeons' satisfaction was higher in the PVB group compared to ICB and patients' satisfaction was higher in the PVB group compared to ICB and TCB group (Fig. 5). Hemodynamic and functional data as well as cardiac biomarkers are shown in Additional file 1: Tables S1, S2 and Fig. S1. The length of hospital stay was 7.7 ± 4.7 days in the DCB group, 5.2 ± 1.1 days in the ICB group and 5.3 ± 0.9 days in the PVB group ($p = 0.610$). There were no in-hospital deaths observed.

Ropivacaine plasma concentration

The ropivacaine plasma concentration is shown in Fig. 6. The plasma concentration of ropivacaine was significantly higher in the DCB and PVB group compared to the ICB group (DCB vs. ICB, $p < 0.001$; DCB vs. PVB, $p = 0.001$; ICB vs. PVB, $p = 0.008$; respectively). There was no adverse event related to the systemic plasma level of ropivacaine in all groups.

Neurological complications

No patient suffered from new intra- or postoperative central neurological deficits. Horner syndrome, hypoglossal

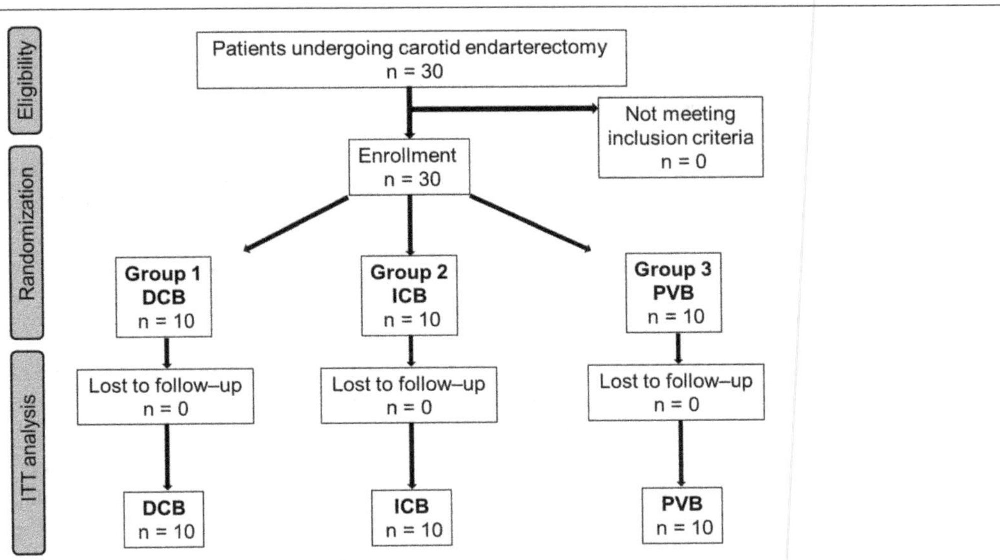

Fig. 3 Flow chart of enrolled patients. ITT: intention-to-treat analysis, DCB: deep cervical block, ICB: intermediate cervical block, PVB: intermediate cervical block with perivascular infiltration of the internal carotid artery

Table 2 Baseline characteristics

	DCB (n = 10)	ICB (n = 10)	PVB (n = 10)
Age [years]	67 ± 10	70 ± 9	72 ± 8
Sex male	7 (70.0)	9 (90.0)	8 (80.0)
female	3 (30.0)	1 (10.0)	2 (20.0)
Bodyweight [kg]	72 ± 8	83 ± 8	84 ± 9
Body height [cm]	167 ± 8	174 ± 8	170 ± 6
BMI [kg/m²]	25.9 ± 1.6	27.3 ± 2.2	29.1 ± 3.4
Stenosis			
Grade [%]	81 ± 7	82 ± 6	82 ± 9
Sight left	5 (50.0)	5 (50.0)	5 (50.0)
right	5 (50.0)	5 (50.0)	5 (50.0)
asymptomatic	6 (60.0)	6 (60.0)	7 (70.0)
symptomatic	4 (40.0)	4 (40.0)	3 (30.0)
ASA II	6 (60.0)	6 (60.0)	5 (50.0)
III	4 (40.0)	4 (40.0)	5 (50.0)
Comorbidities			
Arterial hypertension	10 (100.0)	10 (100.0)	10 (100.0)
Diabetes mellitus	4 (40.0)	4 (40.0)	5 (50.0)
Hyperlipoproteinema	10 (100.0)	9 (90.0)	10 (100.0)
PAOD	6 (60.0)	1 (10.0)	7 (70.0)
CAD	4 (40.0)	4 (40.0)	5 (50.0)
AMI	1 (10.0)	1 (10.0)	2 (20.0)
Stent	2 (20.0)	2 (20.0)	2 (20.0)
CABG	1 (10.0)	0 (0.0)	3 (30.0)
Artrial fibrillation	1 (10.0)	0 (0.0)	0 (0.0)
COPD	2 (20.0)	2 (20.0)	1 (10.0)
CKD	3 (30.0)	2 (20.0)	1 (10.0)
Nicotine abuse	7 (70.0	7 (70.0	3 (30.0)
Alcohol abuse	5 (50.0)	3 (30.0)	0 (0.0)

Values are given as mean ± standard deviation or absolute number and percentage. *AMI* acute myocardial infarction in medical history, *ASA* American Society of Anesthesiology physic status, *BMI* body mass index, *CAD* coronary artery disease, *CABG* coronary artery bypass graft, *CKD* chronic kidney disease, *COPD* chronic obstructive pulmonary disease, *DCB* deep cervical block, *ICB* intermediate cervical block, *PAOD* peripheral artery occlusive disease, *PVB* intermediate cervical block with perivascular infiltration of the internal carotid artery

nerve or permanent facial nerve paralysis were not observed in any patient. Hemi-diaphragmatic impairment caused by phrenic nerve paralysis was associated with a more frequent occurrence in the DCB group ($p = 0.022$, Fig. 7). None of these patients with hemi-diaphragmatic paralysis showed signs of respiratory distress.

Discussion

Major findings

The major findings of the present study are:

1. The plasma level of local anesthetic was significantly higher in the DCB group and PVB group compared to ICB alone, without causing adverse events.
2. Impairment of ventilation due to hemi-diaphragmatic paralysis was frequently observed in the DCB group.
3. The PVB is a feasible regional anesthetic technique providing sufficient analgesia for CEA in all of the desired dermatomes C2-C4.

This is the first trial comparing ropivacaine plasma levels with PVB, DCB and ICB. Regional anesthesia and CEA were performed by senior physicians. We tried to reduce bias by blinding the patients, the surgeons and outcome assessors to groups. In addition to improve adherence to blinding, the anesthesiologist performing the cervical block did not treat the patient during surgery. Adherence to allocation concealment and blinding of participants, study personnel and outcome assessors were maintained throughout the trial.

Regional anesthesia in CEA

The implementation of ultrasound in regional anesthesia has increased safety and efficacy by direct visualization of the target structure and the needle tip as well as by observation of local anesthetic spread during injection. Despite these advantages, even the ultrasound guided regional anesthetic techniques require a high level of local anesthetic infiltration by surgeons [14–16]. In our opinion, an important reason for the high rate of local anesthetic supplementation is the complex innervations of the neurovascular sheath by the vagal and glossopharyngeal nerve. In several previous studies, ultrasound guided perivascular infiltration of the ICA decreased the necessity of local anesthetic supplementation by surgeons and increased the efficacy of regional anesthesia [8, 17, 18]. However, the influence of perivascular infiltration on local anesthetic plasma concentration or the risk of phrenic nerve paralysis were not compared so far.

Ropivacaine plasma levels

The plasma concentration of local anesthetic depends on different conditions. Particularly, the type of local anesthetic as well as the vascularization of the puncture site are important factors of local anesthetic absorption. Ropivacaine is associated with low lipid solubility and provides a better neurological and cardiac toxicity profile than bupivacaine. Additionally, the vasoconstrictive effetcs of ropivacaine delays the absorption of the local anesthetic and may therefore be particularly suitable for regional anesthetic techniques in highly vascularized regions. Besides this advantages also for ropivacaine severe

Table 3 Supplementation of block with additional local anesthesia by the surgeon and NAS results (0 = no pain −10 = worst imaginable pain)

		DCB (*n* = 10)	ICB (*n* = 10)	PVB (*n* = 10)	*P* value
Duration of block disposition [min]		15.9 ± 2.8	11.5 ± 2.1	14.1 ± 2.0	0.019*
Additional lidocaine [No.,%]		6 (60.0)	8 (80.0)	4 (40.0)	n.a.
Additional lidocaine [mg]		90.0 (50.0, 100.0, 145.0,160.0)	150.0 (50.0, 100.0, 200.0, 300.0)	85.0 (30.0, 35.0, 120.0,120.0)	n.a.
Numeric analog scale*	RA	2 (0, 2, 4, 5)	3 (0, 1, 3, 5)	2 (1, 1, 2, 3)	0.336
	Incision	1 (0, 1, 3, 5)	2 (0, 1, 2, 5)	1 (0, 1, 2, 3)	0.659
	Retractor	1 (0, 1, 2, 4)	2 (0, 1, 3, 3)	1 (0, 1, 2, 3)	0.301
	Dissection	2 (1, 1, 4, 6)	1 (0, 3, 4, 5)	2 (1, 2, 2, 3)	0.061
	Clamping	2 (0, 1, 2, 2)	2 (0, 2, 3, 3)	2 (1, 2, 3, 5)	0.153
	Suture	1 (0, 1, 1, 5)	2 (0, 1, 2, 3)	1 (0, 1, 2, 2)	0.189

Values are given as mean ± standard deviation, median (minimum, 25% percentile, 75% percentile, maximum) or absolute number (percentage) as appropriate. Differences among groups were tested with Kruskal-Wallis followed by Dunn-Bonferroni test. Statistical significance was considered to be at two-sided $p < 0.05$. *DCB* deep cervical block, *ICB* intermediate cervical block, *PVB* intermediate cervical block with perivascular infiltration of the internal carotid artery, *RA* regional anesthesia, *No* number, *n.a* statistics not applicable due to low patient number in the PVB group. *: $p < 0.001$ DCB vs. ICB

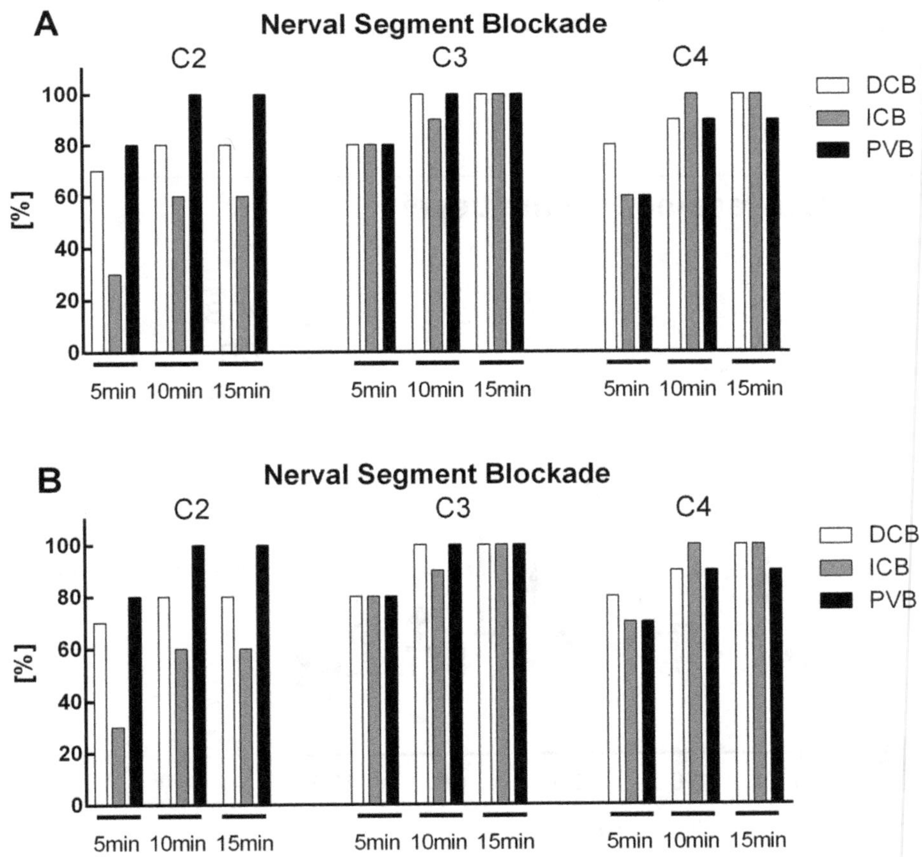

Fig. 4 Block distention in the dermatomes C2 to C4. Block distention was determined using peaked/blunt discrimination (**a**) or warm/cold discrimination (**b**). Values are given as percentage and were measured 5 min, 10 min and 15 min after completion of block placement, respectively. DCB: deep cervical block, ICB: intermediate cervical block, PVB: intermediate cervical block with perivascular infiltration of the internal carotid artery

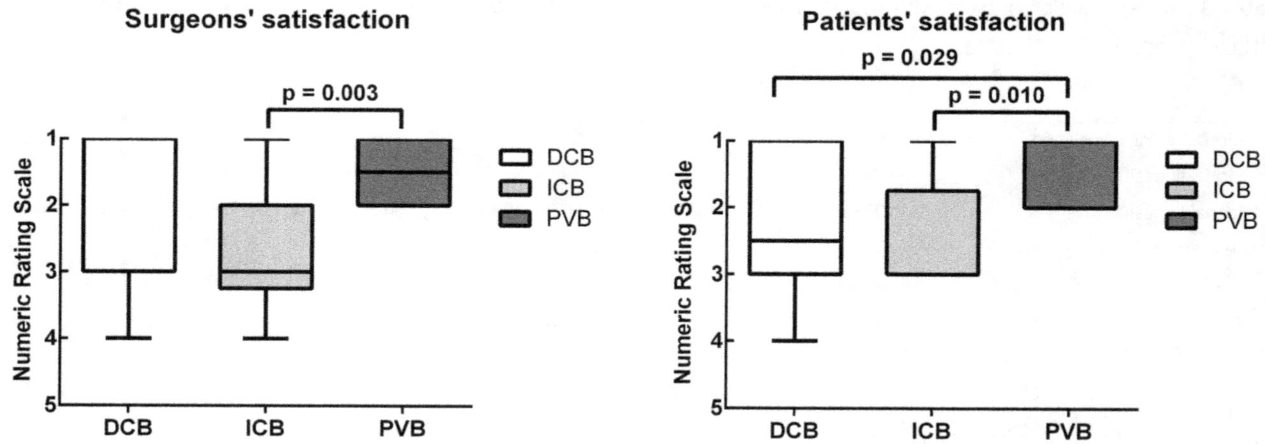

Fig. 5 Surgeons' and Patients' satisfaction. Values are presented as boxplot boxplot (whiskers minimum to maximum) on a numeric rating scale. Grade system: 1-very good, 2-good, 3-reasonable, 4-poor, 5-very poor. Statistical analysis was performed using Kruskal Wallis test followed by Dunn-Bonferroni test for multiple comparison. Statistical significance was considered to be at two-sided $p < 0.05$. DCB: deep cervical block, ICB: intermediate cervical block, PVB: intermediate cervical block with perivascular infiltration of the internal carotid artery

complications up to local anesthetic intoxications with cardiac arrest are reported [19, 20].

In carotid endarterectomy cerebral seizure by local anesthetic intoxication can lead to the inability to properly monitor neurological symptoms and increases the oxygen consumption of the brain. Davies et al. reported two cases of local anesthetic intoxications in 1000 carotid endarterectomies, which equals an incidence of 0.2% [5]. The occurrence of cerebral symptoms depends on the maximum ropivacaine plasma concentration as well as the slope of the plasma level increase.

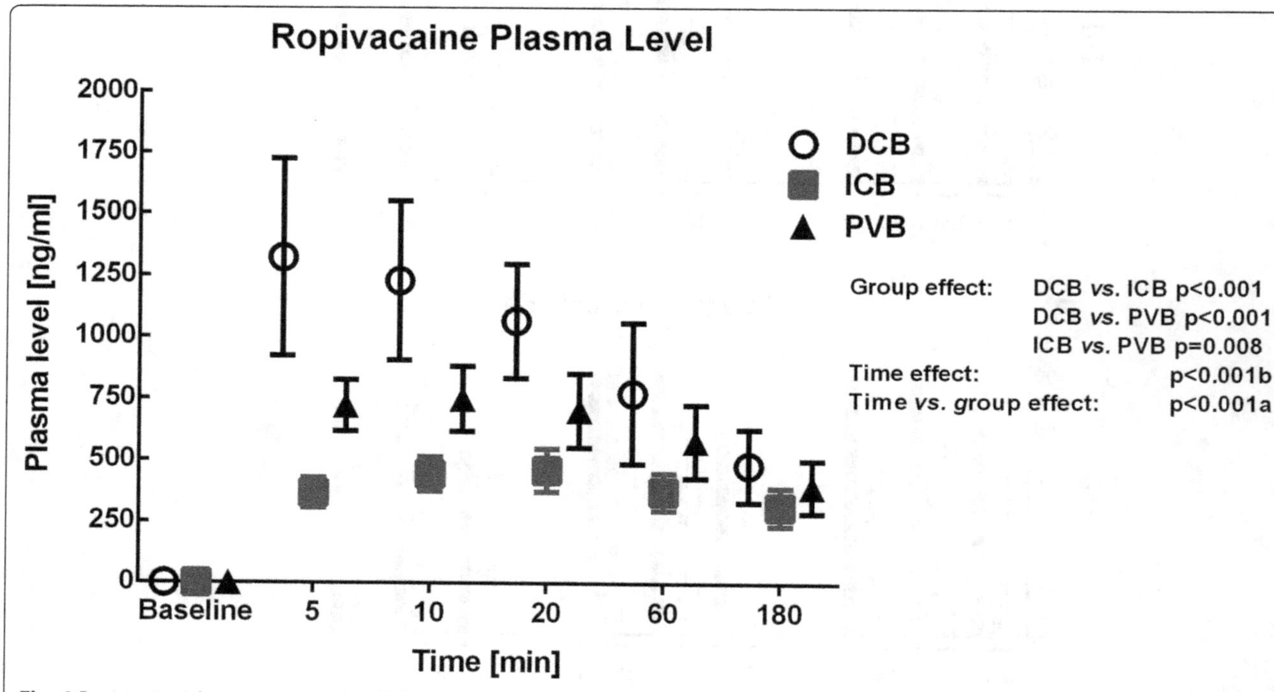

Fig. 6 Ropivacaine plasma concentration. Values are given as mean ± standard deviation. Differences among groups, as well as time and time vs. group effects were tested using a general linear model without a covariate. Statistical significance was considered to be at two-sided $p < 0.05$. DCB: deep cervical block, ICB: intermediate cervical block, PVB: intermediate cervical block with perivascular infiltration of the internal carotid artery

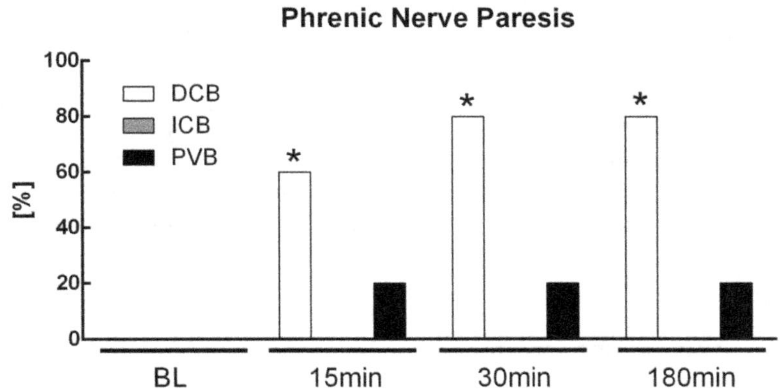

Fig. 7 Incidence of phrenic nerve paralysis. Values are given as percentage at baseline (BL), 5 min, 30 min, and 180 min after completion of block placement, respectively. A Chi-square test with multiple regression approach and Bonferroni post hoc test were performed. Statistical significance was accepted a $p < 0.05$. DCB: deep cervical block, ICB: intermediate cervical block, PVB: intermediate cervical block with perivascular infiltration of the internal carotid artery. *: $p < 0.05$

In the present study, the lowest peak concentrations of ropivacaine (0.3 µg/mL) were measured in the intermediate cervical block group and the highest peak concentrations (2.1 µg/mL) in the deep cervical block group. However, the detected ropivacaine plasma concentrations were well below the threshold for early neurological toxicity symptoms to be 2.2 µg/mL as described by Knudsen et al. [21]. Different groups reported comparable plasma concentrations of ropivacaine after interscalene or deep cervical plexus block [22]. In contrast, few studies examined the ropivacaine plasma concentrations after intermediate cervical block. Koköfer et al. reported plasma concentrations after ultrasound guided triple injection technique (intermediate cervical block, perivascular infiltration and subcutane infiltration) [7]. This group used 20 mL ropivacaine 0.375% or 0.75% for intermediate cervical block and prilocaine 1% for the perivascular infiltration of ICA. Additionally, prilocaine 1% was used also for the subcutaneous infiltration along the anterior border of sternocleidomastoid muscle. The peak plasma levels in the ropivacaine 0.375% group ranged from 4 to 7 µg/mL and in the ropivacaine 0.75% group from 5 to 10 µg/mL. In contrast, the peak plasma levels for intermediate cervical block in our study ranged from 0.3 to 0.6 µg/mL. Several reasons may explain these different results of local anesthetic plasma levels after intermediate cervical plexus block. The use of two different local anesthetics by Koköfer could have led to an increase of ropivacaine plasma concentration. Another cause might be the binding of ropivacaine to α_1-acid glycoprotein, which may markedly affect the pharmacokinetics of ropivacaine [23]. However, α_1-acid glycoprotein levels were measured neither in the present study, nor by Koköfer [7].

The effects of perivascular infiltration on ropivacaine plasma concentration was not examined in any study. Although Koköfer et al. performed a perivascular infiltration, the effect on plasma concentration was not assessed. He used prilocaine 1% for perivascular infiltration as well as for subcutaneous infiltration. In our study, we applied only ropivacaine for all regional anesthetic techniques. The ropivacaine plasma concentrations of the perivascular group were significantly higher than for intermediate block alone. In our opinion, the reason of the higher ropivacaine concentration is the larger volume of local anesthetic applied in the perivascular group compared to the intermediate block alone suggesting similar tissue adsorption characteristics.

The threshold plasma concentration at which central nerve system toxicity occurs may be related more to the rate of increase of the serum concentration rather than to the total amount of drug injected. Wulf and colleagues examined the plasma concentration after combined ilioinguinal-iliohypogastric block with ropivacaine [24]. The peak plasma concentrations of ropivacaine were 1.5 µg/mL and occurred 45 min after injection. In contrast, Rettig et al. examined the plasma concentrations of ropivacaine after brachial plexus blockade using four different approaches [22]. The authors reported the lateral and posterior interscalene block to be associated with earlier (10 and 15 min, respectively) and high peak plasma concentrations of local anesthetic (4,4 µg/mL and 4,5 µg/mL). According to these studies, the increase in plasma concentrations is significantly influenced by the anatomic region of regional anesthesia. In the present study, the fastest increase in ropivacaine concentration was observed in the deep cervical block group. However, no cerebral signs of local anesthetic intoxication were observed. The time to reach the maximum concentration was 5 to 10 min. Similar results were reported by Merle, who found times of 5 to 17 min for the classic deep cervical block [25]. In contrast to deep cervical block, in our study the increase in ropivacaine plasma concentrations was significantly slower (10 to 20 min) for intermediate cervical plexus block alone. Similar results were observed for combination of intermediate cervical block and perivascular infiltration. In this group the time to reach the maximum concentration was 10 to 20 min. In our opinion, the reason of the faster increase in ropivacaine plasma concentration is a pronounced vascularization in the deep cervical space.

Phrenic nerve paralysis

Phrenic nerve paralysis can occur during cervical block due to the close anatomical relation. The phrenic nerve origins mainly from the C4 root, with variable portions from the C3 and C5 root [26]. After formation of the phrenic nerve at the upper lateral border of the anterior scalene muscle the nerve continues caudally between the ventral surface of the anterior scalene muscle and prevertebral fascial layer that covers this muscle and is therefore separated from the brachial plexus only by a thin fascial layer [26]. During regional anesthesia, a perioperative phrenic nerve paralysis can have various causes [27, 28]. Temporary phrenic nerve palsies are most common after cardiac surgery but may also be caused by CEA due to traction or compression as well as local anesthetic supplementation [29].

In the current trial, all patients showed bilateral ventilation before regional anesthesia. In ten patients (DCB: $n = 8$, PVB: $n = 2$) a phrenic nerve paresis was observed. None of these patients suffered from respiratory distress. The high rate of phrenic nerve paralysis in our investigation is not surprising for deep cervical block, where a phrenic nerve paralysis occur in 55 to 61% of the cases [30, 31]. An even higher rate up to 100% of hemi-diaphragmatic paralysis is reported by Urmey et al. for the interscalene brachial plexus block [32, 33]. Despite this high incidence of paralysis of the phrenic nerve, reports of significant shortness of breath or impairment of gas exchange are rare [33–35]. The occurrence of phrenic nerve paresis in the perivascular group is more difficult to explain. The precise anatomy of the deeper neck compartments is complex and has not been completely understood so far. For decades, the concept of impenetrability of the deep fascia of the neck for local anesthetics was indefeasible [36], but has been questioned recently [37, 38]. These doubts are supported by case reports observing complications such as Horner syndrome after superficial blocks [39]. Furthermore, Pandit et al. described in a cadaver study penetration of a superficial injection of methylene blue to the nerve roots in the deep space [40]. Contrary, in another corpse study, Seidel and colleagues observed no spread of methylene blue through the deep cervical fascia [36]. Nevertheless, there were clear methodological differences between these two cadaver studies, especially in the fluid volume administered [36, 40]. In our opinion, larger volumes of local anesthetic may cause higher intra-compartment pressures and therefore enhance a deeper spread of the local anesthetic via the anatomic pathways described by Pandit [38, 40]. This may result in phrenic nerve paresis in the deep cervical compartment. However, further detailed studies are warranted to prove this hypothesis.

Limitations

The present trial has several limitations. First, the present trial was an explorative pilot study. Therefore, no sample size calculation was performed. Second, the hemi-diaphragmatic paresis was diagnosed indirectly through decrease of regional ventilation in one lung via EIT. This functional approach to phrenic nerve paresis was described by Reske and colleagues for interscalene brachial plexus block in a small patient collective [13]. The EIT has the major advantage that the impairment of ventilation could easily be detected at the bedside [41]. Ultrasound imaging of the diaphragm is more observer dependent and can be difficult in obese patients. In contrast, the EIT has also been used in obese patients by Nestler et al. [42]. However, the EIT method for detecting hemi-diaphragmatic paresis has not been validated in a larger patient collective so far. Parallel ultrasound imaging of the diaphragm was not performed in the current trial. Third, the assessment of patient and surgeon satisfaction with the respective block was subjective. The simple grading scale for satisfaction from 1 to 5 was chosen for patients' feasibility. The same grading was used for surgeons' rating with regards to comparability. Fourth, the individual patient pain and convenience level in the operating room may have influenced the surgeons' decision for additional administration of local anesthetic in the operating situs.

Implications for further studies

Future trials investigating the effects of different regional anesthetic techniques such as DCB, ICB and PVB on patient safety, systemic local anesthetic concentration and side effects are warranted. Such a trial should be prospective, randomized, controlled and ideally triple blind focusing for instance on postoperative pulmonary complications caused by phrenic nerve paralysis with dual assessment of diaphragm function by EIT and ultrasound as primary outcome. The present trial may provide a basis for sample size calculation. However, the evaluation of systemic toxic side effects of local anesthetics during regional anesthesia for CEA will be difficult due to the rare occurrence [5]. A prospective observational trial focusing on the occurrence of seizures and new arrhythmias in context to the regional anesthetic technique may help to further investigate these systemic and clinical relevant side effects. The adaptation of the data entry in national or international databases for CEA regarding the specific regional anesthetic technique and type of anesthetic may help researchers to get access to a larger data set for a retrospective trial.

Conclusions

The ultrasound guided intermediate cervical block with perivascular infiltration of the internal carotid artery is a safe and feasible technique for carotid endarterectomy. However, further studies in a larger patient collective are warranted to evaluate rare side effects related to the area of administration and systemic plasma concentration of the local anesthetic.

Abbreviations

CEA: Carotid endarterectomy; CONSORT: Consolidated Standards of Reporting Trials; DCB: Deep cervical block; EIT: Electrical impedance tomography; ICA: Internal carotid artery; ICB: Intermediate cervical block; PVB: Intermediate cervical block with perivascular infiltration of the internal carotid artery; ROI: Region of interest

Acknowledgements

The authors thank the anesthetic and surgical staff of the Department of Visceral, Thoracic and Vascular Surgery, University Hospital Carl Gustav Carus, Technische Universität Dresden, Dresden, Germany. The authors express their special gratitude to Rüdiger Paul, who helped performing regional anesthesia and to Dr. Anja Braune, who developed the Matlab routine for EIT analysis.

Authors' contributions

[TR]1 and CU contributed equally to this manuscript. [TR]1 designed the study protocol, collected data and contributed to manuscript preparation. CU helped with data collection, performed the statistical data analysis and helped preparing the manuscript. JP performed the ropivacaine plasma level measurements and contributed to the manuscript preparation. SL performed carotid surgery and helped preparing the manuscript. [TR]2: helped preparing the manuscript. TK helped preparing the manuscript. PMS helped preparing the manuscript and interpreting the data. SK contributed to manuscript preparation and interpretation of the data. All authors have read and approved the manuscript.

Author details

[1]Department of Anaesthesiology and Critical Care Medicine, University Hospital Carl Gustav Carus Dresden, Technische Universität Dresden, Fetscherstr. 74, 01307 Dresden, Germany. [2]Institute of Legal Medicine, Technische Universität Dresden, Dresden, Germany. [3]Department of Visceral, Thoracic and Vascular Surgery, University Hospital Carl Gustav Carus, Technische Universität Dresden, Dresden, Germany. [4]Department of General Surgery, University Hospital of Friedrich-Alexander-University, Erlangen, Germany.

References

1. Sbarigia E, Schioppa A, Misuraca M, Panico MA, Battocchio C, Maraglino C, Speziale F, Fiorani P. Somatosensory evoked potentials versus locoregional anaesthesia in the monitoring of cerebral function during carotid artery surgery: preliminary results of a prospective study. Eur J Vasc Endovasc Surg. 2001;21(5):413–6.
2. Group GTC, Lewis SC, Warlow CP, Bodenham AR, Colam B, Rothwell PM, Torgerson D, Dellagrammaticas D, Horrocks M, Liapis C, et al. General anaesthesia versus local anaesthesia for carotid surgery (GALA): a multicentre, randomised controlled trial. Lancet. 2008;372(9656):2132–42.
3. Stoneham MD, Doyle AR, Knighton JD, Dorje P, Stanley JC. Prospective, randomized comparison of deep or superficial cervical plexus block for carotid endarterectomy surgery. Anesthesiology. 1998;89(4):907–12.
4. Pandit JJ, Satya-Krishna R, Gration P. Superficial or deep cervical plexus block for carotid endarterectomy: a systematic review of complications. Br J Anaesth. 2007;99(2):159–69.
5. Davies MJ, Silbert BS, Scott DA, Cook RJ, Mooney PH, Blyth C. Superficial and deep cervical plexus block for carotid artery surgery: a prospective study of 1000 blocks. Reg Anesth. 1997;22(5):442–6.
6. Roessel T, Wiessner D, Heller AR, Zimmermann T, Koch T, Litz RJ. High-resolution ultrasound-guided high interscalene plexus block for carotid endarterectomy. Reg Anesth Pain Med. 2007;32(3):247–53.
7. Kokofer A, Nawratil J, Felder TK, Stundner O, Mader N, Gerner P. Ropivacaine 0.375% vs. 0.75% with prilocaine for intermediate cervical plexus block for carotid endarterectomy: a randomised trial. Eur J Anaesthesiol. 2015;32(11): 781–9.
8. Rossel T, Kersting S, Heller AR, Koch T. Combination of high-resolution ultrasound-guided perivascular regional anesthesia of the internal carotid artery and intermediate cervical plexus block for carotid surgery. Ultrasound Med Biol. 2013;39(6):981–6.
9. Karmakar MK, Kwok WH, Ho AM, Tsang K, Chui PT, Gin T. Ultrasound-guided sciatic nerve block: description of a new approach at the subgluteal space. Br J Anaesth. 2007;98(3):390–5.
10. Guntz E, Herman P, Debizet E, Delhaye D, Coulic V, Sosnowski M. Sciatic nerve block in the popliteal fossa: description of a new medial approach. Can J Anaesth. 2004;51(8):817–20.
11. Greher M, Scharbert G, Kamolz LP, Beck H, Gustorff B, Kirchmair L, Kapral S. Ultrasound-guided lumbar facet nerve block: a sonoanatomic study of a new methodologic approach. Anesthesiology. 2004;100(5):1242–8.
12. Eldridge SM, Chan CL, Campbell MJ, Bond CM, Hopewell S, Thabane L, Lancaster GA, Group Pc. CONSORT 2010 statement: extension to randomised pilot and feasibility trials. BMJ. 2016;355:i5239.
13. Wiegel M, Hammermuller S, Wrigge H, Reske AW. Electrical impedance tomography visualizes impaired ventilation due to Hemidiaphragmatic paresis after Interscalene brachial plexus block. Anesthesiology. 2016; 125(4):807.
14. Barone M, Diemunsch P, Baldassarre E, Oben WE, Ciarlo M, Wolter J, Albani A. Carotid endarterectomy with intermediate cervical plexus block. Tex Heart Inst J. 2010;37(3):297–300.
15. Alilet A, Petit P, Devaux B, Joly C, Samain E, Pili-Floury S, Besch G. Ultrasound-guided intermediate cervical block versus superficial cervical block for carotid artery endarterectomy: the randomized-controlled CERVECHO trial. Anaesth Crit Care Pain Med. 2017;36(2):91–5.
16. Calderon AL, Zetlaoui P, Benatir F, Davidson J, Desebbe O, Rahali N, Truc C, Feugier P, Lermusiaux P, Allaouchiche B, et al. Ultrasound-guided intermediate cervical plexus block for carotid endarterectomy using a new anterior approach: a two-Centre prospective observational study. Anaesthesia. 2015;70(4):445–51.
17. Hoefer J, Pierer E, Rantner B, Stadlbauer KH, Fraedrich G, Fritz J, Kleinsasser A, Velik-Salchner C. Ultrasound-guided regional anesthesia for carotid endarterectomy induces early hemodynamic and stress hormone changes. J Vasc Surg. 2015;62(1):57–67.
18. Madro P, Dabrowska A, Jarecki J, Garba P. Anaesthesia for carotid endarterectomy. Ultrasound-guided superficial/intermediate cervical plexus block combined with carotid sheath infiltration. Anaesthesiol Intensive Ther. 2016;48(4):234–8.
19. Sindjelic RP, Vlajkovic GP, Lucic M, Koncar I, Kostic D, Davidovic LB. Incidence of and indications for conversion of cervical plexus block to general anesthesia in patients undergoing carotid surgery: a single center experience. J Cardiovasc Surg. 2015;56(3):441–6.
20. Litz RJ, Popp M, Stehr SN, Koch T. Successful resuscitation of a patient with ropivacaine-induced asystole after axillary plexus block using lipid infusion. Anaesthesia. 2006;61(8):800–1.
21. Knudsen K, Beckman Suurkula M, Blomberg S, Sjovall J, Edvardsson N. Central nervous and cardiovascular effects of i.v. infusions of ropivacaine, bupivacaine and placebo in volunteers. Br J Anaesth. 1997;78(5):507–14.
22. Rettig HC, Lerou JG, Gielen MJ, Boersma E, Burm AG. The pharmacokinetics of ropivacaine after four different techniques of brachial plexus blockade. Anaesthesia. 2007;62(10):1008–14.
23. Simpson D, Curran MP, Oldfield V, Keating GM. Ropivacaine: a review of its use in regional anaesthesia and acute pain management. Drugs. 2005; 65(18):2675–717.

24. Wulf H, Worthmann F, Behnke H, Bohle AS. Pharmacokinetics and pharmacodynamics of ropivacaine 2 mg/mL, 5 mg/mL, or 7.5 mg/mL after ilioinguinal blockade for inguinal hernia repair in adults. Anesth Analg. 1999; 89(6):1471–4.
25. Merle JC, Mazoit JX, Desgranges P, Abhay K, Rezaiguia S, Dhonneur G, Duvaldestin P. A comparison of two techniques for cervical plexus blockade: evaluation of efficacy and systemic toxicity. Anesth Analg. 1999; 89(6):1366–70.
26. Riazi S, Carmichael N, Awad I, Holtby RM, McCartney CJ. Effect of local anaesthetic volume (20 vs 5 ml) on the efficacy and respiratory consequences of ultrasound-guided interscalene brachial plexus block. Br J Anaesth. 2008;101(4):549–56.
27. Wakeno M, Sakamoto S, Asai T, Hirose T, Shingu K. A case of diaphragmatic paralysis in a patient with diabetes mellitus after surgery in prolonged prone position. Masui. 2001;50(9):1019–21.
28. Schram DJ, Vosik W, Cantral D. Diaphragmatic paralysis following cervical chiropractic manipulation: case report and review. Chest. 2001;119(2): 638–40.
29. Kunisawa T, Hanada S, Takeuchi S, Iwasaki H. Transient phrenic nerve paralysis after carotid endarterectomy in a patient with asthma. J Anesth. 2010;24(5):817–8.
30. Emery G, Handley G, Davies MJ, Mooney PH. Incidence of phrenic nerve block and hypercapnia in patients undergoing carotid endarterectomy under cervical plexus block. Anaesth Intensive Care. 1998;26(4):377–81.
31. Castresana MR, Masters RD, Castresana EJ, Stefansson S, Shaker IJ, Newman WH. Incidence and clinical significance of hemidiaphragmatic paresis in patients undergoing carotid endarterectomy during cervical plexus block anesthesia. J Neurosurg Anesthesiol. 1994;6(1):21–3.
32. Urmey WF, Talts KH, Sharrock NE. One hundred percent incidence of hemidiaphragmatic paresis associated with interscalene brachial plexus anesthesia as diagnosed by ultrasonography. Anesth Analg. 1991;72(4): 498–503.
33. Urmey WF, McDonald M. Hemidiaphragmatic paresis during interscalene brachial plexus block: effects on pulmonary function and chest wall mechanics. Anesth Analg. 1992;74(3):352–7.
34. Mian A, Chaudhry I, Huang R, Rizk E, Tubbs RS, Loukas M. Brachial plexus anesthesia: a review of the relevant anatomy, complications, and anatomical variations. Clin Anat. 2014;27(2):210–21.
35. Knoblanche GE. The incidence and aetiology of phrenic nerve blockade associated with supraclavicular brachial plexus block. Anaesth Intensive Care. 1979;7(4):346–9.
36. Seidel R, Schulze M, Zukowski K, Wree A. Ultrasound-guided intermediate cervical plexus block. Anatomical study. Anaesthesist. 2015;64(6):446–50.
37. Nash L, Nicholson HD, Zhang M. Does the investing layer of the deep cervical fascia exist? Anesthesiology. 2005;103(5):962–8.
38. Pandit JJ, Dorje P, Satya-Krishna R. Investing layer of the cervical fascia of the neck may not exist. Anesthesiology. 2006;104(6):1344 author reply 1344-1345.
39. Flores S, Riguzzi C, Herring AA, Nagdev A. Horner's syndrome after superficial cervical plexus block. West J Emerg Med. 2015;16(3):428–31.
40. Pandit JJ, Dutta D, Morris JF. Spread of injectate with superficial cervical plexus block in humans: an anatomical study. Br J Anaesth. 2003;91(5):733–5.
41. Costa EL, Lima RG, Amato MB. Electrical impedance tomography. Curr Opin Crit Care. 2009;15(1):18–24.
42. Nestler C, Simon P, Petroff D, Hammermuller S, Kamrath D, Wolf S, Dietrich A, Camilo LM, Beda A, Carvalho AR, et al. Individualized positive end-expiratory pressure in obese patients during general anaesthesia: a randomized controlled clinical trial using electrical impedance tomography. Br J Anaesth. 2017;119(6):1194–205.

3

What is the role of locoregional anesthesia in breast surgery? A systematic literature review focused on pain intensity, opioid consumption, adverse events, and patient satisfaction

Pasquale Sansone[1*], Luca Gregorio Giaccari[1], Mario Faenza[2], Pasquale Di Costanzo[2], Sara Izzo[2], Caterina Aurilio[1], Francesco Coppolino[1], Maria Beatrice Passavanti[1], Vincenzo Pota[1] and Maria Caterina Pace[1]

Abstract

Background: Breast surgery in the United States is common. Pain affects up to 50% of women undergoing breast surgery and can interfere with postoperative outcomes. General anesthesia is the conventional, most frequently used anaesthetic technique. Various locoregional anesthetic techniques are also used for breast surgeries. A systematic review of the use of locoregional anesthesia for postoperative pain in breast surgery is needed to clarify its role in pain management.

Objectives: To systematically review literature to establish the efficacy and the safety of locoregional anesthesia used in the treatment of pain after breast surgery.

Methods: Embase, MEDLINE, Google Scholar and Cochrane Central Trials Register were systematically searched in Mars 2020 for studies examining locoregional anesthesia for management of pain in adults after breast surgery. The methodological quality of the studies and their results were appraised using the Consensus-based Standards for the Selection of Health Measurement Instruments (COSMIN) checklist and specific measurement properties criteria, respectively.

Results: Nineteen studies evaluating locoregional anesthesia were included: 1058 patients underwent lumpectomy/ mastectomy, 142 breast augmentation and 79 breast reduction. Locoregional anesthesia provides effective anesthesia and analgesia in the perioperative setting, however no statistically significant difference emerged if compared to other techniques. For mastectomy only, the use of locoregional techniques reduces pain in the first hour after the end of the surgery if compared to other procedures ($p = 0.02$). Other potentially beneficial effects of locoregional anesthesia include decreased need for opioids, decreased postoperative nausea and vomiting, fewer complications and increased patient satisfaction. All this improves postoperative recovery and shortens hospitalization stay. In none of these cases, locoregional anesthesia was statistically superior to other techniques.

(Continued on next page)

* Correspondence: pasquale.sansone@unicampania.it
[1]Department of Woman, Child and General and Specialized Surgery, University of Campania "Luigi Vanvitelli", Piazza Luigi Miraglia, 2, Naples, Italy

(Continued from previous page)

Conclusion: The results of our review showed no differences between locoregional anesthesia and other techniques in the management of breast surgery. Locoregional techniques are superior in reducing pain in the first hour after mastectomy.

Keywords: Breast surgery, Mastectomy, Locoregional anesthesia, Pain intensity, Opioid consumption, Adverse events, Patient satisfaction

Background

Rationale

Breast surgery in the United States is common. In 2020, an estimated 276,480 new cases of invasive breast cancer will be diagnosed among women and approximately 80% of patients will have surgery to remove their primary tumour [1]. In addition, an increasing number of women are turning to plastic surgeons for interventions of cosmetic: among these breast augmentation is the first procedure performed in the United States [2].

Pain affects up to 50% of women undergoing breast surgery and can interfere with postoperative outcomes. Breast pain is one of the factors determining patient distress, long hospital stay, and an increase in post-surgical admissions to the hospital [3].

Nociceptive/inflammatory pain is caused by tissue damage, whereas neuropathic pain is the consequence of a central and peripheral nerve damage [4], especially the intercostal nerves from T2 to T6. Neuropathic pain typically begins immediately after breast surgery and can be persistent, sometimes even for months [3].

The pain control is the main objective of anesthesia in breast surgery. The correct management of acute postoperative pain is essential to improve patient outcome and satisfaction.

Various anesthetic agents, devices, and strategies are currently available. For a long time, intravenous analgesia has been the main technique for postoperative pain relief. Over the years, the growing number of surgical procedures for breast cancer and cosmetic treatment has however stimulated the development of new anesthetic techniques with improved pain reduction and safety, and fewer complications.

The international guidelines recommended the use of a multimodal analgesia [5, 6]. Regional anesthesia techniques are effective as a component of multimodal analgesia for management of postoperative pain associated with a number of surgical procedures. These techniques can be administered as a single shot or a continuous catheter, both prior to surgical incision or after surgery [5, 6]. Local anesthetics infiltration also shows benefit for the surgical procedure. Wound infiltration can be performed either as a single injection of local anesthetic typically at the conclusion of surgery or as a continuous infusion of local anesthetic through a catheter at the incision site prior to skin closure [5, 6]. Finally, the international guidelines suggest the use of intravenous (IV) lidocaine, especially in patients underwent open or laparoscopic abdominal surgical procedures [5, 6]. Perioperative lidocaine infusion may be considered for patients undergoing mastectomy [7].

Objectives

We undertook this systematic review to identify the potential clinical role of locoregional anesthesia for breast surgery. We aimed to establish the efficacy and the safety of locoregional anesthesia in the pain management after breast surgery. Postoperative pain severity and opioid consumption during the first 48 h were designated as co-primary outcomes. For secondary objectives, we aimed to examine the effects on the immediate quality of recovery, in relation to adverse effects and patient satisfaction.

Methods

Protocol and registration

We performed a systematic review based on Preferred Reporting Items for Systematic Reviews and Meta-Analyses (PRISMA) statement [8]. Randomized controlled trials that compared the effects of locoregional anesthesia to systemic analgesia alone in patients undergoing breast surgery were sought. Studies were evaluated using a pre-designed protocol. The protocol was not published, and the review was not registered with the International prospective register of systematic reviews (PROSPERO).

Eligibility criteria

The population, intervention, comparison, and outcome (PICO) criteria were applied to the research question (see Table 1). Patients older than 18 years undergoing breast surgery were considered as the population (P); the intervention (I) was postoperative analgesia with locoregional anesthesia techniques; the comparison (C) concept was standard pain treatment provided in each study; pain intensity, opioid consumption, adverse events (AEs), and patient satisfaction were considered the outcomes (O) for this systematic review. We included randomized controlled trials (RCTs) published from 2010 to the present. No language restrictions were placed on study inclusion.

Literature search

We identified the articles by searching electronic databases (Embase, MEDLINE, Google Scholar and Cochrane

Table 1 PICO criteria for including studies

Population	Patients of at least 18 years undergoing breast surgery.
Intervetion	Postoperative analgesia with locoregional anesthesia techniques.
Comparator	Standard pain treatment.
Outcomes	Pain Intensity, Opioid Consumption, Adverse Events, Patient Satisfaction.
Study TYPE	Randomized Controlled Trial.
Time	From 2010 to present.

Central Trials Register). We included other relevant studies from the reference lists of systematic reviews and meta-analyses. These databases were initially searched from Mars 2020.

The search strategy was developed using medical subject headings and keywords relating to the central research question of this paper. Namely, the search terms included in the search strategy covered the following key domains: *"breast augmentation", "breast reduction", "mastectomy", "mastopexy", "local anesthetic agent", "post-operative pain"* and *"randomized clinical trial".*

We applied no language restrictions in searches.

The studies included in this review evaluated adult patients undergoing breast surgery and receiving any type of locoregional anesthesia to treat postoperative pain.

Primary outcomes

Pain scores and opioid consumption in the first 48 h postoperatively were the primary outcomes of interest. Pain intensity was assessed via a Numeric Rating Scale (NRS) at 1, 6, 12, 24 and 48 h after surgery. Pain intensity data assessed by means other than a zero to 10 NRS were converted to this scale. The other primary outcome was the average per patient opioid consumption in the Post-Anesthesia Care Unit (PACU) and in the 48 h after surgery. Opioid consumption was converted to morphine sulfate equivalents [9].

Secondary outcomes

We extracted data on the following secondary outcomes:

1. Adverse Events (AEs) were recorded. Evaluated safety outcomes included postoperative opioid related side-effects (postoperative nausea and vomiting, sedation/respiratory depression, pruritus, hypotension, urinary retention, or constipation), and complications related to the nerve block (pneumothorax, block failure, or local anesthetic systemic toxicity). Complications during wound healing were also analysed.
2. Patient Satisfaction. All measures of patient satisfaction were reported as "satisfied" and "not satisfied".

Selection of studies

Two independent reviewers (P.S. and L.G.G.) initially assessed the results from the literature search based on title and abstract. The full-text citations of potentially eligible articles were subsequently retrieved and reviewed again by the same two independent reviewers. In case of disagreement between the two reviewers on eligibility, a discussion was initiated. If consensus could not be reached after discussion, a third reviewer (M.C.P.) evaluated the study and made the final decision.

The methodological quality of the included studies was evaluated and rated using the COSMIN checklist, based on a 4-point rating scale.

Data extraction and management

A standardized data extraction form was used. Data collected included information relating to:

- Age, weight, height and body mass index (BMI) of participants;
- Number of participants enrolled and completing the study;
- Type of operation;
- Regional anesthesia technique (local anesthetic and dose);
- Pain intensity for all-time points at which it was measured;
- Opioid consumption;
- Patient satisfaction;
- Severity or incidence of adverse events.

Statistical analyses

For continuous outcomes, we extracted the mean and standard deviation (SD). In situations where these are not reported, the median and interquartile range were used to approximate these values. Similarly, in situations where the mean and 95% CI are reported, statistical conversions were used to estimate the mean and SD.

For dichotomous outcomes (side effects, complications), data were converted to overall incidence numbers.

We designated a p value < 0.05 as a threshold of statistical significance for the primary and secondary outcomes. All tests were two-tailed.

Results

Our search strategy identified 40 citations. Searching additional sources yielded an additional 9 potentially eligible citations. Of these, 30 were excluded based on title and abstract screening, because of duplicated papers ($n = 5$), missing outcomes ($n = 7$), or the lack of a standardized pain treatment in the control group ($n = 18$). Thus a total of 19 randomized controlled trials were included in this systematic review. The flow diagram (see Fig. 1) shows the results from the literature search and the study selection process.

The characteristics of included studies and outcomes assessed in this review are presented in Table 2a, b and c.

The surgical procedures performed in the reviewed trials included lumpectomy or mastectomy in 14 of 19 trials [10–23], with additional Sentinel Lymph Node Biopsy (SLNB) or Axillary Lymph Node Dissection (ALND) [10, 12, 14–18, 20, 21, 23]. Three trials included patients undergoing breast augmentation [24–26], and two trials also included patients undergoing breast reduction [27, 28].

The 19 randomized controlled trials involved a total of 1307 patients, of which 749 received nerve blocks, 330 received local infiltration, 115 received IV lidocaine, 73 received infusion of local anesthetic via pump, and 40 received tumescent anesthesia.

According to the COSMIN checklist, all studies included in this review showed an excellent-to-good quality. The majority of clinical trials had a low risk of bias.

Lumpectomy/mastectomy

In the included studies 1086 patients underwent lumpectomy/mastectomy. There were no demographic differences between the two groups as shown in Table 3.

The largest studies involved 140 patients (*Mohamed* et al., [17]; *Versyck* et al., [20]), whereas the smallest consisted of 44 patients (*Couceiro* et al., [11]). All analysed studies were conducted in inpatient settings.

Patients underwent mastectomy, while lumpectomy was performed in 4 studies (*Campbell* et al.,[10]; *Cros* et al., [12]; *Gürkan* et al.,[14]; *Versyck* et al., [20]). *Lanier* et al [16] and *Wang* et al [21] reported immediate tissue

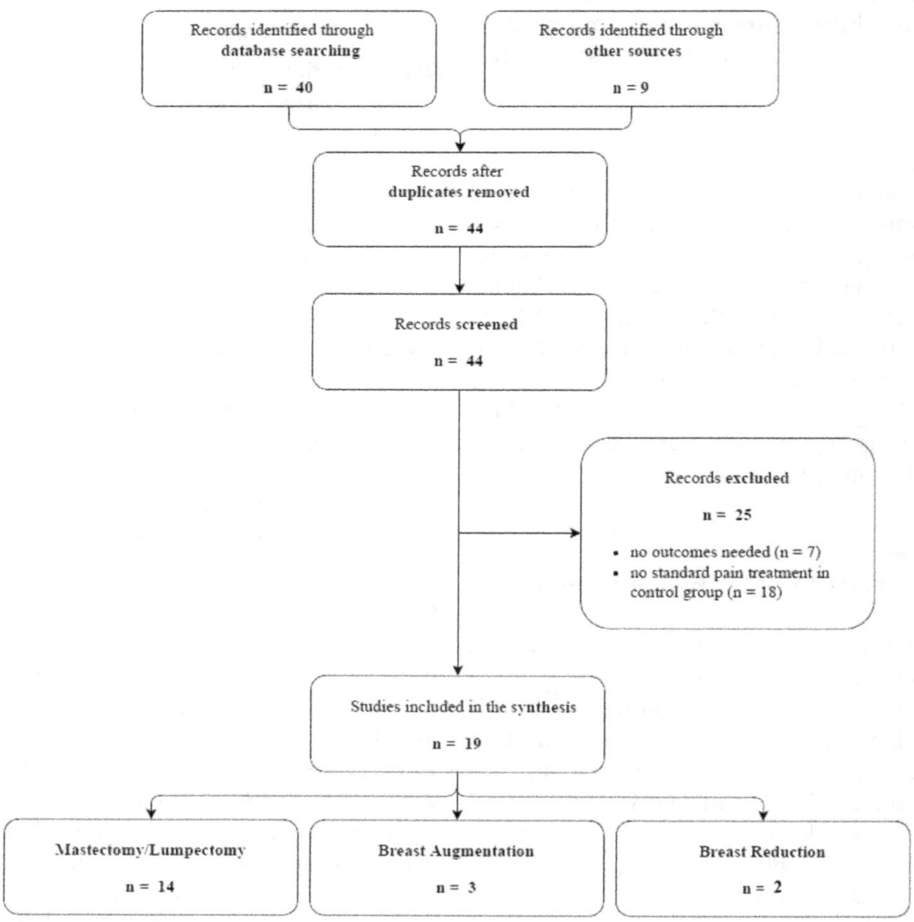

Fig. 1 Flow diagram study selection process

Table 2 Studies characteristics

Author, year	Study	Sites	No.	Type of surgery	Anesthesia	Intervention
A. LUMPECTOMY/MASTECTOMY						
Campbell* et al.,**[10] ***2014	SB-RCT	New Zeland, 1	79	Lumpectomy/Mastectomy ± ALND	?	Local Infiltration
Couceiro* et al.,**[11] ***2014	DB-RCT	Brazil, 1	44	Mastectomy	GA	IV lidocaine
Cros* et al.,**[12] ***2018	DB-RCT	France, 1 Canada, 1	127	Lumpectomy/Mastectomy ± SLNB/ALND	GA	Pecs I
Ferreira Laso* et al.,**[13] ***2014	DB-RCT	Spain, 1	73	Mastectomy	GA	Infusion pump
Gürkan* et al.,**[14] ***2018	SB-RCT	Turkey,?	50	Lumpectomy/Mastectomy ± SLNB/ALND	GA	ESP
Ilfeld* et al.,**[15] ***2014	DB-RCT	US,?	60	Mastectomy ± ALND	Sedation	PVB
Lanier* et al .**[16]2018***	DB-RCT	US,?	45	Mastectomy + reconstruction ± SLNB/ALND	?	Intercostal + pectoral nerve blocks
Mohamed* et al.,**[17] ***2013	DB-RCT	Egypt,?	140	Mastectomy ± ALND	GA	Local infiltration
Neethu* et al.,**[18] ***2018	RCT	India, 1	60	Mastectomy ± SLNB/ALND	GA	Pecs I - II
Terkawi* et al.,**[19]2014***	DB-RCT	US,?	71	Mastectomy	GA	IV lidocaine
Versyck* et al.,**[20] ***2017	DB-RCT	Belgium, 1	140	Mastectomy/tumorectomy ±SLNB/ALND	GA	Pecs II
Wang* et al.,**[21] ***2018	SB-RCT	China,?	64	Mastectomy + reconstruction ± ALND	GA	Pecs II
Wang* et al.,**[22] ***2019	RCT	China,?	61	Mastectomy	GA	Pecs I + SPB
Yao* et al.,**[23] ***2019	DB-RCT	China, 1	72	Mastectomy ± ALND	GA	SPB
B. BREAST AUGMENTATION						
Gardiner* et al.,**[24] ***2012	SB-RCT	Australia,?	40	BA	Sedation	PVB
Picard* et al.,**[25] ***2017	SB-RCT	France,?	72	BA	?	Local infiltration
Schuitemaker* et al.,**[26] ***2019	DB-RCT	Spain,?	30	BA	GA	Pecs II + SPB
C. BREAST REDUCTION						
Christie* et al.,** [27] ***2017	DB-RCT	US, 1	40	BR	GA	Tumescent Anaesthesia
Valente* et al.,**[28] ***2014	DB-RCT	Brazil,?	39	BR	GA	Local infiltration

SB-RCT Single-Blind Randomized Controlled Trial, *DB-RCT* Double-Blind Randomized Controlled Trial, *SLNB* Sentinel Lymph Node Biopsy, *ALND* Axillary Lymph Node Dissection, *GA* General Anesthesia, *Pecs* Pectoralis nerve block, *ESP* Erector Spinae Plane block, *PVB* ParaVertebral Block, *SPB* Serratus Plane Block, *BA* Breast Augmentation, *BR* Breast Reduction;?, not reported

expander or implant based breast reconstruction. Surgical treatment for breast cancer was associated with a sentinel lymph node biopsy (SLNB) or a axillary lymph node dissection (ALND) in 10 papers (*Campbell* et al.,[10]*; Cros* et al.,[12]*; Gürkan* et al.,[14]*; Ilfeld* et al., [15]*; Lanier* et al., [16]*; Mohamed* et al.,[17]*; Neethu* et al., *2018; Versyck* et al. [20]*;Wang* et al., *2018; Yao* et al., *2019*).

Regional anesthetic techniques were performed ten times: the most common procedure was pectoral nerve (Pecs) block type I and II (5 studies: *Cros* et al.,[12]*; Neethu* et al., *2018; Versyck* et al. *2017; Wang* et al., *2018; Wang* et al., *2019*), followed by serratus plane block (SPB) (2 studies: *Wang* et al., *2019; Yao* et al., *2019),* erector spinae plane (ESP) block (*Gürkan* et al., [14]), and paravertebral block (PVB) (*Ilfeld* et al.,[15]). In *Lanier* et al *2018,* intraoperative nerve blocks of intercostal and pectoral nerves were performed under direct visualization by the attending plastic surgeon at the completion of the mastectomy.

Local infiltration was reported in 3 studies. In *Campbell* et al *2014* [10], patients received 20 mL of bupivacaine 0.25% with or without adrenaline to be infiltrated into the breast wound and a further 20 mL of bupivacianee 0.25% with adrenaline to be infiltrated into the axilla wound when applicable. In *Mohamed* et al *2013*, 5 ml of bupivacaine 0.5% with or without clonidine were diluted with saline 0.9% to 15 mL volume and irrigated into the surgical field before skin closure. An infusion pump of levobupivacaine 0.50% for approximately 48 h was evaluated in *Ferreira Laso* et al *2014.*

Couceiro et al [11] and *Terkawi* et al *2014* investigated i.v. lidocaine infusion. In the first paper, a bolus dose of lidocaine was not administered and, after incision, a lidocaine infusion at 3 mg/kg was started. In the other study, lidocaine was administered as a bolus to all patients before anesthetic induction, at a dose of up to 1.5 mg/kg, followed by a lidocaine infusion at 2 mg/kg/h until 2 h after arrival in PACU.

Almost all studies were conducted under general anesthesia, except for *Ilfeld* et al *2014* conducted under sedation. General anesthesia was induced and then maintained with opioids, such as alfentanil (*Ferreira*

Table 3 Personal and clinical characteristics of patients undergoing lumpectomy/mastectomy

	Patients (*n* =)		Age (years)		Weight (kg)		Height (cm)		BMI (kg/m²)	
	Group I	Group C	Group I	Group C	Group I	Group C	Group I	Group C	Group I	Group C
***Campbell* et al., *2014* [10]**	45	34	59.4	61.7	80.7	73.8	163.3	162.3	30.2	28.1
***Couceiro* et al., *2014* [11]**	22	22	47.0	52.4	–	–	–	–	28.1	28.2
***Cros* et al., *2018* [12]**	62	66	60.5	62.0	63.6	65.0	160.0	160.0	24.8	25.6
***Ferreira Laso* et al., *2014* [13]**	34	39	54.8	57.7	67.2	66.7	–	–	–	–
***Gürkan* et al., *2018* [14]**	25	25	49.5	49.8	72.4	73.1	161.0	161.0	27.8	28.2
***Ilfeld* et al., *2014* [15]**	30	30	48.0	49.0	62.0	61.0	165.0	166.0	23.0	24.0
***Lanier* et al., *2018* [16]**	23	22	48.0	50.0	67.0	70.0	160.0	170.0	26.0	26.0
***Mohamed* et al., *2013* [17]**	105	35	39.9	38.9	70.2	69.8	160.6	158.5	27.4	27.9
***Neethu* et al., *2018* [18]**	30	30	50.5	45.6	–	–	–	–	–	–
***Terkawi* et al., *2014* [19]**	34	37	53.0	54.0	–	–	–	–	26.2	28.2
***Versyck* et al., *2017* [20]**	45	40	59.6	58.8	67.3	67.0	165.0	165.0	24.7	24.6
***Wang* et al., *2018* [21]**	30	30	46.8	47.4	–	–	–	–	25.4	24.8
***Wang* et al., *2019* [22]**	32	29	51.3	55.3	58.7	57.6	162.5	161.0	22.3	22.2
***Yao* et al., *2019* [23]**	34	34	46.5	47.7	57.2	56.2	160.9	160.8	22.3	21.9
TOTAL	**585**	**473**	**51.05 ± 5.6**	**52.16 ± 6.3**	**66.65 ± 6.5**	**66.03 ± 5.8**	**162.04 ± 1.8**	**162.74 ± 3.3**	**25.71 ± 2.3**	**25.83 ± 2.2**

Laso et al., *2014*), fentanyl (*Couceiro* et al., [11]; *Gürkan* et al., *2018; Ilfeld* et al., *2014; Mohamed* et al., *2013; Neethu* et al., *2018; Terkawi* et al., *2014; Wang* et al., *2018*), remifentanil (*Wang* et al., *2019*) and sufentanil (*Versyck* et al., *2017; Wang* et al., *2019; Yao* et al., *2019*). For the postoperative pain management, four studies (*Couceiro* et al., [11]; *Cros* et al.,[12]; *Ferreira Laso* et al., *2014; Ilfeld* et al., *2014*) provided infiltration of the chest wall ipsilateral to the mastectomy with local anesthetic; acetaminophen and other NSAIDs were systematically administered. Two studies did not report the anesthesia protocol (*Campbell* et al., *2014* [10]; *Lanier* et al., *2018*).

Pain intensity

Different investigators recorded this outcome on different scales and at different intervals. We normalized all NRS to a zero to 10 range (see Table 4). The majority of authors reported pain intensity at 1, 6, 12, 24 and 48 h after surgery.

As shown in Fig. 2, the average NRS score was 1.83 ± 0.81 at 1 h, 2.02 ± 1.03 at 6 h, 1.92 ± 1.57 at 12 h, 1.74 ± 1.29 at 24 h and 1.51 ± 1.03 at 48 h in the intervention group; in the placebo group NRS scores were recorded of 3.36 ± 1.65 at 1 h, 3.10 ± 1.29 at 6 h, 2.35 ± 1.14 at 12 h, 2.37 ± 1.27 at 24 h and 2.77 ± 1.12 at 48 h.

One study, *Couceiro* et al [11], did not report NRS at any interval: only 2 (9.09%) vs 3 (13.6%) patients in the lidocaine and placebo groups, respectively, experienced severe to very severe pain 24 h after surgery.

Opioid consumption

The most frequently used opioids were codeine (*Campbell* et al., *2014* [10]; *Couceiro* et al., [11]), fentanyl (*Neethu* et al., *2018*), oxycodone (*Campbell* et al., *2014*) [10], piritramide (*Versyck* et al. *2017*), tramadol (*Campbell* et al., *2014* [10]; *Mohamed* et al., *2013; Versyck* et al. *2017*), and sufentanil (*Yao* et al., *2019*). Morphine was used in the other studies.

At discharge from PACU, the overall mean amounts of morphine consumed in the intervention and placebo groups were 3.0 ± 3.63 mg and 4.87 ± 5.76 mg, respectively, with the difference being not statistically significant ($p = 0.51$).

After 48 h, the overall mean amounts of morphine consumed in the intervention and placebo groups were,

Table 4 NRS at 1, 6, 12, 24 and 48 h after lumpectomy/mastectomy

	Up to 1 h		Up to 6 h		Up to 12 h		Up to 24 h		Up to 48 h	
	Group I	Group C	Group I	Group C	Group I	Group C	Group I	Group C	Group I	Group C
Campbell et al., *2014* [10]	–	–	1.75	2	–	–	2.3	1.7	1.8	1.25
Couceiro et al., *2014* [11]	–	–	–	–	–	–	–	–	–	–
Cros et al., *2018* [12]	3	3	–	–	–	–	–	–	–	–
Ferreira Laso et al., *2014* [13]	1.6	6.7	–	–	–	–	0.8	4.2	0.4	3.3
Gürkan et al., *2018* [14]	2	2	2	2	0	1	0	1	–	–
Ilfeld et al., *2014* [15]	–	–	–	–	–	–	3.6	3.7	–	–
Lanier et al., *2018* [16]	3	5	4	5	5	4	4	4	–	–
Mohamed et al., *2013* [17]	2.67	3.7	2.43	3.6	2.53	3.8	2.43	3.7	2.43	3.8
Neethu et al., *2018* [18]	1.78	3.08	0.43	0.76	1.20	1.40	0.5	0.53	–	–
Terkawi et al., *2014* [19]	–	–	2.94	3.88	–	–	2.91	2.66	2.72	3.9
Versyck et al., *2017* [20]	0.38	0.20	–	–	–	–	–	–	–	–
Wang et al., *2018* [21]	1.65	4.3	2.45	3.9	1.8	1.9	1	1	–	–
Wang et al., *2019* [22]	1	3	0.8	4.4	1	2	0.5	1.8	0.2	1.6
Yao et al., *2019* [23]	1.3	2.7	1.4	2.4	–	–	1.2	1.8	–	–
TOTAL	**1.83 ± 0.81**	**3.36 ± 1.65**	**2.02 ± 1.03**	**3.10 ± 1.29**	**1.92 ± 1.57**	**2.35 ± 1.14**	**1.74 ± 1.29**	**2.37 ± 1.27**	**1.51 ± 1.03**	**2.77 ± 1.12**
p	**0.02***		**0.08**		**0.63**		**0.29**		**0.13**	

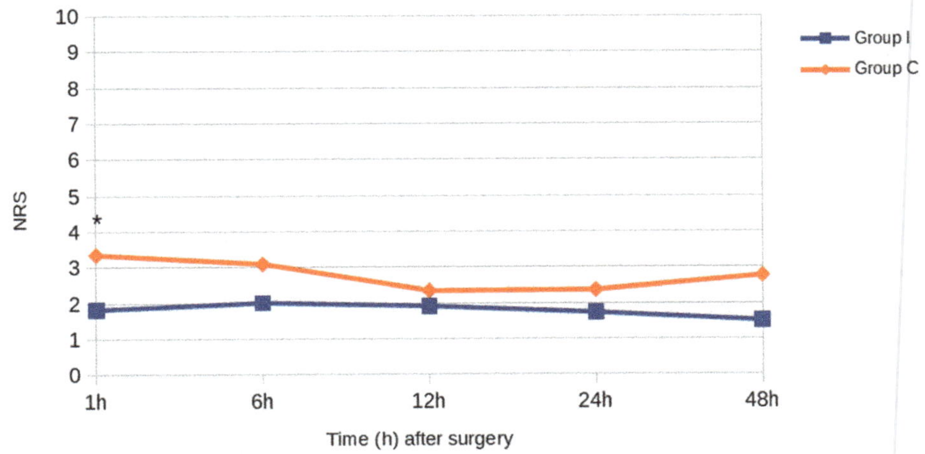

Fig. 2 NRS at 1, 6, 12, 24 and 48 h after lumpectomy/mastectomy

respectively, 2.68 ± 0.88 mg and 4.94 ± 4.61 mg ($p = 0.18$). Among regional anesthetic techniques, postoperative opioid consumption for the first 48 h was respectively 2.14 ± 1.52 mg and 4.84 ± 4.63 mg; no statistically significant difference was observed ($p = 0.16$). The average per patient opioid consumption up to 48 h after surgery was 1.33 ± 1.49 mg vs 3.01 ± 3.05 mg ($p = 0.52$) among patients treated with local infiltration.

Table 5 shows the mean amounts of morphine consumed in the intervention and placebo groups.

In *Couceiro* et al [11], opioid consumption in the first 24 h after surgery was similar in the lidocaine and placebo groups.

Adverse events (AEs)

An adverse event is defined as any undesirable experience associated with the use of a medical product in a patient. A total of 379 AEs were recorded. Three studies (*Couceiro* et al., [11]; *Ilfeld* et al., *2014; Versyck* et al., *2017)* did not report the number of AEs. The most frequently reported AEs were nausea, vomiting and postoperative nausea and vomiting (PONV), pruritus, dizziness, haematoma/bleeding, seroma and bruising (see Table 6 and Fig. 3). Some studies did not specify the timing of adverse events.

Nausea, vomiting and PONV

Nausea, vomiting and PONV were the most frequent AEs (235 events, 62% of AEs). 96 vs 139 episodes were respectively recorded in intervention vs placebo group ($p = 0.25$). In 9 studies (*Cros* et al.,[12]; *Ferreira Laso* et al., *2014; Gürkan* et al., *2018; Lanier* et al., *2018; Neethu* et al., *2018; Terkawi* et al., *2014; Versyck* et al. *2017; Wang* et al., *2018; Yao* et al., *2019*) prophylaxis was administered; in the others studies prescription of antiemetic drugs was missed or not reported.

Pruritus

A total of 23 cases of pruritus was reported in two studies (*Ferreira Laso* et al., *2014; Wang* et al., *2019*). No statistically significant difference was observed (7 vs 16, $p = 0.47$).

Dizziness

Fifteen episodes were recorded among patients not receiving treatment; only two patients reported dizziness in the intervention group. No statistically significant difference ($p = 0.06$) was observed in these 3 studies (*Ferreira Laso* et al., *2014; Wang* et al., *2019; Yao* et al., *2019*).

Haematoma/bleeding

Three studies (*Campbell* et al., *2014* [10]; *Cros* et al.,[12]; *Ferreira Laso* et al.) reported a total of 21 episodes (10 vs 11, $p = 0.85$).

Seroma

Seroma was found in 10 cases in the intervention group vs 11 cases in the placebo group (*Campbell* et al., *2014* [10]; *Ferreira Laso* et al., *2014*) with no statistically significant difference ($p = 0.91$).

Table 5 Average per patient opioid consumption in PACU and up to 48 h after lumpectomy/mastectomy

	PACU			Up to 48 h		
	Group I	Group C	p	Group I	Group C	p
Campbell* et al., *2014 [10]	–	–		3.42	7.33[a]	
Couceiro* et al., *2014 [11]	–	–		–	–	
Cros* et al., *2018 [12]	1.5	3		1.5	3	
Ferreira Laso* et al., *2014 [13]	0	0.7[a]		0	0.7[a]	
Gürkan* et al., *2018 [14]	1	1		5	16[a]	
Ilfeld* et al., *2014 [15]	1	2.4[a]		2.5	5.7	
Lanier* et al., *2018 [16]	8	17		4	5.18	
Mohamed* et al., *2013 [17]	–	–		0.58	1[a]	
Neethu* et al., *2018 [18]	–	–		1.46	2.03[a]	
Terkawi* et al., *2014 [19]	9.35	9.69		11.02	11.61	
Versyck* et al., *2017 [20]	0.18	0.33[a]		0.20	0.37[a]	
Wang* et al., *2018 [21]	–	–		1.75	5.42[a]	
Wang* et al., *2019 [22]	–	–		–	–	
Yao* et al., *2019 [23]	–	–		0.73	1.03[a]	
TOTAL	**3.0 ± 3.63**	**4.87 ± 5.76**	**0.51**	**2.68 ± 0.88**	**4.94 ± 4.61**	**0.18**

[a] Difference statistically significant

Table 6 Number of adverse events (AEs) after lumpectomy/mastectomy

AEs	Group I (*n* =)	Group C (*n* =)	*p*
Nausea/Vomiting/PONV	96	139	0.25
Pruritus	7	16	0.47
Hypotension	5	2	0.25
Hypertension	0	1	0.32
Dizzness	2	15	0.06
Bradycardia	2	0	0.32
Hematoma/Bleeding	10	11	0.85
Seroma	10	11	0.91
Alteration of healing	2	3	0.78
Infection	3	2	0.69
DVT	1	1	1.00
PTE	1	1	1.00
Acute respiratory infection	1	1	1.00
Bruising	23	13	0.70
TOTAL	**163**	**216**	**0.74**

Bruising

Campbell et al *2014* [10] reported 36 episodes of bruising (20 vs 16, $p = 0.70$).

Others

Haemodynamic changes were rarely reported. Hypotension was reported in 3 studies (*Cros* et al., [12]; *Ferreira Laso* et al., *2014; Mohamed* et al., *2013*) for a total of 7 AEs (5 vs 2, $p = 0.25$). *Ferreira Laso* et al *2014* reported a case of hypertension. Two episodes of bradycardia were reported from *Mohamed* et al *2013.*

Infection was observed, respectively, 3 vs 2 times in intervention and placebo groups in two studies (*Campbell* et al., *2014* [10]; *Ferreira Laso* et al.); no statistically significant difference was noticed ($p = 0.69$). Deep vein thrombosis (DVT), pulmonary thromboembolism (PTE) and acute respiratory infection were equally distributed (1 vs 1, $p = 1.0$) in *Ferreira Laso* et al *2014.*

Patient satisfaction

Patient satisfaction results were presented as different degrees of subjective satisfaction levels. We normalized all of them to "satisfied / not satisfied".

Only 5 studies (*Cros* et al.,[12]; *Ferreira Laso* et al., *2014; Lanier* et al., *2018; Neethu* et al., *2018; Wang* et al., *2019;*) were available for analysis of satisfaction (see Table 7 and Fig. 4).

Among the intervention group, there were 164 satisfied patients vs 14 not satisfied patients; in the placebo group 149 patients were satisfied and 40 not satisfied. No statistically significant difference was observed between the two groups (satisfied, $p = 0.28$; not satisfied, $p = 0.14$).

In *Versyck* et al *2017,* both patient-groups were very satisfied with their management; while in *Yao* et al *2019,* patient satisfaction scores were higher in the SPB group.

Breast augmentation

One hundred forty-two patients underwent breast augmentation. As shown in Table 8, the groups were similar in age, weight, height and body mass index.

All patients underwent subpectoral bilateral cosmetic breast augmentation.

Regional anesthetic techniques were performed in two studies: PVB in *Gardiner* et al [24]; association of Pecs type II and PSB in *Schuitemaker* et al [26]. In the other study, *Picard* et al [25], a local infiltration was performed.

Patients received general anesthesia in *Schuitemaker* et al [26], and sedation in *Gardiner* et al [24]. In both studies patients received fentanyl. *Picard* et al [25] did not report the anesthesia protocol.

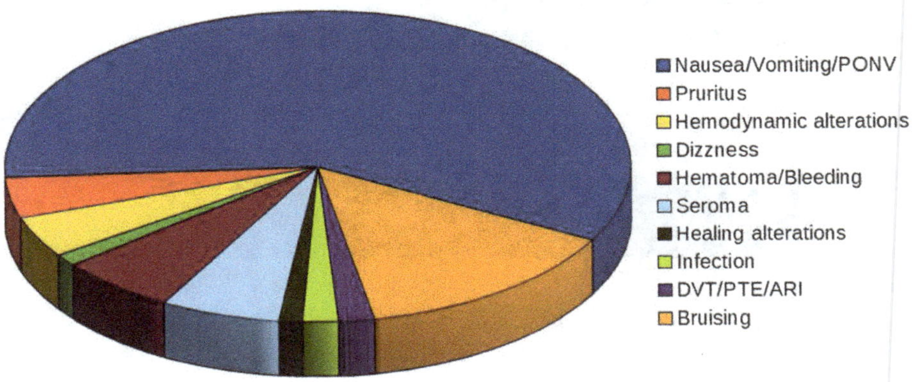

Fig. 3 Distribution of adverse events (AEs) among intervention group (lumpectomy/mastectomy)

Table 7 Patient satisfaction after lumpectomy/mastectomy

	Group I		Group C	
	Satisfied	Not satisfied	Satisfied	Not satisfied
Campbell et al., *2014* [10]	–	–	–	–
Couceiro et al., *201 4*[11]	–	–	–	–
Cros et al., *2018* [12]	*61*	*1*	*64*	*1*
Ferreira Laso et al., *2014* [13]	*32*	*2*	*37*	*2*
Gürkan et al., *2018* [14]	–	–	–	–
Ilfeld et al., *2014* [15]	–	–	–	–
Lanier et al., *2018* [16]	*23*	0	23	0
Mohamed et al., *2013* [17]	–	–	–	–
Neethu et al., *2018* [18]	*25*	*5*	*10*	*20*
Terkawi et al., *2014* [19]	–	–	–	–
Versyck et al., *2017*[a] [20]	–	–	–	–
Wang et al., *2018* [21]	–	–	–	–
Wang et al., *2019* [22]	*23*	*6*	*15*	*17*
Yao et al., *2019*[b] [23]	–	–	–	–
TOTAL	***164***	***14***	***149***	***40***

[a] Both patient-groups were very satisfied about their management (9.6 ± 0.6 and 9.1 ± 1.8 on a 10-point scale, $p = 0.21$)
[b]Patient satisfaction scores were higher in the SPB group

Pain intensity

Different investigators recorded this outcome on different scales and at different intervals. We normalized all NRS to a zero to 10 range (see Table 9). The majority of authors reported pain intensity at 1, 6, 24 and 72 h after surgery.

As shown in Fig. 5, the average NRS scores were 3.4 ± 0.5 at 1 h, 3.0 at 6 h, 3.65 ± 1.15 at 24 h and 3.05 ± 0.25 at 72 h in the intervention group; in the placebo group NRS scores were recorded of 5.25 ± 0.05 at 1 h, 3.0 at 6 h, 3.65 ± 1.15 at 24 h and 4.2 ± 0.5 at 72 h.

Opioid consumption

In *Gardiner* et al [24], 6 patients in the placebo group required supplementary opioid use. No patient received opioids in the intervention group.

After 24 h in *Schuitemaker* et al [26], the overall mean amounts of morphine consumed in the intervention and placebo groups were 0.2 ± 0.8 mg and 0.6 ± 1.2 mg, respectively, with the difference being not statistically significant ($p = 0.29$).

No data on opioid consumption was available in *Picard* et al [25].

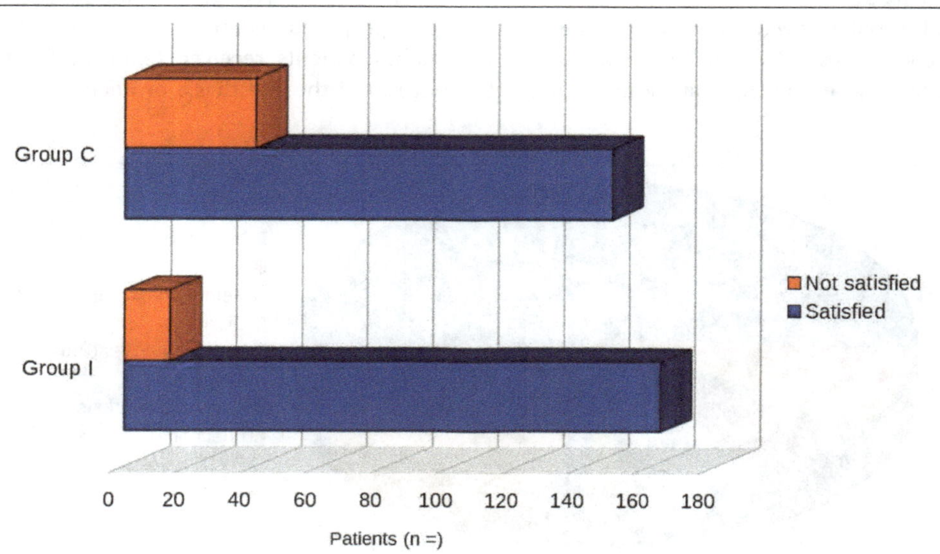

Fig. 4 Patient satisfaction after lumpectomy/mastectomy

Table 8 Personal and clinical characteristics of patients undergoing breast augmentation

	Patients (*n* =)		Age (years)		Weight (kg)		Height (cm)		BMI (kg/m^2)	
	Group I	Group C	Group I	Group C	Group I	Group C	Group I	Group C	Group I	Group C
Gardiner et al., *2012* [24]	20	20	33.4	34.9	–	–	–	–	20.5	20.1
Picard et al., *2017* [25]	29	43	32.4	34.6	–	–	–	–	–	–
Schuitemaker et al., *2019* [26]	15	15	33.0	33.0	52.0	54.0	163.0	163.0	20.0	20.0
TOTAL	**64**	**78**	**32.93 ± 0.41**	**34.16 ± 0.83**	**52.0**	**54.0**	**163.0**	**163.0**	**20.25 ± 0.25**	**20.05 ± 20.04**

Adverse events (AEs)

A total of 19 (9 vs 10) AEs were recorded.

Gardiner et al [24] reported 12 episodes of nausea and vomiting (5 vs 7, $p = 0.36$). In this study, hypotension occurred 3 times among patients in the intervention group and once in the placebo group. A single case of bradycardia occurred in both groups.

No differences were observed between groups concerning the appearance of AEs in *Schuitemaker* et al [26].

No adverse effects were reported in *Picard* et al *2017.*

Patient satisfaction

Only *Schuitemaker* et al [26] reported data about patient satisfaction: after 24 h, 80% vs 53% of patients in intervention and placebo groups were satisfied.

Breast reduction

Seventy-nine patients underwent breast reduction. The mean age was 38.28 ± 2.71 years vs 38.78 ± 3.21 years (see Table 10).

All patients underwent breast reduction surgery.

Tumescent anesthesia was performed in *Christie* et al *2017;* in *Valente* et al *2014* [28], patients received local infiltration. All patients in these studies underwent general anesthesia.

Pain intensity

Different investigators recorded this outcome on different scales and at different intervals. We normalized all NRS to a zero to 10 range (see Table 11). The authors reported pain intensity at 24 h after surgery.

The average NRS score was 2.55 ± 1.72 in the intervention group; in the placebo group a NRS score was recorded of 2.85 ± 1.14 ($p = 0.89$).

Opioid consumption

After 24 h in *Christie* et al *2017,* the overall mean amounts of morphine consumed in the intervention and placebo groups were 0.58 mg and 0.64 mg, respectively, with the difference being not statistically significant ($p = 0.71$).

No data on opioid consumption is available in *Valente* et al *2014* [28].

Adverse events (AEs)

There was no significant difference in occurrence of nausea or vomiting in the first 24 h between the two groups in *Christie* et al *2017.* No adverse effects were reported in *Valente* et al *2014* [28].

Patient satisfaction

The level of satisfaction was not reported in these studies.

Discussion

Our systematic review is the first to demonstrate the analgesic benefits of locoregional anesthesia following breast surgery, and to demonstrate the clinical utility of these techniques. For perioperative and postoperative analgesia, locoregional anaesthesia can be used as a standalone anaesthetic technique, or in association with sedation or general anaesthesia. In almost all the studies of this review, locoregional anesthesia was performed to reduce pain as an "adjuvant technique".

Table 9 NRS at 1, 6, 24 and 72 h after breast augmentation

	Up to 1 h		Up to 6 h		Up to 24 h		Up to 72 h	
	Group I	Group C	Group I	Group C	Group I	Group C	Group I	Group C
Gardiner et al., *2012* [24]	3.9	5.2	–	–	–	–	3.3	4.7
Picard et al., *2017* [25]	–	–	–	–	4.8	5.1	2.8	3.7
Schuitemaker et al., *2019* [26]	2.9	5.3	3.0	3.0	2.5	3.0	–	–
TOTAL	**3.4 ± 0.5**	**5.25 ± 0.05**	**3.0**	**3.0**	**3.65 ± 1.15**	**4.05 ± 1.05**	**3.05 ± 0.25**	**4.2 ± 0.5**
p	**0.06**		**–**		**0.82**		**0.17**	

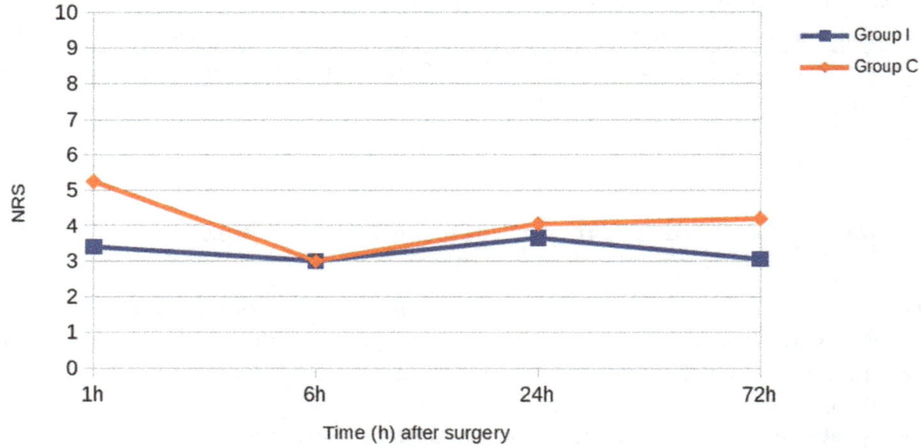

Fig. 5 NRS at 1, 6, 24 and 72 h after breast augmentation

Lumpectomy/mastectomy

Pain intensity

Pain intensity on a numeric rating scale (NRS) was lower in the intervention group than in the placebo group at 1, 6, 12, 24 and 48 h after surgery. The difference of NRS at 1 h between the groups was statistically significant ($p = 0.02$); no statically significant difference was reported at other intervals.

In the first hour after surgery, all patients in the intervention group reported NRS lower than 4; instead in the placebo group, two studies (*Ferreira Laso* et al., *2014; Wang* et al., *2018*) experienced, respectively, a mean pain intensity of 6.7 and 4.3. In the placebo group we also found NRS higher than 4 in *Wang* et al *2019* after 6 h and in *Ferreira Laso* et al *2014* after 24 h.

We considered NRS lower than 4 as an optimal cut-off point between mild and moderate pain. This cut-off was identified as the tolerable pain threshold [29].

Opioid consumption

Postoperative use of opioids was lower in the interventional group both upon discharge from the PACU and after 48 h, although there was no statistically significant difference. The difference in opioid use was statistically significant in three studies (*Ferreira Laso* et al., *2014; Ilfeld* et al., *2014; Versyck* et al. *2017*) at the time of discharge from the PACU. Eight studies (*Campbell* et al., *2014* [10]; *Ferreira Laso* et al., *2014; Gürkan* et al., *2018; Mohamed* et al., *2013; Neethu* et al., *2018; Versyck* et al. *2017; Wang* et al., *2018; Yao* et al., *2019*) reached statistical significance after 48 h from surgery.

Safety

No statistically significant difference was noticed ($p = 0.74$) between interventional and placebo groups. Among the intervention group a total of 163 AEs was reported. Nausea, vomiting or PONV were the most common (59%), followed by bruising (14%), haematoma/bleeding (6%), seroma (6%), pruritus (4%) and haemodynamic alterations (4%), such as hypotension, hypertension or bradycardia.

Patient satisfaction

Patient satisfaction was high, with minimum 92% of satisfaction among patients treated with locoregional anesthesia. The satisfaction rate was also high in the placebo group (79%).

Breast augmentation

Pain intensity on a numeric rating scale (NRS) was lower in the intervention group than in the placebo group at 1, 6, 24 and 72 h after surgery. No statically significant difference was reported at these intervals.

Postoperative use of opioids was lower in the interventional group after 24 h, although there was no statistically significant difference.

Table 10 Personal and clinical characteristics of patients undergoing breast reduction

	Patients, n		*Age, years*		*Weight, kg*		*Height, cm*		*BMI, kg/m²*	
	Group I	*Group C*	*Group I*	*Group C*	*Group I*	*Group C*	*Group I*	*Group C*	*Group I*	*Group C*
Christie* et al., *2017 [27]	20	20	41.0	42.0	–	–	–	–	33.0	31.0
Valente* et al., *2014 [28]	18	20	35.57	35.57	–	–	–	–	–	–
TOTAL	**38**	**40**	**38.28 ± 2.71**	**38.78 ± 3.21**	**–**	**–**	**–**	**–**	**33.0**	**31.0**

Table 11 NRS at 24 h after breast reduction

	Up to 24 h	
	Group I	Group C
Christie et al., *2017* [27]	4.28	4.00
Valente et al., *2014* [28]	0.83	1.71
TOTAL	**2.55 ± 1.72**	**2.85 ± 1.14**
p	**0.89**	

Concerning safety, no difference was noticed between interventional and placebo groups.

Breast reduction

Pain intensity on a numeric rating scale (NRS) was lower in the intervention group than in the placebo group after 24 h. No statically significant difference was reported.

Postoperative use of opioids was lower in the interventional group after 24 h, although there was no statistically significant difference.

No difference was noticed between interventional and placebo groups about AEs incidence.

General anesthesia is the conventional, most frequently used anesthetic technique. Various locoregional anesthetic techniques are also used for breast surgeries. These include local wound infiltration [30], tumescent anesthesia [31], regional anesthetic techniques, such as pectoral nerve (Pecs) blocks type 1 and 2 [32, 33], serratus plane block (SPB) [34], and parasternal block (PSB) [35], pain pump [36, 37], and intravenous regional block [7, 38].

We considered continuous IV infusion of lidocaine for our review. Various are the reasons that led us to consider this technique. Local anesthetics exert their pharmacological action through the block of sodium channels in neural tissues, thereby interrupting neuronal transmission. This action is best demonstrated when the drug comes directly in contact of neural tissues. However, the systemic effects of lidocaine are also probably or at least partially, related to this mechanism [39]. The IV lidocaine shares many of the effects of local anesthetics when used in regional anesthesia techniques. It can lead to better postoperative analgesia, reduced opioid consumption and improved intestinal motility [40]. In addition to the analgesic action, local anesthetics have anti-inflammatory action, justifying also the use of intravenous lidocaine to modulate the inflammatory response resulting from postoperative pain [41].

Locoregional anesthesia provides effective anesthesia and analgesia in the perioperative setting. The beneficial analgesic effect of the regional block is well known, and also confirmed in our analysis. After mastectomy, the use of locoregional anesthesia techniques seems to reduce pain especially in the first hour after the end of the surgery.

Other potentially beneficial effects of locoregional anaesthesia and analgesia on other perioperative outcomes include decreased need for opioids for controlling postoperative pain, decreased postoperative nausea and vomiting, fewer complications and increased patient satisfaction. In our review, there was no statistically significant difference between the analysed anesthesia techniques.

The effective management and relief of postoperative pain plays a vital role in overall surgical outcome. Untreated pain has been linked to prolonged hospital stays, deep venous thrombosis, pulmonary embolism, pneumonia, bowel dysmotility, insomnia, and impaired wound healing [42]. Reduced occurrence of nausea and vomiting is related to better analgesia and opioids/inhalational anaesthetics sparing effect by regional blocks [43, 44]. All this improves post-operative recovery and shortens hospitalization stay.

Limitations

Our review has several limitations. First, some outcomes were characterized by high levels of heterogeneity. Reasons for this may be attributable to subtle variations in surgical technique and differences in anesthetic and analgesic regimens. Second, for 3 studies included in this review (*Campbell* et al *2014* [10], *Lanier* et al *2018* and *Picard* et al [25]), it is not possible to assess whether only regional anesthesia for breast surgery was performed. The impact of locoregional anesthesia on nociception as a "pure" or "adjuvant" technique is different, notably because of the different dosage of local anesthetics. We decided not to exclude these studies and to accept the possible bias during the analysis. Third, many of the included studies had small sample sizes, which decreases their effect and limits external validity. Fourth, another major limitation of this review was the large and unexplained statistical heterogeneity between the studies. Finally, we included two studies (*Couceiro* et al [11]; *Terkawi* et al *2014*) analysing the use of i.v. lidocaine. Systemic lidocaine is not "really" a locoregional anesthesia technique, nevertheless we decided to include it in our review accepting the possible bias arising from systemic effects of this local anesthetic.

All these limitations reduced the quality of the evidence for most of the outcomes.

Conclusion

In this systematic review we found evidence for an effect of locoregional anesthesia on the pain due to breast surgery as one the major predefined outcomes. The difference of NRS at 1 h between the groups was statistically significant among patients who underwent lumpectomy/mastectomy; no statically significant difference was reported at other intervals.

The postoperative opioids consumption, the incidence of PONV and other AEs, and the patient satisfaction were not different among patients who underwent locoregional anesthesia or conventional analgesia.

Abbreviations
AEs: Adverse Events; ALND: Axillary Lymph Node Dissection; BMI: Body Mass Index; DVT: Deep Vein Thrombosis; ESP: Erector Spinae Plane; IV: Intravenous; NRS: Numeric Rating Scale; PACU: Post-Anesthesia Care Unit; Pecs: Pectoralis nerve; PONV: Postoperative Nausea and Vomiting; PTE: Pulmonary Thromboembolism; PVB: Paravertebral Block; SLNB: Sentinel Lymph Node Biopsy; SPB: Serratus Plane Block

Acknowledgements
Not applicable.

Disclosures
Pasquale Sansone, Luca G. Giaccari, Mario Faenza, Pasquale Di Costanzo, Sara Izzo, Caterina Aurilio, Francesco Coppolino, Maria Beatrice Passavanti, Vincenzo Pota and Maria Caterina Pace have nothing to disclose.

Authors' contributions
PS helped design the study, conduct the study, analyse the data, and write the manuscript; LGG helped design the study, conduct the study, analyse the data, and write the manuscript; MF helped design the study and analyse the data; PDC helped design the study and analyse the data; SI helped design the study and analyse the data; CA helped design the study and analyse the data; FC helped design the study and analyse the data; MBP helped design the study and analyse the data; VP helped design the study and analyse the data; MCP helped design the study, conduct the study and analyse the data. All authors have read and approved the manuscript.

Author details
[1]Department of Woman, Child and General and Specialized Surgery, University of Campania "Luigi Vanvitelli", Piazza Luigi Miraglia, 2, Naples, Italy. [2]Multidisciplinary Department of Medical Surgical and Dental Sciences – Plastic Surgery Unit, University of Campania "Luigi Vanvitelli", Naples, Italy.

References

1. Siegel RL, Miller KD, Jemal A. Cancer statistics, 2020. CA A Cancer J Clin. 2000;70:7–30.
2. American Society of Plastic Surgeons. Plastic Surgery Statistics Report. https://www.plasticsurgery.org/documents/News/Statistics/2018/plastic-surgery-statistics-full-report-2018.pdf. Accessed 13 Apr 2020.
3. Broyles JM, Tuffaha SH, Williams EH, Glickman L, George TA, Lee DA. Pain after breast surgery: etiology, diagnosis, and definitive management. Microsurgery. 2016;36(7):535–8.
4. Pace MC, Mazzariello L, Passavanti MB, Sansone P, Barbarisi M, Aurilio C. Neurobiology of pain. J Cell Physiol. 2006;209(1):8–12.
5. Chou R, Gordon DB, de Leon-Casasola OA, et al. Management of Postoperative Pain: a clinical practice guideline from the American pain society, the American Society of Regional Anesthesia and Pain Medicine, and the American Society of Anesthesiologists' committee on regional anesthesia, executive committee, and administrative council. J Pain. 2016; 17(2):131–57.
6. Wick EC, Grant MC, Wu CL. Postoperative multimodal analgesia pain management with nonopioid analgesics and techniques: a review. JAMA Surg. 2017;152(7):691–7.
7. Dunn LK, Durieux ME. Perioperative Use of Intravenous Lidocaine. Anesthesiology. 2017;126(4):729–37.
8. Moher D, Liberati A, Tetzlaff J, Altman DG, The PRISMA Group. Preferred Reporting Items for Systematic Reviews and Meta-Analyses: The PRISMA Statement. BMJ. 2009;339:b2535.
9. Equivalent Opioid Calculator (EOC). Available at http://clincalc.com/Opioids/. Accessed 6 Apr 2020.
10. Campbell I, Cavanagh S, Creighton J, et al. Local anaesthetic in breast surgery. ANZ J Surg. 2015;85:353–7.
11. Couceiro TC, Lima LC, Burle LM, Valença MM. Intravenous lidocaine for postmastectomy pain treatment: randomized, blind, placebo controlled clinical trial. Braz J Anesthesiol. 2015;65(3):207–12.
12. Cros J, Sengès P, Kaprelian S, et al. Pectoral I block does not improve postoperative analgesia after breast Cancer surgery: a randomized, double-blind, dual-centered controlled trial. Reg Anesth Pain Med. 2018;43:596–604.
13. Ferreira Laso L, Lopez-Picado A, Lamata L, et al. Postoperative Analgesia by Infusion of Local Anesthetic into the Surgical Wound after Modified Radical Mastectomy. Plast Reconstr Surg. 2014;134(6):p862e–70e.
14. Gürkan Y, Aksu C, Kuş A, Yörükoğlu UH, Kılıç CT. Ultrasound guided erector spinae plane block reduces postoperative opioid consumption following breast surgery: a randomized controlled study. J Clin Anesth. 2018;50:65–8.
15. Ilfeld BM, Madison SJ, Suresh PJ, et al. Treatment of postmastectomy pain with ambulatory continuous paravertebral nerve blocks: a randomized, triple-masked, placebo-controlled study. Reg Anesth Pain Med. 2014;39(2):89–96.
16. Lanier ST, Lewis KC, Kendall MC, et al. Intraoperative nerve blocks fail to improve quality of recovery after tissue expander breast reconstruction: a prospective, double-blinded, randomized, Placebo-Controlled Clinical Trial. Plast Reconstr Surg. 2018;141(3):590–7.
17. Mohamed SA, Abdel-Ghaffar HS. Effect of the addition of clonidine to locally administered bupivacaine on acute and chronic postmastectomy pain. J Clin Anesth. 2013;25(1):20–7.
18. Neethu M, Pandey RK, Sharma A, et al. Pectoral nerve blocks to improve analgesia after breast cancer surgery: a prospective, randomized and controlled trial. J Clin Anesth. 2018;45:12–7.
19. Terkawi AS, Durieux ME, Gottschalk A, et al. Effect of intravenous Lidocaine on postoperative recovery of patients undergoing mastectomy: a double-blind, placebo-controlled randomized trial. Reg Anesth Pain Med. 2014;39: 472–7.
20. Versyck B, van Geffen CJ, Van Houwe P. Prospective double blind randomized placebo-controlled clinical trial of the pectoral nerves (Pecs) block type II. J Clin Anesth. 2017;40:46–50.
21. Wang K, Zhang X, Zhang T, et al. The efficacy of ultrasound-guided type II pectoral nerve blocks in perioperative pain Management for Immediate Reconstruction after Modified Radical Mastectomy: a prospective, Randomized Study. Clin J Pain. 2018;34(3):231–6.
22. Wang W, Song W, Yang C, et al. Ultrasound-guided pectoral nerve block I and Serratus-intercostal plane block alleviate postoperative pain in patients undergoing modified radical mastectomy. Pain Physician. 2019;22(4):E315–23.
23. Yao Y, Li J, Hu H, Xu T, Chen Y. Ultrasound-guided serratus plane block enhances pain relief and quality of recovery after breast cancer surgery. Eur J Anaesthesiol. 2019;36(6):436–41.
24. Gardiner S, Rudkin G, Cooter R, Field J, Bond M. Paravertebral blockade for day-case breast augmentation. Anesth Analg. 2012;115(5):1053–9.
25. Picard F, Niddam J, De Runz A, Chaouat M, Mimoun M, Boccara D. Intraoperative instillation of ropivacaine during the placement of sub-muscular cosmetic breast implants: is there a clinical benefit? Ann Chir Plast Esthet. 2018;63(1):20–4.
26. Schuitemaker RJB, Sala-Blanch AP, Sánchez Cohen LA, López-Pantaleon JT, Mayoral R, Cubero M. Analgesic efficacy of modified pectoral block plus serratus plane block in breast augmentation surgery: a randomised, controlled, triple-blind clinical trial. Rev Esp Anestesiol Reanim. 2019;66(2):62–71.
27. Christie BM, Kapur S, Kempton SJ, Hanson SE, Ma Y, Rao VK. A Prospective Randomized Trial Comparing the Effects of Lidocaine in Breast Reduction Surgery. Plast Reconstr Surg. 2017;139(5):1074e–9e.
28. Valente DS. Preemptive analgesia with bupivacaine in reduction Mammaplasty. Plast Reconstr Surg. 2014;134(4):581–6.
29. Gerbershagen HJ, Rothaug J, Kalkman CJ, Meissner W. Determination of moderate-to-severe postoperative pain on the numeric rating scale: a cut-off point analysis applying four different methods. Br J Anaesth. 2011;107(4): 619–26.
30. Mustoe TA, Buck DW, Lalonde DH. The safe management of anesthesia, sedation and pain in plastic surgery. Plast Reconstr Surg J. 2010;126(4): 165e–76e.
31. Khater A, Mazy A, Gad M, Taha Abd Eldayem O, Hegazy M. Tumescent mastectomy: the current indications and operative tips and tricks. Breast Cancer Targets Ther. 2017;9:237–43.
32. Blanco R. The 'pecs block': a novel technique for providing analgesia after breast surgery. Anaesthesia. 2011;66:840–52.
33. Blanco R, Fajardo M, Parras MT. Ultrasound description of Pecs II (modified Pecs I): a novel approach to breast surgery. Rev Esp Anestesiol Reanim. 2012;59:470–5.
34. Blanco R, Parras T, McDonnell JG, Prats-Galino A. Serratus plane block: a novel ultrasound-guided thoracic wall nerve block. Anaesthesia. 2013;68(11): 1107–13.
35. Fusco P, Scimia P, Petrucci E, DI Carlo S, Marinangeli F. The ultrasound-guided parasternal block: a novel approach for anesthesia and analgesia in breast cancer surgery. Minerva Anestesiol. 2017;83(2):221–2.

36. Chandran GJ, Lalonde DH. A review of pain pumps in plastic surgery. Can J Plast Surg. 2010;18(1):15–8.
37. Monahan AM, Ilfeld BM. Continuous peripheral nerve blocks. In: Hadzic A, editor. Hadzic's textbook of regional anesthesia and acute pain management. 2th ed. United States: McGraw Hill Companies; 2017. p. 1180–6.
38. Chang YC, Liu CL, Liu TP, Yang PS, Chen MJ, Cheng SP. Effect of perioperative intravenous lidocaine infusion on acute and chronic pain after breast surgery: a meta-analysis of randomized controlled trials. Pain Pract. 2017;17(3):336–43.
39. de Oliveira CM, Issy AM, Sakata RK. Intraoperative intravenous lidocaine. Rev Bras Anestesiol. 2010;60(3):325–33.
40. Kranke P, Jokinen J, Pace NL, et al. Continuous intravenous perioperative lidocaine infusion for postoperative pain and recovery. Cochrane Database Syst Rev. 2015;7:CD009642.
41. Clarke C, McConachie I, Banner R. Lidocaine infusion as a rescue analgesic in the perioperative setting. Pain Res Manag. 2008;13:421–3.
42. Carr DB, Goudas L. Acute pain. Lancet. 1999;353:2051.
43. Calì Cassi L, Biffoli F, Francesconi D, Petrella G, Buonomo O. Anesthesia and analgesia in breast surgery: the benefits of peripheral nerve block. Eur Rev Med Pharmacol Sci. 2017;21:1341–5.
44. Becker DE. Nausea, vomiting, and hiccups: a review of mechanisms and treatment. Anesth Prog. 2010;57:150–6.

4

Comparison of ropivacaine combined with sufentanil for epidural anesthesia and spinal-epidural anesthesia in labor analgesia

Yanshuang Wang and Mingjun Xu*

Abstract

Background: To compare the application and efficacy of ropivacaine combined with sufentanil for continuous epidural anesthesia (CEA) and combined spinal-epidural anesthesia (CSEA) in labor analgesia.

Methods: Three hundred sixty pregnant women requesting labor analgesia from October 2017 to August 2018 were selected retrospectively. According to the anesthetic method, subjects were divided into CSEA group and CEA group. Ropivacaine combined with sufentanil were used in all subjects. The labor time, visual analogue scale (VAS), Apgar score of newborn, adverse pregnancy outcomes and adverse drug reactions were observed.

Results: There was no significant difference in pre-analgesia (T_0) VAS scores between the two groups ($P > 0.05$). VAS scores of first stage of labor (T_1), second stage of labor (T_2) and third stage of labor (T_3) in CSEA group were significantly lower than CEA group ($P < 0.01$). The onset time, T_1 and total labor time in CSEA group were significantly shorter than CEA group ($P < 0.01$). There were no significant differences between T2 and T3 ($P > 0.05$). There were no significant differences in adverse pregnancy outcomes and Apgar scores at 1, 5 and 10 min after birth between the two groups ($P >$ 0.05). The incidence of adverse drug outcomes in CSEA group was significantly lower than CEA group ($P < 0.01$). Maternal satisfaction in CSEA group was significantly higher than CEA group ($P < 0.01$).

Conclusion: Considering ropivacaine combined with sufentanil for CSEA achieved a shorter onset time and labor period, significant analgesic effect, lower adverse drug reactions rates and higher subject satisfaction than CEA, it may be worthy of clinical promotion and application.

Keywords: Ropivacaine, Sufentanil, Continuous epidural anesthesia, Combined spinal-epidural anesthesia, Labor analgesia

Background

Childbirth is usually the most challenging and painful experience of a mother's life [1]. Fear of childbirth has increased the cesarean delivery rate. Due to the fact that natural vaginal delivery has many advantages compared with cesarean section and promotion of natural vaginal delivery is considered important by the health care systems, labor analgesia has become a key concern for both puerperal and clinical anesthesiologists [2].

At present, labor analgesia methods include non-pharmacological analgesia and pharmacological analgesia. Non-pharmacological analgesia mainly includes acupuncture, massage, yoga and hydrotherapy and the analgesic effect of which is poor although there is no maternal and fetal injury [3]. For pharmacological analgesia, there are intramuscular analgesics, intravenous analgesics, and spinal analgesia. Among them, intraspinal labor analgesia is the best method for clinical application of analgesia, including continuous epidural analgesia (CEA), combined spinal-epidural anesthesia (CSEA) and continuous spinal anesthesia [4, 5]. Epidural analgesia is considered as a widely practiced analgesic technique in clinic worldwide [6]. An ideal labor analgesia method should exhibit good analgesic effect, increase subject satisfaction and comfort, and reduce the incidence of

* Correspondence: xumingjun88@yeah.net
Department of Anesthesiology, Beijing Obstetrics and Gynecology Hospital, Capital Medical University, Beijing 100029, China

adverse pregnancy outcomes and adverse drug reactions without affecting the progress of labor [7].

In recent years, with the development of anesthesia technology, combined spinal-epidural anesthesia has increasingly used in labor analgesia because it combines the advantages of epidural anesthesia and spinal anesthesia, including rapid onset, significant analgesic effect, lower drug dosage and fewer side effects [8, 9]. However, there are few reports on the specific anesthesia methods and medication regimens of combined spinal-epidural anesthesia, which is not conducive to guiding clinical work. Here, we compared the clinical effects of combined spinal-epidural anesthesia and continuous epidural anesthesia, to provide guidance for clinical work.

Methods

Study design and population

In this retrospective, single-center case-control analysis, a total of 360 cases of voluntary acceptance of painless childbirth pregnant from October 2017 to August 2018 in the Beijing Obstetrics and Gynecology Hospital were selected in this study retrospectively. The inclusion criteria were: (1) primiparous women; (2) at first full-term pregnancy, singleton pregnancies; and (3) cephalic, and had no spinal deformity. Exclusion criteria were: (1) pregnant women who had contraindication to epidural anesthesia; (2) pregnant women who had signs of fetal distress; (3) pregant women with contraindications for vaginal delivery. The subjects were divided into observation group and control group according to anesthetic method ($n = 180$ in each group, control: case were 1:1). For the observation group, combined spinal-epidural anesthesia (CSEA group) was used. Cases in control group received continuous epidural anesthesia (CEA group). Ropivacaine combined with sufentanil were used in all subjects. All subjects were American Society of Anesthesiologists (ASA) physical status class I or II. One hundred forty-two subjects in CSEA group and 133 subjects in CEA group were class I and 18 subjects in CSEA group and 27 subjects in CEA group were class II.

Anesthetic method

After entering the clinical delivery, the routine monitoring was established for all women, including blood pressure (BP), heart rate (HR), pulse oximetry (SpO2) and electrocardiography (ECG). Oxygen therapy by nasal catheter venous access and fetal heart monitoring was given. In terms of labor analgesia, the impact on the patient's circulation and other aspects is very small since the dosage of CSEA injected into the subarachnoid space is only 1/5–1/10 of normal CSEA anesthesia. In addition, CEA and CSEA were performed in patients with normal coagulation function. Therefore, there is no obvious tendency in the selection of indications. Both CEA and CSEA were routinely used in our department and the method was chosen according to the anesthesiologist's personal anesthesia operation habits.

For CEA group, pregnant women were placed in the left lateral position. After successful epidural puncture at L2–3 or L3–4 interspace, 3 mL of 0.5% ropivacaine (Naropin; AstraZeneca Co., Ltd.; 10 ml/100 mg; Registration number: H20140763) were slowly injected. If no occurrence of adverse reactions were observed 10 min later, pre-configured 10 mL of analgesic pump solution were given from the epidural space and epidural analgesia analgesia pump (PCEA) was then connected. The formula of analgesic pump solution was: 10 ml of 1% ropivacaine combined with 0.3–0.4 μg/ml sufentanil (Eurocept BV Trapgans 51,244 RL Ankeveen, The Netherlands; 75 μg/1 ml; Batch number: 170553) diluted to 100 ml with 0.9% sterile saline. The analgesic pump parameters were set as follows: continuous background infusion of 5 ml/h, single additional dose (PCA) of 7 ml/time, interval lockout time of 15 min and total amount of 100 ml.

For pregnant women in CSEA group, after successful epidural puncture at L2–3 or L3–4 interspace, a 25-G lumbar puncture needle was inserted through the epidural needle (Xinxiang Camel Medical Devices Co., Ltd.; Batch number: 1310015). After the cerebrospinal fluid was seen 2–3 mg of 0.1% ropivacaine (diluted to 2–3 ml with sterile saline) was then injected into the subarachnoid space. After 3–4 cm of epidural catheter was set to the head side, subjects in both groups were placed in the supine position. Ten minutes later, epidural analgesia analgesia pump (PCEA) was connected after no occurrence of adverse reactions were observed. The formula of analgesic pump solution and analgesic pump parameters were the same as CEA group.

For both groups, the heart rate, blood pressure and fetal heart rate of the pregnant women were closely monitored during the process of analgesia and childbirth. After the uterine cervix was opened, the pump fluid infusion was stopped, and the epidural catheter was pulled out 2 h after delivery.

Observation indexes

The onset time of analgesia, T1, T2, T3, total labor time and doses of ropivacaine and sufentanil in two groups were recorded. Pain was assessed by visual analog scale (VAS) [10] scores at four time points: (1) T_0, stage before analgesia; (2) T_1, from the beginning of uterine contractions to cervical dilatation of 10 cm; (3) T_2, from cervical dilatation of 10 cm to the delivery of the baby; (4) T_3, From the delivery of the baby to the delivery of the placenta. The T_0, T_1, T_2 and T_3 in this study were defined according to the guidelines from the National Institute for Health and Clinical Excellence [11].

The Apgar scores were assessed at 1, 5, and 10 min after birth [12]. Apgar scores of 8–10 points were considered normal for newborns; 4–7 points indicated mild asphyxia; and 0–3 points suggested severe asphyxia.

Maternal satisfaction evaluation were performed based on subjects' feelings during different labor periods on labor analgesia (80–100: very satisfactory; 60–80: general satisfactory; below 60: unsatisfactory).

Finally, the adverse pregnancy outcomes and adverse drug reactions were observed.

Statistical analysis

All statistical analyses were conducted with SPSS software, version 18.0 (SPSS Inc., Chicago, USA). PP plot (probability-probability plot) indicates the normal distribution of data. Values are presented as mean ± standard deviation (SD) or number (percentage) at appropriate. Quantitative variables (VAS scores, labor time, apgar scores and doses of ropivacaine and sufentanil) were compared by *Student's t test* and χ2 test was used for categorical variables (adverse pregnancy outcomes and adverse drug reactions). Repeated-measures ANOVA were used for the comparison of different time points within the group. All reported *P* values are two-sided, and *P* value of less than 0.05 was considered statistically significant.

Results

There were no significant differences with regard to age, height, weight, BMI and duration of pregnancy between CSEA group and CEA group ($P > 0.05$) (Table 1).

VAS scores in two groups

There was no significant differenceregarding VAS scores at T_0 between two groups ($P > 0.05$). In two groups, VAS scores at T_1, T_2 and T_3 were significantly lowercompared with T_0 in the same group ($P < 0.01$). VAS scores at T_1, T_2 and T_3 in CSEA group were significantly lower compared with those in CEA group at the same time ($P < 0.01$) (Table 2).

Table 1 Clinical characteristics of subjects (mean ± SD)

	CEA (*n* = 180)	CSEA (*n* = 180)	*P* value
Age, years	26.8 ± 4.2	27.1 ± 3.9	0.483
Height, cm	160.4 ± 4.3	161.3 ± 4.6	0.056
Weight, kg	65.4 ± 16.2	66.3 ± 15.6	0.592
BMI, kg/m^2	22.3 ± 3.4	22.2 ± 3.1	0.771
Duration of pregnancy, weeks	38.5 ± 1.3	38.3 ± 1.4	0.161

BMI Body Mass Index. *P* value of comparison between CSEA and CEA groups

Table 2 Comparison of pain VAS scores at different times in two groups (mean ± SD)

	CEA (*n* = 180)	CSEA (*n* = 180)
T_0 (min)	8.32 ± 1.37	8.36 ± 1.35
T_1(min)	3.35 ± 0.64*	3.02 ± 0.67$^{*\#}$
T_2 (min)	4.22 ± 0.87*	3.84 ± 0.83$^{*\#}$
T_3 (min)	6.84 ± 1.26*	5.31 ± 1.12$^{*\#}$

$^*P < 0.01$, vs T_0; $^\#P < 0.01$, vs CEA group

Labor time in two groups

The onset time, T_1 and total labor time in CSEA group were significantly shorter than those in CEA group ($P < 0.01$). However, there was no significant difference regarding labor time at T_2 and T_3 between two groups ($P > 0.05$) (Table 3).

Apgar scores in two groups

There were no significant differences in Apgar scores at 1, 5, and 10 min after birth between the two groups ($P > 0.05$) (Table 4).

Adverse pregnancy outcomes in two groups

There were no significant differences in adverse pregnancy outcomes after labor analgesia between the two groups ($P > 0.05$) (Table 5), including obstetric apparatus, cesarean, 24 h postpartum hemorrhage and episiotomy.

Doses of drugs and adverse drug reactions in two groups

Doses of ropivacaine and sufentanil in CSEA group were significantly lower than that in CEA group ($P < 0.01$) (Table 6). There were no significant differences in the rates of uroschesis and respiratory depression between two groups ($P > 0.05$). However, the rates of nausea, vomiting, pruritus and total adverse drug reactions in CSEA group were significantly lower than these in CEA group ($P < 0.01$). Besides, subject satisfaction in CSEA group were significantly higher than that in CEA group ($P < 0.01$) (Table 7).

Discussion

Under the different combinations of ropivacaine and sufentanil, the observation and analysis of the two anesthesia methods in this study showed that CSEA was

Table 3 Comparison of labor time in two groups (mean ± SD)

	CEA (*n* = 180)	CSEA (*n* = 180)	*P* value
Onset time (min)	6.32 ± 3.45	3.21 ± 1.42	< 0.001
T_1(min)	524.33 ± 126.46	468.32 ± 114.10	< 0.001
T_2(min)	48.24 ± 10.34	46.09 ± 11.22	0.060
T_3(min)	7.38 ± 0.76	7.24 ± 0.83	0.096
Total labor time (min)	578.29 ± 132.08	512.67 ± 124.38	< 0.001

Table 4 The Apgar scores at 1, 5, and 10 min after birth in two groups (mean ± SD)

	CEA (*n* = 180)	CSEA (*n* = 180)	*P* value
1 min after birth	8.47 ± 0.34	8.41 ± 0.35	0.099
5 min after birth	8.85 ± 0.41	8.83 ± 0.42	0.647
10 min after birth	9.52 ± 0.38	9.48 ± 0.33	0.278

superior to CEA in analgesic effect and maternal satisfaction.

CSEA refers to a method of injecting a small amount of anesthetic drug into the subarachnoid space after successful epidural puncture [13]. Currently, the combination of local anesthetic and opioid is the common compatibility program for CSEA, including bupivacaine, ropivacaine, fentanyl and sufentanil [14, 15]. Ropivacaine (1-propyl-2′, 6′-pipecoloxylidide, chemical structure) is an amino acid local anesthetic and was recently introduced for labor analgesia, since it has less cardiac toxicity and provide more differential block between sensory and motor [7, 16]. For opioids, the analgesic effect of sufentanil is 3 to 5 times more potent than fentanyl due to the strong affinity for opioid receptors [17, 18].

Clinically, ropivacaine combined with low-dose sufentanil has been widely used in labor analgesia [19]. The combination of the two drugs allows use of lower doses of both drugs, thus decreasing the rate and severity of adverse effects [20]. However, previous studies [21, 22] have shown that ropivacaine combined with sufentanil injected into the subarachnoid space after the spinal anesthesia pierced the dura mater resulted in a higher pruritus rates than ropivacaine alone. In this study, ropivacaine combined with sufentanil were used for CEA group. While for CSEA group, ropivacaine were used alone before epidural catheter were placed and ropivacaine combined with sufentanil were used thereafter. As a result, better analgesic effect was achieved in CSEA group compared with CEA group according to the VAS scores. Besides, the overall incidence of adverse drug reactions in CSEA group was lower than CEA group, including the lower nausea and vomiting rates and pruritus rates. The reduced dose of sufentanil were responsible for this result since complications of anesthetics were dose-dependent [18, 23]. Additionally, delaying sufentanil injection may exert the maximum effect of ropivacaine, which has long analgesic duration, less adverse drug reactions and differential block between sensory and motor [24].

Table 5 Comparison of adverse pregnancy outcomes in two groups (mean ± SD)

	CEA (*n* = 180)	CSEA (*n* = 180)	*P* value
Obstetric apparatus, n (%)	7 (3.89)	8 (4.45)	0.792
Cesarean, n (%)	18 (10.00)	22 (12.22)	0.499
24 h postpartum hemorrhage, n (%)	6 (3.33)	5 (2.78)	0.759
Episiotomy, n (%)	22 (12.22)	16 (8.89)	0.303
Total adverse pregnancy outcomes, n (%)	44 (24.44)	41 (22.78)	0.709

Table 6 Doses of Ropivacaine and Sufentanil in each group. (mean ± SD)

	CEA (*n* = 180)	CSEA (*n* = 180)	*P* value
Ropivacaine	39.88 ± 4.52	38.42 ± 3.16	< 0.001
Sufentanil	19.98 ± 6.66	16.01 ± 5.26	< 0.001

In this study, CSEA group has a relative shorter onset time compared with CEA group, which is inconsistent with a previous study [25], showing that there were no differences between groups for onset time and analgesia evaluation. We assume that this possibly due to the different doses of ropivacaine and sufentanil in both studies. We found no statistically significant differences with regard to the Apgar scores of the newborns at 1, 5 and 10 min and adverse pregnancy outcomes between the two groups suggesting that CSEA could achieve the same newborn conditions as CEA with lower doses of ropivacaine and sufentanil. Maternal satisfaction were improved due to the fewer adverse drug reactions associated with intrathecal sufentanil that can be disconcerting for subjects.

The limitation of this study was that pregnant women with contraindication to epidural anesthesia were not suitable for this method. Therefore, more studies should be carried out in the future to further improve the labor analgesia method.

Conclusion

CSEA group in this study achieved better analgesic effect, lower onset time and fewer adverse drug reactions compared with CEA group. Thus, CSEA method with our block method and doses may provide some reference for clinical labor analgesia.

Table 7 Comparison of adverse drug reactions in two groups

	CEA (*n* = 180)	CSEA (*n* = 180)	*P* value
Nausea and vomiting, n (%)	20 (11.11)	8 (4.44)	0.018
Pruritus, n (%)	12 (6.67)	4 (2.22)	0.041
Uroschesis, n (%)	8 (4.44)	4 (2.22)	0.240
Respiratory depression, n (%)	4 (2.22)	2 (1.11)	0.410
Total adverse drug reactions, n (%)	44 (24.44)	18 (10.00)	< 0.001
Subject satisfaction, n (%)	120 (66.67)	150 (83.33)	< 0.001

Acknowledgments
None.

Authors' contributions
JX and YW conceived the project and analyzed the data. YW designed the experiments and performed the experiments. JX wrote the paper. Both authors have read and approved the manuscript, and ensure that this is the case.

References

1. Chajut E, Caspi A, Chen R, Hod M, Ariely D. In pain thou shalt bring forth children: the peak-and-end rule in recall of labor pain. Psychol Sci. 2014;25: 2266–71.
2. Attar AS, Feizabadi AS, Jarahi L, Feizabadi LS, Sheybani S. Effect of Entonox on reducing the need for Pethidine and the relevant Fetal and maternal complications for painless labor. Electron Physician. 2016;8:3325–32.
3. Koyyalamudi V, Sidhu G, Cornett EM, Nguyen V, Labrie-Brown C, Fox CJ, Kaye AD. New labor pain treatment options. Curr Pain Headache Rep. 2016; 20:11.
4. Simmons SW, Taghizadeh N, Dennis AT, Hughes D, Cyna AM. Combined spinal-epidural versus epidural analgesia in labour. Cochrane Database Syst Rev. 2012;10:Cd003401.
5. McKenzie CP, Carvalho B, Riley ET. The Wiley spinal catheter-over-needle system for continuous spinal Anesthesia: a case series of 5 Cesarean deliveries complicated by Paresthesias and headaches. Reg Anesth Pain Med. 2016;41:405–10.
6. Bos EME, Hollmann MW, Lirk P. Safety and efficacy of epidural analgesia. Curr Opin Anaesthesiol. 2017;30:736–42.
7. Chen SY, Lin PL, Yang YH, Yang YM, Lee CN, Fan SZ, Chen LK. The effects of different epidural analgesia formulas on labor and mode of delivery in nulliparous women. Taiwan J Obstet Gynecol. 2014;53:8–11.
8. Matsumine R, Sumikura H. Analgesic treatment of vaginal delivery for late termination and intrauterine fetal demise during the second or third trimester of pregnancy. J Anesth. 2013;27:320–1.
9. Feng BB, Wang L, Zhai JJ. Investigation on delivery analgesia effect of combined spinal epidural anesthesia plus doula and safety of mother and baby. Clin Exp Obstet Gynecol. 2013;40:574–8.
10. Patrick DW, Ronald M. Textbook of PAIN. New York: Chruchill Livingstone; 1985. p. 377–86.
11. Bick D. Caesarean section. Clinical guideline. National Collaborating Centre for Women's and Children's health: commissioned by the National Institute for clinical excellence. Worldviews Evid-Based Nurs. 2004;1:198–9.
12. Apgar V. A proposal for a new method of evaluation of the newborn infant. Curr Res Anesth Analg. 1953;32:260–7.
13. Okutomi T, Saito M, Mochizuki J, Kuczkowski KM. Combined spinal-epidural analgesia for labor pain: best timing of epidural infusion following spinal dose. Arch Gynecol Obstet. 2009;279:329–34.
14. Lv BS, Wang W, Wang ZQ, Wang XW, Wang JH, Fang F, Mi WD. Efficacy and safety of local anesthetics bupivacaine, ropivacaine and levobupivacaine in combination with sufentanil in epidural anesthesia for labor and delivery: a meta-analysis. Curr Med Res Opin. 2014;30:2279–89.
15. Shah OM, Bhat KM. Comparison of the efficacy and safety of morphine and fentanyl as adjuvants to bupivacaine in providing operative Anesthesia and postoperative analgesia in Subumblical surgeries using combined spinal epidural technique. Anesth Essays Res. 2017;11:913–20.
16. Zhao L, Wang Y, Zhai Y, Wang Z, Liu J, Zhai G. Ropivacaine loaded microemulsion and microemulsion-based gel for transdermal delivery: preparation, optimization, and evaluation. Int J Pharm. 2014;477:47–56.
17. Li B, Wang H, Gao C. Bupivacaine in combination with fentanyl or sufentanil in epidural/intrathecal analgesia for labor: a meta-analysis. J Clin Pharmacol. 2015;55:584–91.
18. Coleman L, Carvalho B, Lipman S, Schmiesing C, Riley E. Accidental intrathecal sufentanil overdose during combined spinal-epidural analgesia for labor. Int J Obstet Anesth. 2009;18:78–80.
19. Bremerich DH, Waibel HJ, Mierdl S, Meininger D, Byhahn C, Zwissler BC, Ackermann HH. Comparison of continuous background infusion plus demand dose and demand-only parturient-controlled epidural analgesia (PCEA) using ropivacaine combined with sufentanil for labor and delivery. Int J Obstet Anesth. 2005;14:114–20.
20. Lee AI, McCarthy RJ, Toledo P, Jones MJ, White N, Wong CA. Epidural labor analgesia-fentanyl dose and breastfeeding success: a randomized clinical trial. Anesthesiology. 2017;127:614–24.
21. Li Y, Hu C, Fan Y, Wang H, Xu H. Epidural analgesia with amide local anesthetics, bupivacaine, and ropivacaine in combination with fentanyl for labor pain relief: a meta-analysis. Med Sci Monit. 2015;21:921–8.
22. Ortner CM, Posch M, Roessler B, Faybik P, Rutzler K, Grabovica J, Kimberger O, Gustorff B. On the ropivacaine-reducing effect of low-dose sufentanil in intrathecal labor analgesia. Acta Anaesthesiol Scand. 2010;54:1000–6.
23. Zhang L, Shu R, Zhao Q, Li Y, Wang C, Wang H, Yu Y, Wang G. Preoperative but not postoperative Flurbiprofen Axetil alleviates Remifentanil-induced Hyperalgesia after laparoscopic Gynecological surgery: a prospective, randomized, double-blinded, trial. Clin J Pain. 2017;33:435–42.
24. Ngan Kee WD, Ng FF, Khaw KS, Tang SPY, Koo AGP. Dose-response curves for Intrathecal bupivacaine, Levobupivacaine, and Ropivacaine given for labor analgesia in nulliparous women. Reg Anesth Pain Med. 2017;42: 788–92.
25. Nakamura G, Ganem EM, Rugolo LM, Castiglia YM. Effects on mother and fetus of epidural and combined spinal-epidural techniques for labor analgesia. Rev Assoc Med Bras (1992). 2009;55:405–9.

Intravenous dexmedetomidine versus tramadol for treatment of shivering after spinal anesthesia

Jinguo Wang[1], Zaitang Wang[2], Junyan Liu[1] and Na Wang[3*]

Abstract

Background: Shivering is a frequent complication after spinal anesthesia. Increasing studies have compared the effect of intravenous dexmedetomidine and intravenous tramadol on shivering after spinal anesthesia, hence we performed a meta-analysis of randomized controlled trials to compare dexmedetomidine with tramadol on the treatment of post-spinal anesthesia shivering.

Methods: PubMed, Embase, Cochrane library, Web of Science and Google Scholar were searched to find the eligible studies comparing the effect of dexmedetomidine and tramadol on the treatment of shivering after spinal anesthesia. Mean difference (MD) or risk ratio (RR) along with 95% confidence interval (CI) was used to analyze the outcomes. I^2 test was conducted to assess the heterogeneity of the included trials. We utilized Review Manager 5.3 to perform statistical analyses.

Results: Thirteen randomized controlled trials including 864 subjects were included. Dexmedetomidine had higher effective rate of shivering control (RR =1.03; 95%CI [1.01, 1.06], $P = 0.01$, $I^2 = 14\%$), shorter time to cease shivering (MD = -2.14; 95%CI [− 2.79, − 1.49], $P < 0.00001$, $I^2 = 98\%$), lower recurrent rate of shivering (RR = 0.45; 95%CI [0.27, 0.73], $P = 0.001$, $I^2 = 0\%$), lower incidences of nausea (RR = 0.10; 95%CI [0.05, 0.19], $P < 0.00001$, $I^2 = 48\%$), and vomiting (RR = 0.13; 95%CI [0.06, 0.30], $P < 0.00001$, $I^2 = 0\%$), higher incidence of sedation (RR = 2.48; 95%CI [1.32, 4.65], $P = 0.005$, $I^2 = 82\%$), hypotension (RR = 2.50; 95%CI [1.24, 5.03], $P = 0.01$, $I^2 = 0\%$) and bradycardia (RR = 4.78; 95%CI [1.76, 13.00], $P = 0.002$, $I^2 = 0\%$), compared with tramadol.

Conclusions: Dexmedetomidine is superior to tramadol for shivering treatment, due to higher effective rate of shivering control, earlier onset of action and lesser recurrence of shivering with higher incidence of sedation and lower incidences of nausea and vomiting. However, dexmedetomidine is also associated with higher incidences of hypotension and bradycardia than tramadol.

Keywords: Dexmedetomidine, Tramadol, Postanesthesia shivering, Meta-analysis

* Correspondence: wangna080613@163.com
[3]Department of Anesthesiology, The First Hospital of Jilin University, No.1 Xinmin Street, Changchun, Jilin 130021, China

Background

Shivering is a common perioperative complication because of postanesthesia hypothermia [1]. Spinal anesthesia has impairment of shivering in the block area and greater heat loss than general anesthesia because of abnormal heat loss owing to vasodilatation [2, 3]. Shivering can cause severe consequences, such as arterial hypoxia and myocardial ischemia by increasing oxygen consumption [4, 5]. Tramadol is commonly used for the treatment of shivering in clinical practice. However, tramadol can lead to nausea and vomiting which is very distressing for the patient. Therefore, it is necessary to find a better drug with fewer side effects. Dexmedetomidine, an alpha 2-adrenergic agonist, has been confirmed the effect on treatment and prevention of shivering in various surgeries by reducing the shivering threshold [6].

There are no large-sample clinical trials evaluating the advantages or disadvantages between dexmedetomidine and tramadol on post-spinal anesthesia shivering. Therefore, we conduct a meta-analysis of randomized controlled trials (RCTs) to compare the effect of intravenous dexmedetomidine and tramadol on post-spinal anesthesia shivering.

Methods

Literature review

Relevant articles were found by searching PubMed, Cochrane library, Web of Science and Google Scholar by two investigators independently. The terms used for searching included: "Dex", "Dexmedetomidine", "Tramadol", "Anesthesia, Spinal", "Injections, Spinal" and "Shivering" through March 2020, without limits. Furthermore,

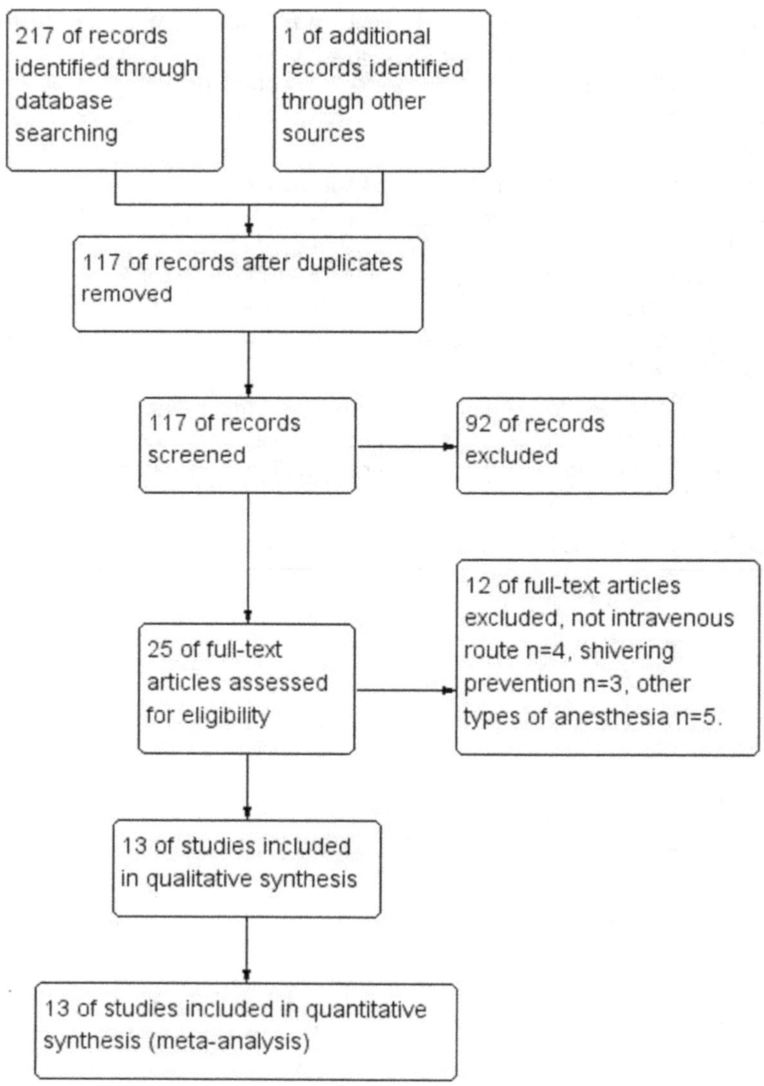

Fig. 1 The flow chart of study selection

Table 1 Characteristics of the included studies

Author Date	Dosage	Study type	Jadad Score	Sample size D/T	Patient characteristics; Surgical setting	Type of anesthesia; Drug for anesthesia	Definition of shivering	Outcomesmeasures
Kundra 2017	Dexmedetomidine 0.5 μg/kg, tramadol 0.5 mg/kg	RCT	5	50/50	18–65 yr, ASA: I-II; Orthopedic, general, or urological surgery	Spinal anesthesia; 0.5% bupivacaine	Grade 3 or 4	①②③④⑤⑥⑦⑧
Venkatraman 2016	Dexmedetomidine 0.5 μg/kg, tramadol 1 mg/kg	RCT	5	30/30	18–70 yr, ASA: I-II; No mention	Spinal anesthesia; To achieve sensory level of at least T10	Grades 2 to 4	①②③⑤⑥⑦⑧
Mittal 2014	Dexmedetomidine 0.5 μg/kg; tramadol 0.5 mg/kg	RCT	4	25/25	18–65 yr, ASA: I-II; Lower abdominal, lower limb, orthopaedic and plastic surgeries	Spinal anesthesia; 0.5% heavy bupivacaine 15 mg.	Grade 3 or 4	①②③④⑤⑥⑦⑧
Fern 2015	Dexmedetomidine 0.5 μg/kg; tramadol 0.5 mg/kg	RCT	3	20/20	18–70 yr, ASA: I-II; Elective orthopaedic, gynaecology or general surgery	Combined spinal and epidural anesthesia; 0.5% hyperbaric bupivacaine 15 mg.	Grade 3 or 4	①②⑥⑦⑧
Keerthi 2017	Dexmedetomidine 0.5 μg/kg; tramadol 0.5 mg/kg	RCT	4	32 /32	18–60 yr, ASA: I-II; Lower abdomen and lower limb surgery	Spinal anesthesia; 0.5% hyperbaric bupivacaine 2.8 to 3 ml	Grades 2 to 4	①②③④⑤⑥⑦⑧
Ramesh 2019	Dexmedetomidine 0.5 μg/kg; tramadol 0.5 mg/kg	RCT	3	30/30	18–65 yr, ASA: I-II; Elective lower limb surgery	Spinal anesthesia; 0.5% hyperbaric bupivacaine 12.5 mg	Grade 3 for at least 2 min	①②③④⑤⑧
Verma 2018	Dexmedetomidine 0.5 μg/kg; tramadol 0.5 mg/kg	RCT	4	60/60	18–65 yr, ASA: I-II; Elective lower limb, lower abdominal, gynaecological procedures, caesarean sections	Spinal anesthesia; No mention	Grade 3 or 4	①②③④⑤⑥⑦⑧
Prasad 2018	Dexmedetomidine 0.5 μg/kg; tramadol 0.5 mg/kg	RCT	5	25/25	18–40 yr, ASA: I-II; Caesarean section	Spinal anesthesia; 0.5% hyperbaric bupivacaine	Grade 3 or 4	①②③④⑤⑥⑦⑧
Kumar 2016	Dexmedetomidine 0.6 μg/kg; tramadol 1.0 mg/kg	RCT	3	20/20	18–60 yr, ASA: I-II; Elective lower abdominal surgeries and lower limb surgeries	Spinal anesthesia; 0.5% hyperbaric bupivacaine 15 mg	Grade 3	①②③⑥⑦
Verma 2016	Dexmedetomidine 0.5 μg/kg; tramadol 2 mg/kg	RCT	4	30/30	18–45 yr, ASA: I-II; Elective abdominal, gynecological and orthopedic surgeries	Spinal anesthesia; 0.5% hyperbaric bupivacaine 15 mg	Grades 2 to 4	①②③④⑤⑥⑦
Singla 2017	Dexmedetomidine 0.5 μg/kg; tramadol 0.5 mg/kg	RCT	4	50/50	18–65 yr, ASA: I-II; Various surgeries under spinal anesthesia	Spinal anesthesia; 0.5% hyperbaric bupivacaine 3–3.6 ml	Grades 2 to 4	①②③⑥⑦⑧
Singh 2016	Dexmedetomidine 0.5 μg/kg; tramadol 0.5 mg/kg	RCT	4	30/30	20–50 yr, ASA: I-II; Elective lower abdominal, lower limb orthopaedic and gynaecological surgeries	Spinal anesthesia; 0.5% hyperbaric bupivacaine 15 mg	Grade 3	①②③④⑤⑥⑦⑧
Aasim 2016	Dexmedetomidine 0.5 μg/kg; tramadol 0.5 mg/kg	RCT	5	30/30	18–65 yr, ASA: I-II; Various surgeries under spinal anesthesia	Spinal anesthesia; 0.5% hyperbaric bupivacaine 15 mg	Grade 3	①②③④⑤⑥⑦⑧

RCT randomized controlled trial, *ASA* American Society of Anesthesiologists. ①: Effective rate of shivering treatment, ②: Time to cease shivering, ③: recurrent rate of shivering, ④: the incidence of nausea, ⑤: the incidence of vomiting, ⑥: the incidence of bradycardia, ⑦: the incidence of hypotension, ⑧: sedation score

the researchers looked through the references of the relative papers to find additional studies.

Inclusion criteria of studies

Inclusion criteria were as follows: 1) the patients underwent an operation under spinal anesthesia or combined spinal and epidural anesthesia; 2) the comparison was between intravenous dexmedetomidine and tramadol about the treatment effect of shivering; 3) the incidence of side effects was reported in both dexmedetomidine and tramadol groups; 4) the study was a RCT. Meeting papers, correspondences and editorials were excluded.

Data extraction

Data were collected independently by two researchers, including patient characteristics, types of surgery, anesthetic type, the drugs for spinal anesthesia, doses of the study drugs, shivering degree, efficacy of shivering treatment, incidence of recurrent shivering and adverse effects. Shivering was graded using a four point scale as per Wrench in all included papers [7]. Any disaccord was further settled by the third researcher.

Evaluation of risk of bias and the study quality

Two researchers independently evaluated the risk of bias and the qualities of all included studies according to Cochrane Handbook v5.0.2 and 5 point Jadad scale [8]. Each of the following items of risk of bias was graded as "high risk of bias", "uncertain risk of bias" or "low risk of bias": random sequence generation, allocation concealment, blinding of participants and personnel, blinding of outcome assessment, incomplete outcome data, selective reporting and other bias. Disputes were settled by discussion, if necessary, a third investigator helped to make a decision.

Statistical analysis

Review Manager 5.3 (Cochrane Collaboration, Copenhagen, Denmark) was utilized to perform all statistical analyses. For dichotomous data, risk ratio (RR) with 95% confidence interval (CI) was calculated with the Mantel-Haenszel method. Mean difference was used for continuous variables. If there was significant heterogeneity ($I^2 > 50\%$), we tried to find possible reasons of heterogeneity, and then sensitivity analysis was performed with fixed effect model.

Results

Figure 1 showed the flow chart of this meta-analysis. Thirteen studies were included, involving 864 patients (432 received dexmedetomidine and 432 tramadol) [9–21]. The characteristics of the identified clinical trials were displayed in Tables 1. Surgeries were performed under spinal anesthesia in 12 studies [9–20] and under combined spinal and epidural anesthesia in one study [21]. In the included studies, 7 compared dexmedetomidine with tramadol [9–15] and the other 6 compared dexmedetomidine with tramadol and clonidine [16–18, 20], pethidine [21] or butorphanol [19]. Because our study only compared dexmedetomidine with tramadol, clonidine, pethidine and butorphanol were neglected. The risk-of-bias plot was formed utilizing Review Manager 5.3. (Fig. 2).

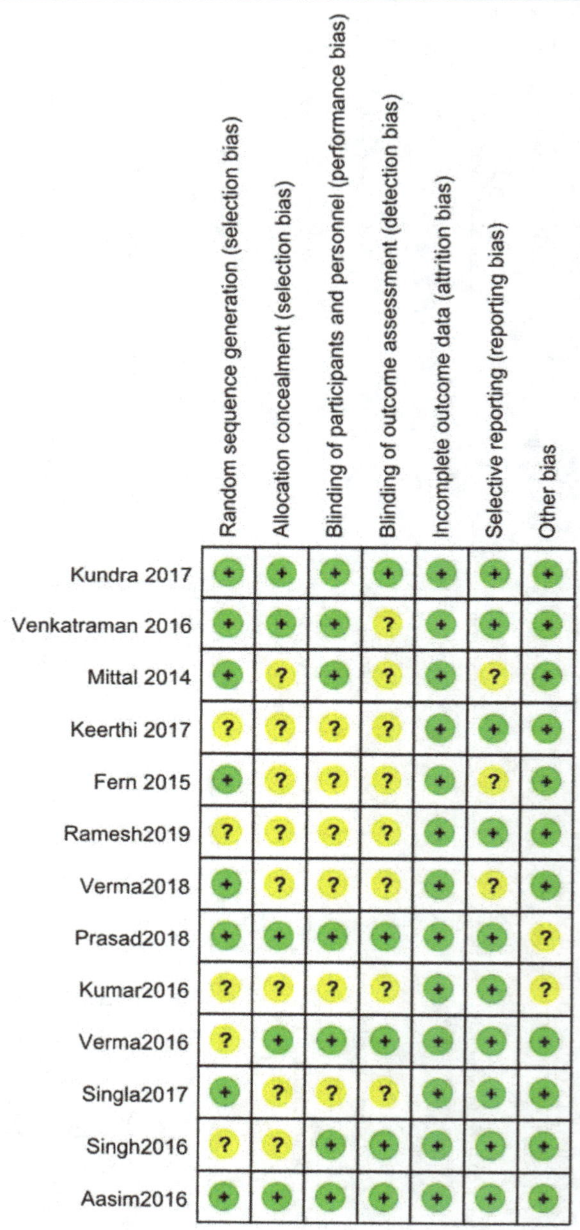

Fig. 2 The risk of bias assessment of the included studies. Note: There was no high risk of bias found in these studies

Study or Subgroup	Dexmedetomidine Events	Dexmedetomidine Total	Tramadol Events	Tramadol Total	Weight	Risk Ratio M-H, Fixed, 95% CI
Kundra 2017	50	50	50	50	11.9%	1.00 [0.96, 1.04]
Venkatraman 2016	30	30	29	30	7.0%	1.03 [0.94, 1.13]
Mittal 2014	25	25	25	25	6.0%	1.00 [0.93, 1.08]
Keerthi 2017	32	32	32	32	7.7%	1.00 [0.94, 1.06]
Fern 2015	20	20	17	20	4.1%	1.17 [0.96, 1.43]
Ramesh2019	30	30	30	30	7.2%	1.00 [0.94, 1.07]
Verma2018	59	60	52	60	12.3%	1.13 [1.02, 1.26]
Prasad2018	25	25	25	25	6.0%	1.00 [0.93, 1.08]
Kumar2016	20	20	20	20	4.8%	1.00 [0.91, 1.10]
Verma2016	29	30	30	30	7.2%	0.97 [0.88, 1.06]
Singla2017	50	50	49	50	11.7%	1.02 [0.97, 1.08]
Singh2016	30	30	28	30	6.7%	1.07 [0.96, 1.20]
Aasim2016	30	30	30	30	7.2%	1.00 [0.94, 1.07]
Total (95% CI)		**432**		**432**	**100.0%**	**1.03 [1.01, 1.06]**
Total events	430		417			

Heterogeneity: Chi² = 13.88, df = 12 (P = 0.31); I² = 14%
Test for overall effect: Z = 2.45 (P = 0.01)

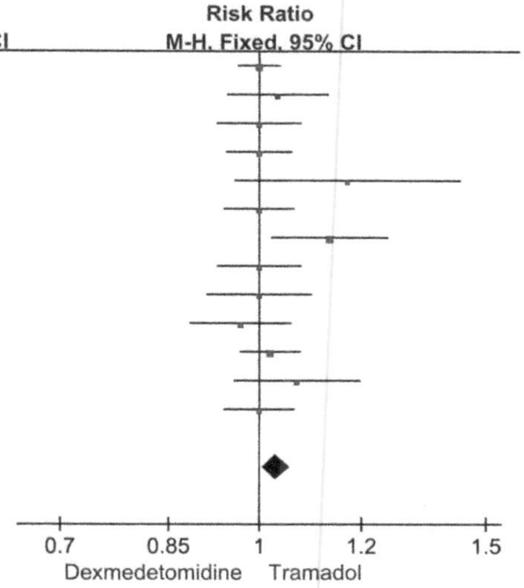

Fig. 3 Forest plot for effective rate of shivering. Abbreviations: CI, confidence interval; M-H, Mantel-Haenszel

Effective rate

All eligible RCTs reported the effective rate of shivering control [9–21]. The value of $I^2 = 0\%$ indicated no heterogeneity among the included studies. Dexmedetomidine had higher effective rate of shivering control than tramadol (RR =1.03; 95% CI [1.01, 1.06], $P = 0.01$, $I^2 = 14\%$). (Fig. 3).

Time to cease shivering

Twelve included RCTs compared time to cease shivering of dexmedetomidine and tramadol [9–16, 18–21]. The random effect model was utilized, because a high heterogeneity was detected ($I^2 = 98\%$). The result showed that dexmedetomidine was associated with shorter time to cease shivering than tramadol (MD = -2.14; 95%CI [−2.79, −1.49], $P < 0.00001$, $I^2 = 98\%$). (Fig. 4) Sensitivity analysis was performed for time to cease shivering by excluding single study sequentially, but no source of heterogeneity was detected.

Recurrent rate of shivering

There were 12 studies reporting the recurrent rate of shivering [9–20]. The value of $I^2 = 0\%$ indicated no heterogeneity. The result of this study indicated that the recurrent rate of shivering of tramadol was significantly higher than that of dexmedetomidine (RR = 0.45; 95%CI [0.27, 0.73], $P = 0.001$, $I^2 = 0\%$). (Fig. 5).

Nausea and vomiting

Ten papers recorded nausea, [9–13, 15, 18–21] and 10 recorded vomiting [9–13, 15, 16, 18–20]. Four out of

Study or Subgroup	Dexmedetomidine Mean	Dexmedetomidine SD	Dexmedetomidine Total	Tramadol Mean	Tramadol SD	Tramadol Total	Weight	Mean Difference IV, Random, 95% CI
Kundra 2017	2.9	0.24	50	4.62	0.39	50	9.5%	-1.72 [-1.85, -1.59]
Venkatraman 2016	5.7	0.79	30	6.76	0.93	30	9.2%	-1.06 [-1.50, -0.62]
Mittal 2014	2.52	0.44	25	5.92	0.81	25	9.3%	-3.40 [-3.76, -3.04]
Keerthi 2017	3.12	0.9	32	5.03	1.15	32	9.0%	-1.91 [-2.42, -1.40]
Fern 2015	7.3	3.8	20	5.9	2.1	20	5.3%	1.40 [-0.50, 3.30]
Ramesh2019	2.87	0.27	30	4.62	0.41	30	9.5%	-1.75 [-1.93, -1.57]
Verma2018	2.95	1.18	60	7.15	1.77	60	9.0%	-4.20 [-4.74, -3.66]
Prasad2018	3.8	1.12	25	5.12	1.27	25	8.7%	-1.32 [-1.98, -0.66]
Verma2016	1.54	0.53	30	1.89	0.53	30	9.4%	-0.35 [-0.62, -0.08]
Singla2017	8.74	5.54	50	14.08	11.83	50	2.4%	-5.34 [-8.96, -1.72]
Singh2016	2.48	0.36	30	5.93	0.54	30	9.4%	-3.45 [-3.68, -3.22]
Aasim2016	2.5	0.44	30	5.96	0.81	30	9.3%	-3.46 [-3.79, -3.13]
Total (95% CI)			**412**			**412**	**100.0%**	**-2.14 [-2.79, -1.49]**

Heterogeneity: Tau² = 1.15; Chi² = 556.02, df = 11 (P < 0.00001); I² = 98%
Test for overall effect: Z = 6.47 (P < 0.00001)

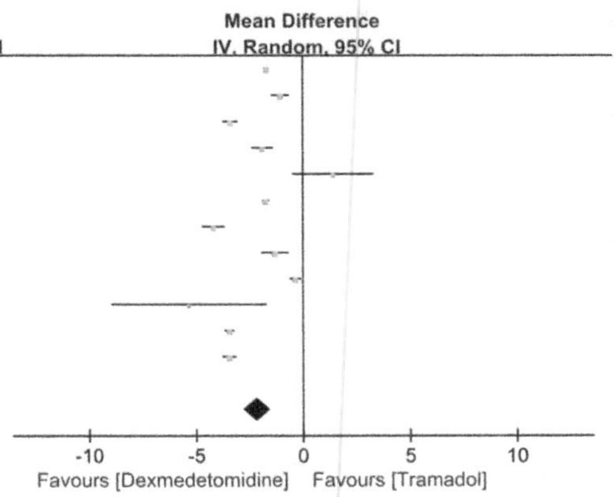

Fig. 4 Forest plot for time to cease shivering in minutes. Abbreviations: SD, standard deviation; CI, confidence interval; IV, inverse variance

Study or Subgroup	Dexmedetomidine Events	Dexmedetomidine Total	Tramadol Events	Tramadol Total	Weight	Risk Ratio M-H, Fixed, 95% CI
Kundra 2017	3	50	8	50	17.0%	0.38 [0.11, 1.33]
Venkatraman 2016	1	30	7	30	14.9%	0.14 [0.02, 1.09]
Mittal 2014	1	25	2	25	4.3%	0.50 [0.05, 5.17]
Keerthi 2017	0	32	3	32	7.4%	0.14 [0.01, 2.66]
Ramesh2019	2	30	5	30	10.6%	0.40 [0.08, 1.90]
Verma2018	3	60	5	60	10.6%	0.60 [0.15, 2.40]
Prasad2018	2	25	4	25	8.5%	0.50 [0.10, 2.49]
Kumar2016	2	20	4	20	8.5%	0.50 [0.10, 2.43]
Verma2016	3	30	0	30	1.1%	7.00 [0.38, 129.93]
Singla2017	0	50	1	50	3.2%	0.33 [0.01, 7.99]
Singh2016	0	30	3	30	7.4%	0.14 [0.01, 2.65]
Aasim2016	2	30	3	30	6.4%	0.67 [0.12, 3.71]
Total (95% CI)		**412**		**412**	**100.0%**	**0.45 [0.27, 0.73]**
Total events	19		45			

Heterogeneity: Chi² = 6.34, df = 11 (P = 0.85); I² = 0%

Test for overall effect: Z = 3.19 (P = 0.001)

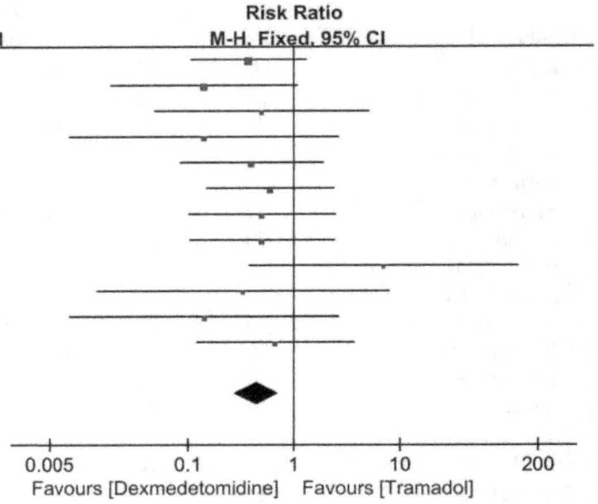

Fig. 5 Forest plot comparing recurrent rate of shivering. Abbreviations: CI, confidence interval; M-H, Mantel-Haenszel

332 patients receiving dexmedetomidine experienced nausea, and 80 out of 332 patients receiving tramadol experienced nausea. There were 342 patients receiving dexmedetomidine (1 with vomiting) and 342 patients receiving tramadol (41 with vomiting). Dexmedetomidine had lower incidences of nausea and vomiting than tramadol (Nausea: RR = 0.10; 95%CI [0.05, 0.19], $P < 0.00001$, $I^2 = 48\%$; Vomiting: RR = 0.13; 95% CI [0.06, 0.30], $P < 0.00001$, $I^2 = 0\%$). (Figs. 6 and 7).

Hypotension and bradycardia

The incidences of hypotension and bradycardia were recorded in all of the included RCTs, but one [13]. There were 402 patients receiving dexmedetomidine (24 experienced hypotension and 19 had bradycardia) and 402 patients receiving tramadol (9 experienced hypotension and 2 had bradycardia).

Dexmedetomidine was associated with higher incidence of hypotension (RR = 2.50; 95%CI [1.24, 5.03], $P = 0.01$, $I^2 = 0\%$), and bradycardia (RR = 4.78; 95%CI [1.76, 13.00], $P = 0.002$, $I^2 = 0\%$). (Figs. 8 and 9).

Sedation

Ten studies reported the incidence of sedation which we defined as being drowsy and responding to verbal or physical stimuli [9–16, 19, 20]. The value of $I^2 = 82\%$ indicated high heterogeneity. The incidence of sedation of dexmedetomidine was significantly higher than that of tramadol (RR = 2.48; 95%CI [1.32, 4.65], $P = 0.005$, $I^2 = 82\%$). (Fig. 10).

Sensitivity analysis was performed for the incidence of sedation by excluding single study sequentially, but no source of high heterogeneity was detected. There were no patients with over sedation reported in the included

Study or Subgroup	Dexmedetomidine Events	Dexmedetomidine Total	Tramadol Events	Tramadol Total	Weight	Risk Ratio M-H, Fixed, 95% CI
Kundra 2017	0	50	14	50	17.3%	0.03 [0.00, 0.56]
Mittal 2014	0	25	7	25	8.9%	0.07 [0.00, 1.11]
Keerthi 2017	0	32	10	32	12.5%	0.05 [0.00, 0.78]
Fern 2015	0	20	0	20		Not estimable
Ramesh2019	0	30	8	30	10.1%	0.06 [0.00, 0.98]
Verma2018	0	60	15	60	18.5%	0.03 [0.00, 0.53]
Prasad2018	0	25	4	25	5.4%	0.11 [0.01, 1.96]
Verma2016	4	30	3	30	3.6%	1.33 [0.33, 5.45]
Singh2016	0	30	11	30	13.7%	0.04 [0.00, 0.71]
Aasim2016	0	30	8	30	10.1%	0.06 [0.00, 0.98]
Total (95% CI)		**332**		**332**	**100.0%**	**0.10 [0.05, 0.19]**
Total events	4		80			

Heterogeneity: Chi² = 15.40, df = 8 (P = 0.05); I² = 48%

Test for overall effect: Z = 6.46 (P < 0.00001)

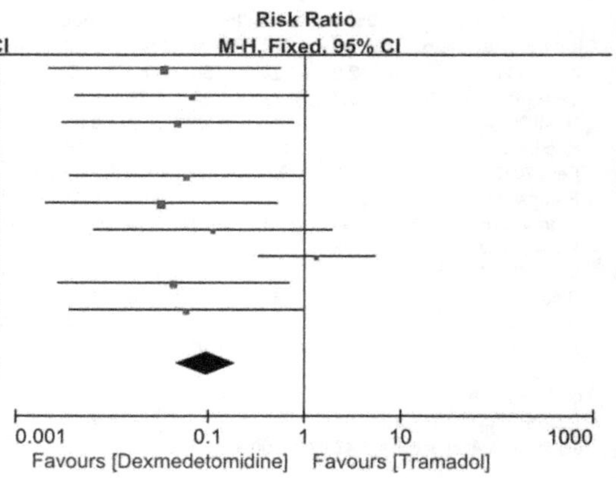

Fig. 6 Forest plot comparing the incidence of nausea. Abbreviations: CI, confidence interval; M-H, Mantel-Haenszel

Study or Subgroup	Dexmedetomidine Events	Dexmedetomidine Total	Tramadol Events	Tramadol Total	Weight	Risk Ratio M-H, Fixed, 95% CI
Kundra 2017	0	50	4	50	9.8%	0.11 [0.01, 2.01]
Venkatraman 2016	0	30	4	30	9.8%	0.11 [0.01, 1.98]
Mittal 2014	0	25	5	25	12.0%	0.09 [0.01, 1.56]
Keerthi 2017	0	32	1	32	3.3%	0.33 [0.01, 7.89]
Ramesh2019	0	30	2	30	5.4%	0.20 [0.01, 4.00]
Verma2018	0	60	8	60	18.5%	0.06 [0.00, 1.00]
Prasad2018	0	25	3	25	7.6%	0.14 [0.01, 2.63]
Verma2016	1	30	0	30	1.1%	3.00 [0.13, 70.83]
Singh2016	0	30	8	30	18.5%	0.06 [0.00, 0.98]
Aasim2016	0	30	6	30	14.1%	0.08 [0.00, 1.31]
Total (95% CI)		**342**		**342**	**100.0%**	**0.13 [0.06, 0.30]**
Total events	1		41			

Heterogeneity: Chi² = 5.03, df = 9 (P = 0.83); I² = 0%

Test for overall effect: Z = 4.76 (P < 0.00001)

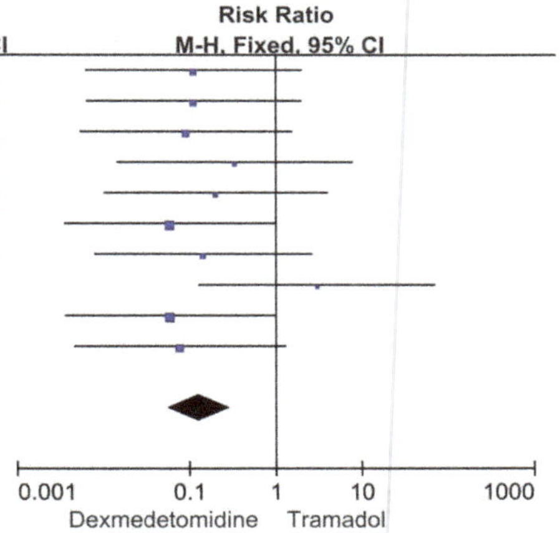

Fig. 7 Forest plot comparing the incidence of vomiting. Abbreviations: CI, confidence interval; M-H, Mantel-Haenszel

studies. Over sedation was defined as no response to physical stimuli.

Publication bias

Figure 11 showed that no publication bias was detected for recurrent rate of shivering.

Discussion

In this meta-analysis, we compare the efficacy of intravenous dexmedetomidine and tramadol on the treatment of shivering after spinal anesthesia in adult patients. Dexmedetomidine is associated with higher effective rate of shivering control, shorter time to cease shivering, lesser recurrence of shivering, lower incidences of nausea and vomiting, higher incidences of hypotension, bradycardia and sedation than tramadol.

In this meta-analysis, dexmedetomidine has shorter time to cease shivering and a higher incidence of sedation than tramadol. But these outcomes have high heterogeneities, which are possibly associated with the following: 1) Inclusion criteria for shivering degree are different among the included studies, shivering degrees of 2 to 4 are included in 4 RCTs [14, 16, 18, 19] and shivering degrees of 3 or 4 in the other 9 RCTs [9–13, 15, 17, 20, 21]. 2) The types and doses of local anesthetics for spinal anesthesia are different among the studies; 3) The types and duration of the surgeries are different.

In this study, tramadol is associated with significantly higher incidences of nausea and vomiting than dexmedetomidine. Nausea and vomiting is very distressing for the patient. Moreover, vomiting may cause rare but

Study or Subgroup	Dexmedetomidine Events	Dexmedetomidine Total	Tramadol Events	Tramadol Total	Weight	Risk Ratio M-H, Fixed, 95% CI
Kundra 2017	0	50	0	50		Not estimable
Venkatraman 2016	6	30	2	30	20.0%	3.00 [0.66, 13.69]
Mittal 2014	0	25	0	25		Not estimable
Keerthi 2017	3	32	0	32	5.0%	7.00 [0.38, 130.26]
Fern 2015	5	20	2	20	20.0%	2.50 [0.55, 11.41]
Verma2018	3	60	0	60	5.0%	7.00 [0.37, 132.66]
Prasad2018	0	25	0	25		Not estimable
Kumar2016	0	20	0	20		Not estimable
Verma2016	6	30	3	30	30.0%	2.00 [0.55, 7.27]
Singla2017	1	50	2	50	20.0%	0.50 [0.05, 5.34]
Singh2016	0	30	0	30		Not estimable
Aasim2016	0	30	0	30		Not estimable
Total (95% CI)		**402**		**402**	**100.0%**	**2.50 [1.24, 5.03]**
Total events	24		9			

Heterogeneity: Chi² = 2.89, df = 5 (P = 0.72); I² = 0%

Test for overall effect: Z = 2.57 (P = 0.01)

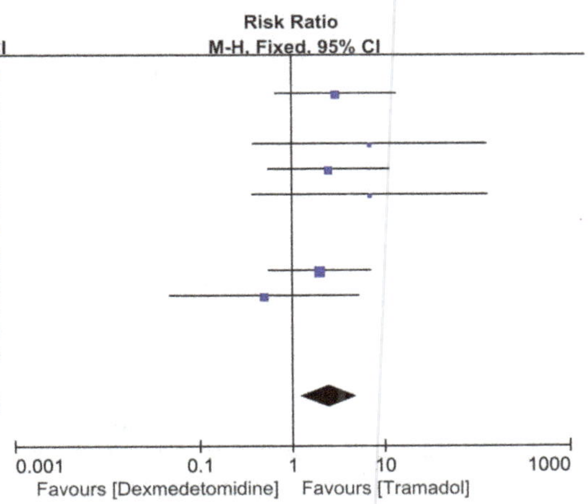

Fig. 8 Forest plot comparing the incidence of hypotension. Abbreviations: CI, confidence interval; M-H, Mantel-Haenszel

Study or Subgroup	Dexmedetomidine Events	Dexmedetomidine Total	Tramadol Events	Tramadol Total	Weight	Risk Ratio M-H, Fixed, 95% CI
Kundra 2017	1	50	0	50	11.1%	3.00 [0.13, 71.92]
Venkatraman 2016	1	30	0	30	11.1%	3.00 [0.13, 70.83]
Mittal 2014	0	25	0	25		Not estimable
Keerthi 2017	5	32	0	32	11.1%	11.00 [0.63, 191.04]
Fern 2015	4	20	0	20	11.1%	9.00 [0.52, 156.91]
Verma2018	3	60	0	60	11.1%	7.00 [0.37, 132.66]
Prasad2018	0	25	0	25		Not estimable
Kumar2016	0	20	0	20		Not estimable
Verma2016	2	30	1	30	22.2%	2.00 [0.19, 20.90]
Singla2017	3	50	1	50	22.2%	3.00 [0.32, 27.87]
Singh2016	0	30	0	30		Not estimable
Aasim2016	0	30	0	30		Not estimable
Total (95% CI)		**402**		**402**	**100.0%**	**4.78 [1.76, 13.00]**
Total events	19		2			

Heterogeneity: $Chi^2 = 1.44$, $df = 6$ ($P = 0.96$); $I^2 = 0\%$

Test for overall effect: $Z = 3.06$ ($P = 0.002$)

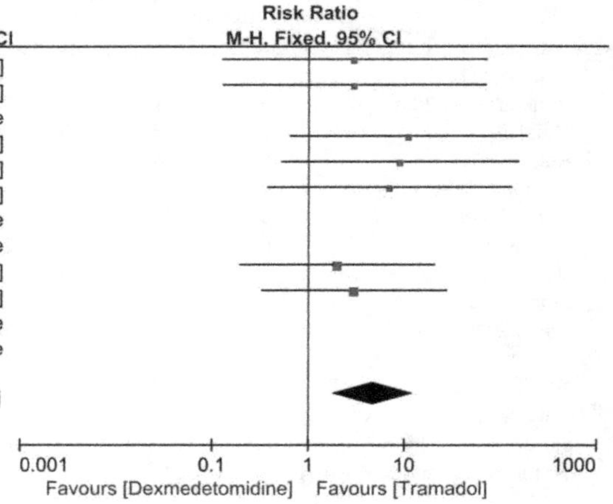

Fig. 9 Forest plot comparing the incidence of bradycardia. Abbreviations: CI, confidence interval; M-H, Mantel-Haenszel

serious consequences, such as aspiration, esophageal rupture, subcutaneous emphysema or pneumothorax [22]. However, dexmedetomidine has significantly higher incidences of hypotension and bradycardia compared to tramadol. Dexmedetomidine has an inherent property of postsynaptic activation of alpha 2-adrenoceptors in the central nervous system to decrease heart rate and blood pressure. We can't assess the clinically significance of hypotension and bradycardia, because of lack of research data.

Tramadol is a well-established agent in treatment of shivering. The mechanism of anti-shivering action of tramadol may be its opioid or serotonergic and noradrenergic activity or both [23–25]. Dexmedetomidine, an alpha-2 adrenoceptor agonist, has antihypertensive, sedative, analgesic and anti-shivering properties [26]. The anti-shivering effects of alpha adrenoceptor agonists are mediated by binding to alpha receptors that mediate the vasoconstriction. In addition, it has hypothalamic thermoregulatory effects of reducing the vasoconstriction and shivering thresholds [27]. It suggests that dexmedetomidine acts on the central thermoregulatory system rather than preventing shivering peripherally [28]. The effect of dexmedetomidine on treatment of shivering has been confirmed in the previous studies [29–31]. Dexmedetomidine and tramadol are not only effective for shivering treatment, but also effective for shivering prevention [32–34].

The sedation achieved is better in patients receiving dexmedetomidine than patients receiving tramadol. None of patients experiencing over sedation or respiratory depression is reported in the included studies [9–21]. Since the surgery is done under spinal anesthesia, the sedation seen with dexmedetomidine is beneficial for the surgeon, anesthetist as well as the patient, because it provides comfort and amnesia to the patient, cardiorespiratory stability and good surgical conditions during

Study or Subgroup	Dexmedetomidine Events	Dexmedetomidine Total	Tramadol Events	Tramadol Total	Weight	Risk Ratio M-H, Random, 95% CI
Kundra 2017	50	50	0	50	3.9%	101.00 [6.40, 1593.11]
Venkatraman 2016	28	30	18	30	14.5%	1.56 [1.14, 2.12]
Mittal 2014	6	25	7	25	11.3%	0.86 [0.34, 2.19]
Keerthi 2017	22	32	1	32	6.2%	22.00 [3.15, 153.58]
Ramesh2019	5	30	2	30	7.8%	2.50 [0.53, 11.89]
Verma2018	47	60	14	60	13.9%	3.36 [2.08, 5.41]
Prasad2018	5	25	4	25	9.8%	1.25 [0.38, 4.12]
Singla2017	14	50	2	50	8.5%	7.00 [1.68, 29.22]
Singh2016	16	30	10	30	13.2%	1.60 [0.87, 2.94]
Aasim2016	6	30	6	30	10.9%	1.00 [0.36, 2.75]
Total (95% CI)		**362**		**362**	**100.0%**	**2.48 [1.32, 4.65]**
Total events	199		64			

Heterogeneity: $Tau^2 = 0.69$; $Chi^2 = 49.40$, $df = 9$ ($P < 0.00001$); $I^2 = 82\%$

Test for overall effect: $Z = 2.82$ ($P = 0.005$)

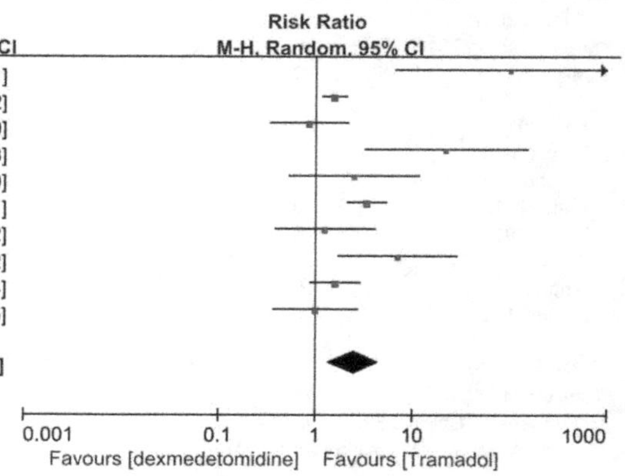

Fig. 10 Forest plot comparing the incidence of sedation. Abbreviations: CI, confidence interval; M-H, Mantel-Haenszel

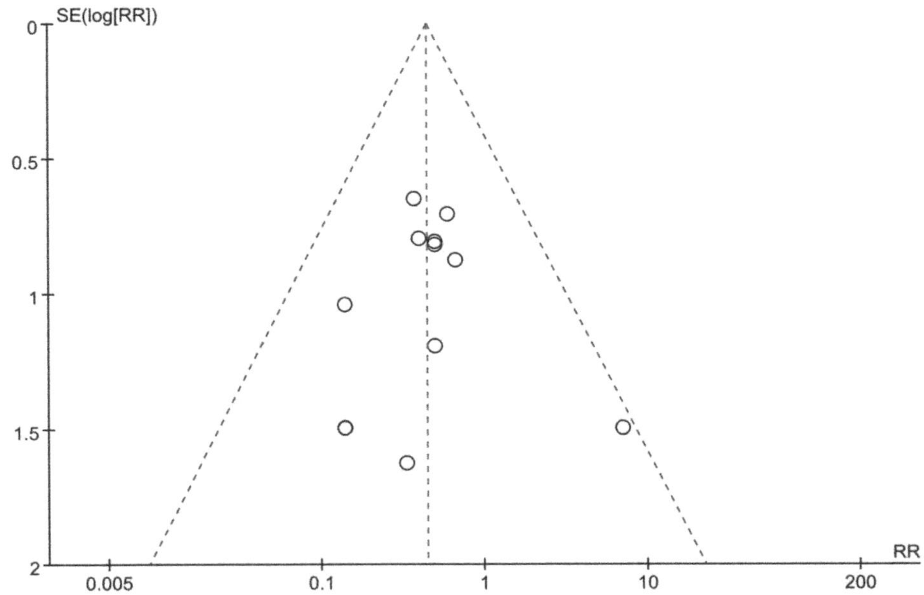

Fig. 11 Funnel plot of recurrent rate of shivering

surgery. Therefore, dexmedetomidine may be a good choice for shivering control after spinal anesthesia because of its dual effects of anti-shivering and sedation.

There are two limitations in this study. First of all, there is a high heterogeneity regarding time to cease shivering and the incidence of sedation. Secondly, intravenous dexmedetomidine causes hypotension and bradycardia, but we haven't analyzed whether it is clinically significant, due to lack of research data. Therefore, more RCTs are required for further study.

Conclusions

Dexmedetomidine is superior to tramadol for shivering treatment, due to higher effective rate of shivering control, earlier onset of action and lesser recurrence of shivering with higher incidence of sedation and lower incidences of nausea and vomiting. However, dexmedetomidine is also associated with higher incidences of hypotension and bradycardia than tramadol.

Abbreviations

MD: Mean difference; RR: Relative risk; CI: Confidence interval; RCT: Randomized controlled trials

Acknowledgements

Not applicable.

Authors' contributions

NW and JW conceived the study, participated in the design, collected the data, performed statistical analyses, and drafted the manuscript. NW, JW and ZW participated in the design, collected the data, and helped to draft the manuscript. ZW and JL helped to perform statistical analyses and to revise it critically for important intellectual content. All authors read and approved the final manuscript.

Author details

[1]Department of Urology, The First Hospital of Jilin University, No.1 Xinmin Street, Changchun, Jilin 130021, China. [2]Department of Taxation, School of Public Economics and Administration of Shanghai University of Finance and Economics, NO.777, Guoding Road, Yangpu District, Shanghai 200433, China. [3]Department of Anesthesiology, The First Hospital of Jilin University, No.1 Xinmin Street, Changchun, Jilin 130021, China.

References

1. Shukla U, Malhotra K, Prabhakar T. A comparative study of the effect of clonidine and tramadol on post-spinal anaesthesia shivering. Indian J Anaesth. 2011;55:242–6.
2. Alfonsi P. Postanaesthetic shivering. Epidemiology, pathophysiology and approaches to prevention and management. Minerva Anestesiol. 2003;69: 438–42.
3. Crowley LJ, Buggy DJ. Shivering and neuraxial anesthesia. Reg Anesth Pain Med. 2008;33:241–52.
4. Giesbrecht GG, Sessler DI, Mekjavić IB, Schroeder M, Bristow GK. Treatment of mild immersion hypothermia by direct body-to-body contact. J Appl Physiol. 1994;76:2373–9.
5. Ciofolo MJ, Clergue F, Devilliers C, Ben Ammar M, Viars P. Changes in ventilation, oxygen uptake, and carbon dioxide output during recovery from isoflurane anesthesia. Anesthesiology. 1989;70:737–41.
6. Blaine Easley R, Brady KM, Tobias JD. Dexmedetomidine for the treatment of postanesthesia shivering in children. Pediatric Anaesth. 2007;17:341–6.
7. Wrench IJ, Singh P, Dennis AR, Mahajan RP, Crossley AW. The minimum effective doses of pethidine and doxapram in the treatment of post-anaesthetic shivering. Anaesthesia. 1997;52:32–6.
8. Jadad AR, Moore RA, Carroll D, Jenkinson C, Reynolds DJ, Gavaghan DJ, et al. Assessing the quality of reports of randomized clinical trials: is blinding necessary? Control Clin Trials. 1996;17:1–12.
9. Kundra TS, Kuthiala G, Shrivastava A, Kaur P. A comparative study on the efficacy of dexmedetomidine and tramadol on post-spinal anesthesia shivering. Saudi J Anaesth. 2017;11:2–8.
10. Mittal G, Gupta K, Katyal S, Kaushal S. Randomised double-blind comparative study of dexmedetomidine and tramadol for post-spinal anaesthesia shivering. Indian J Anaesth. 2014;58:257–62.
11. Verma A, Bhandari D, Dhande P, Jain S, Tidke S. Comparative evaluation of dexmedetomidine and tramadol for attenuation of post-Spinal anaesthesia shivering. J Clin Diagn Res. 2018;12:UC01–4.

12. Prasad P. Comparison of tramadol and dexmedetomidine for treatment of shivering during spinal anaesthesia in caesarean section. J Evolution Med Dent Sci. 2019;7:5601–3.
13. Ramesh K, Bhushanam KN, Sharma BA, Kumar SSS. A clinical comparative study between intra venous dexmedetomidine and tramadol for control of post spinal anesthesia shivering. J Dent Med Sci. 2019;18:26–31.
14. Singla A, Chaudhari M, Patel A. Efficacy and safety of tramadol and dexmedetomidine in treatment of shivering following spinal anaesthesia: a randomized controlled study. J Med Sci Clin Res. 2017;5:20338–44.
15. Aasim SA, Reddy AS, Reddy V, reddy M, Chandrakanth C. Randomised double-blind comparative study of tramadol and dexmedetomidine for post-spinal anaesthesia shivering. J Chalmeda Anand Rao Institut Med Sci. 2016;11:18–21.
16. Venkatraman R, Karthik K, Pushparani A, Mahalakshmi A. A prospective, randomized, double-blinded control study on comparison of tramadol, clonidine and dexmedetomidine for post spinal anesthesia shivering. Rev Bras Anestesiol. 2016;68:42–8.
17. Kumar YD, Kumar TR, Sasi RK, Prachi P. A clinical comparative study of dexmedetomidine, clonidine and tramadol in post spinal shivering in lower limb and lower abdominal surgeries. J Dent Med Sci. 2016;15:50–4.
18. Verma NK, Kumar M. Comparison of clonidine, dexmedetomidine and tramadol for control of post spinal shivering: A randomized double blind clinical study. Int J Life Sci Scienti Res. 2016;2:658–64.
19. Keerthi P, Kamath SS. Comparative study of dexmedetomidine, butorphanol and tramadol for post-spinal anesthesia shivering. Res J Pharmaceutical Biological Chemical Sci. 2017;8:1801–9.
20. Singh A, Gupta KK, Solanki SL, Kumar M. A prospective randomized double blind comparative study of clonidine, dexmedtomidine and tramadol for treatment of shivering under spinal anaesthesia. Ind J Public Health Res Dev. 2016;7:114–9.
21. Fern L, Misiran K. Comparison of dexmedetomidine, pethidine and tramadol in the treatment of post-neuraxial anaesthesia shivering. South Afr J Anaesth Analg. 2015;21:21–6.
22. Apfel CC. Postoperative nausea and vomiting. Miller's Anaesthesia. 7th ed. New York: Churchill Livingstone; 2010.
23. Lee CR, McTavish D, Sorkin EM. Tramadol. A preliminary review of its pharmacodynamic and pharmacokinetic properties, and therapeutic potential in acute and chronic pain states. Drugs. 1993;46:313–40.
24. Mathews S, Al Mulla A, Varghese PK, Radim K, Mumtaz S. Postanaesthetic shivering-a new look at tramadol. Anaesthesia. 2002;57:394–8.
25. Tsai YC, Chu KS. A comparison of tramadol, amitriptyline, and meperidine for postepidural anesthetic shivering in parturients. Anesth Analg. 2001;93: 1288–92.
26. Grewal A. Dexmedetomidine: new avenues. J Anaesthesiol Clin Pharmacol. 2011;27:297–302.
27. Bajwa SJ, Bajwa SK, Kaur J, Singh G, Arora V, Gupta S, et al. Dexmedetomidine and clonidine in epidural anaesthesia: a comparative evaluation. Indian J Anaesth. 2011;55:116–21.
28. Talke P, Tayefeh F, Sessler DI, Jeffrey R, Noursalehi M, Richardson C. Dexmedetomidine does not alter the sweating threshold, but comparably and linearly decreases the vasoconstriction and shivering thresholds. Anesthesiology. 1997;87:835–41.
29. Bajwa SJ, Gupta S, Kaur J, Singh A, Parmar S. Reduction in the incidence of shivering with perioperative dexmedetomidine: a randomized prospective study. J Anaesthesiol Clin Pharmacol. 2012;28:86–91.
30. Usta B, Gozdemir M, Demircioglu RI, Muslu B, Sert H, Yaldiz A. Dexmedetomidine for the prevention of shivering during spinal anesthesia. Clinics (Sao Paulo). 2011;66:1187–91.
31. Moawad HES, Elawdy MM. Efficacy of intrathecal dexmedetomidine in prevention of shivering in patients undergoing transurethral prostatectomy: a randomized controlled trial. Egypt J Anaesth. 2015;31:178–81.
32. Ameta N, Jacob M, Hasnain S, Ramesh G. Comparison of prophylactic use of ketamine, tramadol, and dexmedetomidine for prevention of shivering after spinal anesthesia. J Anaesthesiol Clin Pharmacol. 2018;34:352–6.
33. Bozgeyik S, Mizrak A, Kılıç E, Yendi F, Ugur BK. The effects of preemptive tramadol and dexmedetomidine on shivering during arthroscopy. Saudi J Anaesth. 2014;8:238–43.
34. Singh S, Verma VK, Prasad C, Prakash J. Randomised double-blind comparative study of dexmedetomidine and tramadol for prevention of perioperative shivering in transurethral resection of prostate under spinal anaesthesia. J Evolution Med Dent. 2016;5:572–5.

6

Landmark-guided versus modified ultrasound-assisted paramedian techniques in combined spinal-epidural anesthesia for elderly patients with hip fractures

Bo Qu[1], Luying Chen[1], Yuling Zhang[1], Mengting Jiang[1], Caineng Wu[2], Wuhua Ma[2] and Yuhui Li[2*]

Abstract

Background: Combined spinal-epidural (CSE) anesthesia is considerably challenging for elderly patients with hip fractures due to spine degeneration and limitations in positioning. This study aimed to investigate the ability of a modified preprocedural ultrasound-guided technique to improve the success rate and efficacy of CSE anesthesia for elderly patients with hip fractures.

Methods: This prospective, single-blinded, parallel-group randomized controlled trial included 80 patients (aged ≥65 years) who were scheduled for elective hip fracture surgery with CSE anesthesia. Patients were randomly allocated into landmark group ($n = 40$) or the ultrasound group ($n = 40$). The primary outcome was first-pass success rate. Secondary outcomes included first-attempt success rate; number of needle insertion attempts; number of needle passes; locating, puncture, and total time; level of block; procedural adverse reactions and postoperative complications; and patient satisfaction score. Patients were blinded to group allocation.

Results: Eighty patients completed the study and were included in the final analysis. The first-pass success rates for the landmark and ultrasound groups were 20 and 70%, respectively ($P < 0.001$). The first-attempt success rates in the landmark and ultrasound groups were 42.5 and 85%, respectively ($P < 0.001$). The median number of attempts was lower in ultrasound-assisted group (1 [1, 1]) than landmark-guided group (2 [1, 2]), $P < 0.001$). The median number of needle passes was lower in ultrasound group (1 [1, 2]) than in landmark-guided group (3 [2, 4], $P < 0.001$). The locating time ($P < 0.001$) and total time ($P = 0.001$) were longer in the ultrasound group, while puncture time was shorter ($P = 0.003$). No significant difference was found regarding the incidence of adverse reactions and complications. More patients in the ultrasound group had a high satisfaction score of 4–5 ($P = 0.007$). Interestingly, subgroup analysis demonstrated benefits for ultrasound in patients with scoliosis.

(Continued on next page)

* Correspondence: liliuyuhui@126.com; liyuhui1531@gzucm.edu.cn
[2]Department of Anesthesiology, The First Affiliated Hospital of Guangzhou University of Chinese Medicine, Guangzhou 510405, Guangdong, China

(Continued from previous page)
Conclusions: Modified ultrasound-assisted CSE anesthesia increases first-pass and first-attempt success rates, and reduces needle insertion attempts, passes, and puncture time for elderly patients with hip fracture, especially those with scoliosis. This technique improves patient satisfaction and warrants consideration for application in clinical practice.
Keywords: Combined spinal-epidural anesthesia, Ultrasonography, Aged, Hip fractures

Background

Hip fracture is the second leading cause of hospitalization in the elderly population, its incidence is increasing with age [1–3]. Compared with general anesthesia, patients who receive combined spinal-epidural (CSE) anesthesia for hip surgery have a lower 30-day mortality [4, 5] and shorter hospital stays [1, 4, 6]. Traditional CSE anesthesia relied on the palpation of surface landmarks to identify the intervertebral levels; however, the possible occurrence of spine degeneration, supraspinous and interspinous ligament calcification, narrowing of intervertebral space, lumbar scoliosis, and deformities may make the identification of the intervertebral space unreliable and cause difficulties in needle insertion [7–10] In addition, the limitation in body positioning in patients with hip fracture may limit the opening of intervertebral space, and make the puncture challenging in traditional landmark-guided technique [11, 12].

The ultrasound-assisted CSE anesthesia technique provides improved precision and efficacy, overcoming the technical difficulties of performing neuraxial blocks [13–17] for obese [18, 19], obstetric [20–23], and aged patients [12, 24, 25], as well as patients with difficult-to-detect and abnormal anatomical surface landmarks [9, 26]. However, few studies have focused on ultrasound-assisted CSE anesthesia in elderly patients who have difficulty achieving optimal body positioning. The paramedian technique is the preferred choice of CSE anesthesia for the elderly. However, its success requires proper cephalad [27] and medial needle angulation [28]. Previous studies have determined the optimal needle insertion point and depth via ultrasonography; however, the ideal needle angulation has not been investigated to date [24, 29]. Furthermore, while the ultrasound-assisted central neuraxial block has been conventionally applied in spinal anesthesia with either a midline [22] or paramedian approach [24, 29, 30], and in CSE anesthesia with a midline approach [23], few studies have investigated the use of a paramedian approach in CSE anesthesia.

The current study aimed to investigate whether the ultrasound-assisted paramedian CSE anesthesia technique, modified with suggested needle insertion angulations and a more caudad needle insertion point, can contribute to an improved first pass success rate than conventional landmark-guided paramedian technique in elderly patients with hip fractures.

Methods

Study design and participants

This prospective, randomized controlled trial was approved by the hospital's Institutional Review Board (Ethics Committee of The First Affiliated Hospital of Guangzhou University of Chinese Medicine; Y [2019]042; February 11, 2019) and written informed consent was obtained from all patients participating in the trial. This study was registered prior to patient enrolment at the Chinese Clinical Trial Register (identifier, ChiCTR1900020819; principal investigator, Y.L.; date of registration, January 20, 2019). The trial was performed from February 2019 to September 2019 in The First Affiliated Hospital of Guangzhou University of Chinese Medicine, Guangzhou, China, and adhered to the applicable Consolidated Standards of Reporting Trials guidelines (Fig. 1).

A total of 80 patients were recruited. The inclusion criteria comprised (1) patients who were scheduled to receive CSE anesthesia for elective hip fracture surgery; (2) age ≥ 65 years; (3) body mass index (BMI) ≤ 30 kg/m^2; and (4) an American Society of Anesthesiologists (ASA) classification of I to III. Exclusion criteria are as follows (1) severe cardiopulmonary diseases; (2) a contraindication to CSE anesthesia (e.g., coagulopathy, hypovolemia, raised intracranial pressure, infection in puncture area, allergy to local anesthetics, or lack of cooperativity); and (3) a history of lumbar surgery.

Randomization

The patients were randomized (using a computer-generated randomized number table) to receive CSE anesthesia using either a landmark-guided technique ($n = 40$) or an ultrasound-assisted technique ($n = 40$). The allocation of patients was determined by sequentially numbered, sealed envelopes after the patients were moved into the operating room. During the procedure, patients were blinded to group allocation.

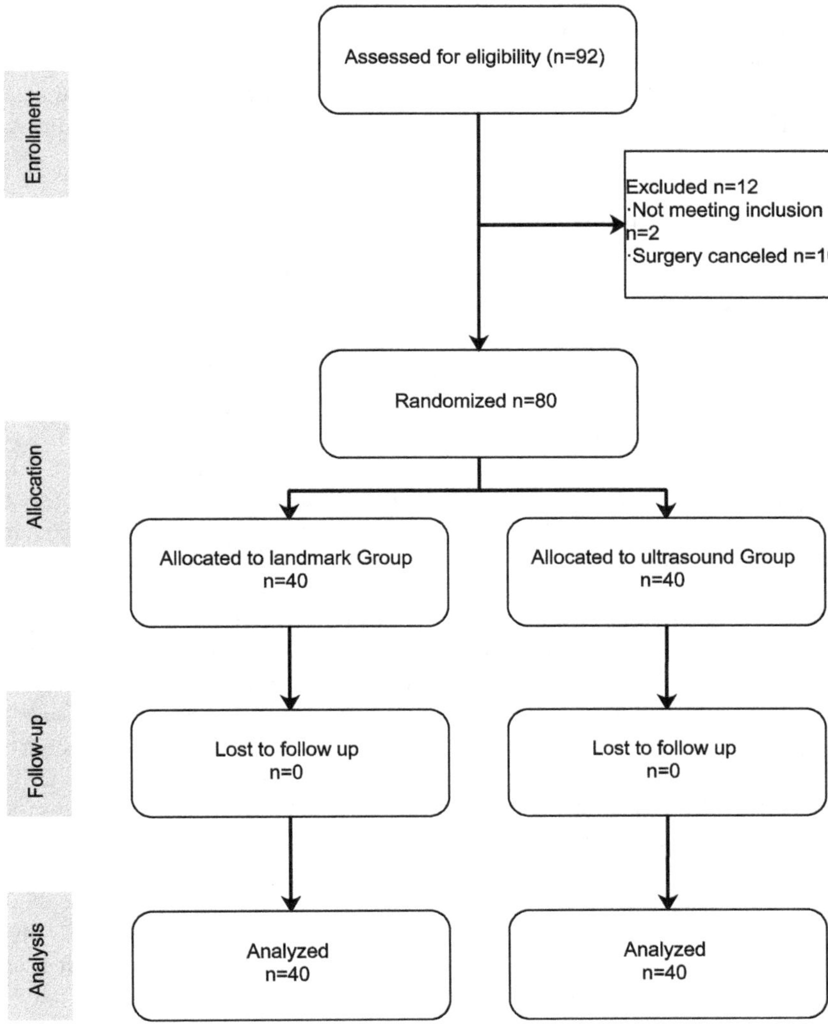

Fig. 1 Consolidated Standards of Reporting Trials diagram showing the progress of patients through the study

Procedures

Three anesthesiologists conducted the trial, and each had previously performed more than 40 ultrasound-assisted neuraxial blocks and ample experiences (> 15 years in average) in conducting CSE anesthesia. In the landmark group, ultrasound and CSE anesthesia were performed by distinct operators, while the whole procedure in the ultrasound group was performed by the same operator.

After the patients were moved to the operating room, routine monitoring (non-invasive blood pressure, 3-lead electrocardiogram, oximetry) and face mask oxygen at a flow rate of 1–2 L/min were applied, and peripheral intravenous access was established. During the whole procedure, no sedative was administered. An ultrasound-guided fascia iliaca compartment block was performed with 20 mL of 0.375% ropivacaine to reduce pain for all patients [31, 32]. After 15 min, the patient was assisted in assuming a lateral decubitus position with the fracture side up. In both groups, the anesthesiologists palpated the surface landmark and graded the ease of palpation using a 3-point scale (easy, moderate, and difficult) as described in a previous study [25].

For the landmark group, the procedure was done following these three steps:

- Identification of the needle insertion point. The needle insertion point was marked on the skin by traditional palpation. The first anesthetist subsequently left the operating room.
- Ultrasound scan. A portable ultrasound machine (Konica Minolta, SONIMAGE HS1, Japan) with a low frequency (2–5 MHz) curved array probe with a depth of 8 cm was used. Due to safety concerns, a second anesthesiologist conducted an ultrasound to check if the skin mark was above the L1-L2

interlaminar space; if so, the anesthetist was required to perform CSE anesthesia at a lower interlaminar space [23]. Ultrasound images were saved.

- Administration of CSE anesthesia. CSE anesthesia was performed by the first anesthesiologist, using the paramedian approach.

For the ultrasound group, the entire procedure was carried out using the following six steps:

- Marking of the midline. The probe was placed at the transverse midline (TM) plane for the evaluation of spine anatomy. The probe was tilted to obtain optimal ultrasound images. Midpoints of the long edge of the ultrasound probe were marked as the midline of the spine.
- Identification of the interlaminar space. The probe was placed at the parasagittal oblique (PSO) plane, 1–2 cm to the midline. The scan was performed upwards from the sacrum; the L5-S1 to L2-L3 interlaminar spaces were identified successively by the "counting-up" approach. The primary and secondary choice of interlaminar space for puncture were determined by the ultrasound image quality and the length of the anterior/posterior complex.
- Identification of the needle insertion point. The probe was adjusted to achieve the best ultrasound image at the determined interlaminar space. Then, the upper edge of the inferior laminar was placed at the center of the ultrasound screen. Skin marks were made at the midpoints of the long and short borders of the probe. The intersection of two connecting lines indicated the needle insertion point.
- Measurement of the suggested insertion angles. The built-in tool in the ultrasound unit was used to measure the maximum cephalad angle ($\angle\alpha$ in Fig. 2a) between (1) the connecting line from the insertion point to the far end of the posterior complex and (2) the midline of the ultrasound screen; 1/2 $\angle\alpha$ was the suggested cephalad angle. The probe's tilt to the median plane indicated the medial angle ($\angle\beta$), and was measured using a 180° protractor (Deli, Shanghai, China) (Fig. 2b).
- Measurement of the needle insertion depth. The distance from the insertion point to the posterior complex, which was the presumed minimum insertion depth, was measured using the ultrasound clipper tool (Fig. 2a).
- Administration of CSE anesthesia. CSE anesthesia was conducted using the paramedian technique according to the marked insertion point, suggested insertion angles, and presumed depth. After the needle reached the subcutaneous tissue and became stable, a low temperature plasma sterilized protractor (Deli, Shanghai, China) was used to correct the needle insertion angle (Fig. 2c). When the puncture was successful, the actual needle insertion angles (cephalad and medial) were measured (Fig. 2d).

In both groups, an aseptic technique was strictly applied throughout the entire process. CSE anesthesia was performed using a needle-through-needle approach, with a 25/16-gauge CSE kit (Kindao Interventional Medical Co., Ltd., Guangzhou, China). When the backflow of clear cerebrospinal fluid was observed, 0.5% ropivacaine (9.75–12.75 mg) was injected. Then, a 20-gauge multi-orifice epidural catheter (Kindao Interventional Medical Co., Ltd., Guangzhou, China) was inserted through the Touhy needle, up to 5 cm into the epidural space. If three attempts failed, the secondary interlaminar space was used. If attempts at two different interlaminar spaces failed, an alternative technique was allowed (palpation, ultrasound guidance, midline approach, another anesthetist). In the event that the alternative technique failed, general anesthesia was induced.

The patient satisfaction score was rated using a 5-point scale (from 1: completely dissatisfied to 5: completely satisfied) after anesthesia [23]. The block level was tested by loss of cold sensation, 15 min after anesthesia. The quality of the ultrasound image was assessed as good (the posterior complex and anterior complex were both visible), moderate (either the posterior complex or anterior complex was visible), or poor (neither the posterior nor anterior complex was visible) [24, 29, 33]. The discrepancy (Δ) between the suggested and actual angle was classified as accurate ($0° \le \Delta \le 5°$), acceptable ($5° < \Delta \le 10°$), or inaccurate ($\Delta > 10°$). During the entire procedure, data were recorded by a research assistant; for all measurements, the mean of three readings was calculated. A postoperative follow-up was conducted within 48 h after the surgery.

Study outcomes

The primary outcome in this study was the first-pass success rate of CSE anesthesia. A first-pass success was defined as the needle reaching the subarachnoid space within a single insertion attempt, without redirection.

Secondary outcomes were as follows:

- First-attempt success rate: defined as the needle reaching the subarachnoid space within a single insertion attempt and allowing redirection.
- Number of needle insertion attempts: each skin puncture was considered as a separate attempt.
- Number of needle passes: total number of insertion attempts and needle redirections.

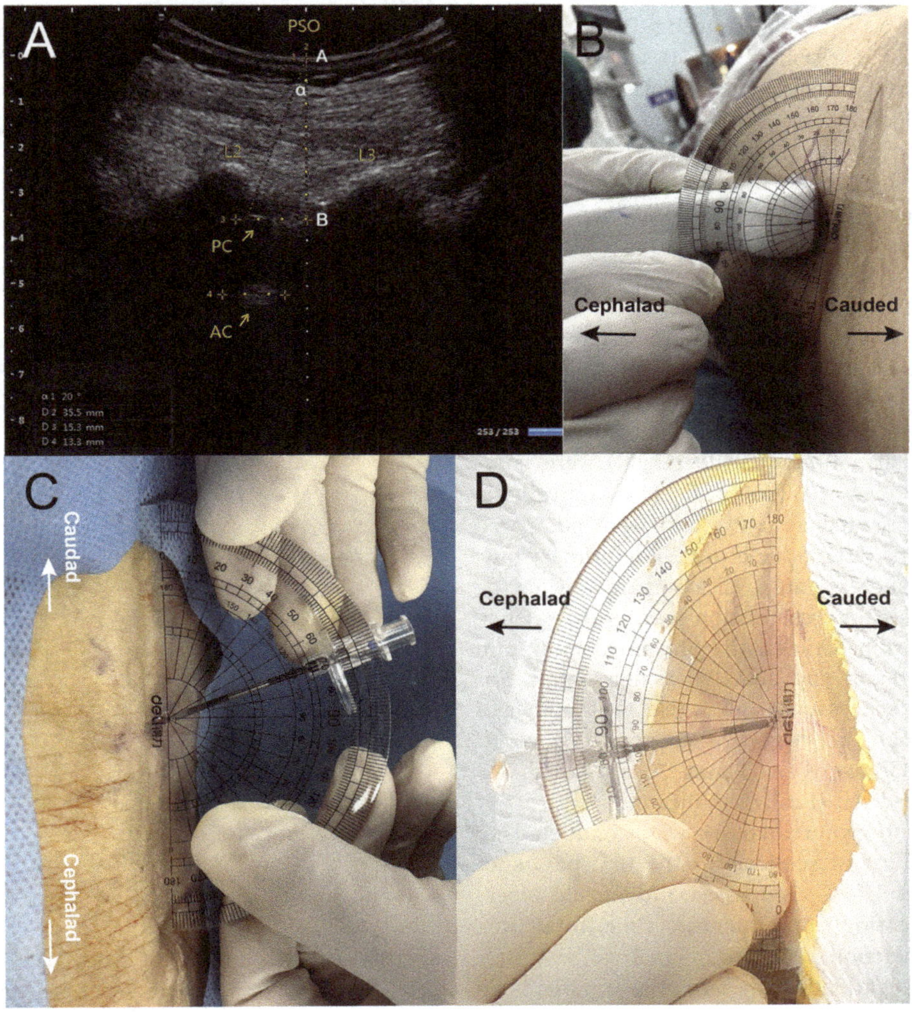

Fig. 2 Measurement and application of the needle angle. **a** An ultrasound image from the paramedian sagittal oblique (PSO) view, which shows the L2-L3 interlaminar space, posterior complex (PC), and anterior complex (AC). ∠α is the measured maximum cephalad angle of the needle. A to B is the distance from the skin to the posterior complex. **b** Measuring the medial angle with a 180° protractor during the paramedian approach, which is the tilting angle of the probe to the median plane. **c** An aseptic 180° protractor was used to assist the cephalad needle insertion angle. **d** After a successful puncture, the actual medial angle was measured with an aseptic 180° protractor

- Locating time: the time from when the operator touched the patient's skin to the marking of the insertion point on the skin (landmark group), and the time from when the probe was placed on the skin to the marking of the insertion point (ultrasound group).
- Puncture time: interval between the contact of the skin with the Touhy needle, and the observation of cerebrospinal fluid from the spinal needle.
- Total time: the sum of the locating time and puncture time.
- Level of block: measured by testing the loss of cold sensation.
- Procedural adverse reactions: radicular pain, bloody tap, unintentional dural puncture.
- Postoperative complications: including paresthesia, backache, and post-dural puncture headache.
- Patient satisfaction score: 1 (completely dissatisfied), 2 (dissatisfied), 3 (moderate), 4 (satisfied), 5 (completely satisfied). It was defined as the overall comfort level the patients experienced during the procedure, which includes (i) the back pain the patients felt, (ii) radicular pain the patient felt (iii) the discomfort due to the repositioning after a failed needle insertion and (iv) the overall anxiety or fear the patients felt. One negative response to these situations will deduct the satisfaction score by one point.

Statistical analysis

The sample size was calculated using PASS software Version 15.0 (NCSS, Kaysville, USA). Based on our pilot study, the first-pass success rates in patients using the conventional palpation and ultrasound-assisted technique were 22 and 59%, respectively. With an α error of 5% and a β error of 10% (90% power), a sample size of 35 patients per group was required. We increased the target sample size to 40 patients per group to allow for dropouts.

Data were analyzed using SPSS 25.0 (IBM Corporation, NY, USA). Continuous data were tested for normality using the Kolmogorov-Smirnov test. Normally distributed data (mean ± standard deviation [SD]) were compared using the Student's t-test. Non-normally distributed data (median [interquartile range]) were compared using the Mann-Whitney U test. Categorical variables were presented as n (%) and were compared using the $\chi2$ test or Fisher's exact test. The primary outcome (first-pass success rate) was compared using the $\chi2$ test. Spearman's rank correlation was used to determine the relationship between the presumed minimum needle insertion depth and actual insertion depth. For the differences in success rates for a selected number of passes and attempts between two groups, 95% confidence intervals (CI) were calculated. A two-tailed $P < 0.05$ was considered statistically significant.

Pre-specified sub-group analysis was conducted to investigate the effect of scoliosis to the first-pass success rate, number of needle passes and needle insertion attempts, locating time, puncture time, total time and patient satisfaction. Sub-group analysis was performed for all 12 patients with scoliosis, 6 patients in each group.

Table 1 Patient characteristics

	Landmark-guided group *n* = 40	Ultrasound-assisted group *n* = 40	*P*-value
Age (y)	82.3 ± 7.1	83.3 ± 6.7	0.549
Height (cm)	156.7 ± 7.0	156.9 ± 7.2	0.925
Weight (kg)	50.6 ± 8.4	53.2 ± 10.1	0.203
BMI (kg/m^2)	20.6 ± 3.0	21.6 ± 3.6	0.176
Sex (male/female)	7/33	10/30	0.412
ASA Classification			0.502
I	0 (0%)	0 (0%)	
II	22 (55%)	19 (47.5%)	
III	18 (45%)	21 (52.5%)	
Degree of back curvature			0.635[a]
Backward	4 (10%)	2 (5%)	
None	33 (82.5%)	36 (90%)	
Forward	3 (7.5%)	2 (5%)	
Scoliosis			1.000
Positive	6 (15%)	6 (15%)	
Negative	34 (85%)	34 (85%)	
Ease of landmark palpation			0.654[a]
Easy	34 (85%)	31 (77.5%)	
Moderate	5 (12.5%)	7 (17.5%)	
Difficult	1 (2.5%)	2 (5%)	

Data are presented as mean ± SD or n (%)

Abbreviations: BMI Body mass index, *SD* Standard deviation, *ASA* American Society of Anesthesiologists

[a]Fisher's exact test

Results

From February to September 2019, 92 elderly patients were recruited and assessed for eligibility. Eighty patients, aged 82.8 ± 6.8 years, were included for random allocation to the landmark ($n = 40$) or ultrasound ($n = 40$) group (Fig. 1). No data were missing, and no patients were lost to follow-up. The reasons for the 12 exclusions were that patients did not meet the inclusion criteria ($n = 2$), or surgery was canceled by the surgical department ($n = 10$).

There were no significant differences between the groups for baseline characteristics (Table 1). A significantly higher first-pass success rate (70% vs. 20%) and success rate within two passes (82.5% vs. 40%) were achieved in the ultrasound group vs. the landmark group (both $P < 0.001$; Table 2). The first attempt success rate in the ultrasound group was twice higher than that in the landmark group (85% vs. 42.5%, $P < 0.001$). However, no difference between the two groups was found for the success rate within two attempts ($P = 0.264$). A significantly lower median number of needle attempts and passes were achieved in the ultrasound group (both $P < 0.001$; Table 2).

Compared with the landmark group, the locating time was much longer while the puncture time was shorter in the ultrasound group. A longer total time for CSE anesthesia was required in the ultrasound group. More patients rated their satisfaction of the CSE anesthesia as 4 or 5 in the ultrasound group (90% vs. 65%, $P = 0.007$, Table 2).

Discrepancies between suggested and actual angles are presented in Table 3. In terms of the cephalad angle, the actual cephalad angle exceeded the measured maximum angle in five cases. A total of 70% cases reached the "accurate" level. For the medial angle, 80% cases reached the "accurate" level.

In all cases, the width of the posterior complex was 0.94 ± 0.22 cm, and that of the anterior complex was 1.24 ± 0.31 cm. The minimum needle insertion depth (measured through ultrasound imaging) had a certain correlation with the actual insertion depth ($r = 0.514$, $P < 0.001$).

Table 2 Comparison of procedure related data

	Landmark- guided group $n = 40$	Ultrasound- assisted group $n = 40$	*P* value	95% CI of differences (%)
First pass success, n (%)	8 (20)	28 (70)	< 0.001	(31.1 to 68.9)
Success within 2 passes, n (%)	16 (40)	33 (82.5)	< 0.001	(23.3 to 61.7)
First attempt success, n (%)	17 (42.5)	34 (85)	< 0.001	(23.6 to 61.4)
Success in 2 attempts, n (%)	34 (85)	38 (95)	0.264[a]	(−3 to 23)
Number of attempts	2 [1 to 2]	1 [1 to 1]	< 0.001	
Number of passes	3 [2 to 4]	1 [1 to 2]	< 0.001	
Locating time(s)	32.5 [21.3 to 40.8]	337.5 [300.0 to 403.8]	< 0.001	
Puncture time(s)	320.0 [223.3 to 583.0]	227.5 [170.0 to 340.0]	0.003	
Total time(s)	440.3 ± 240.1	608.2 ± 196.9	0.001	
Patients' satisfaction;4–5	26 (65.0%)	36 (90.0%)	0.007	(7.5 to 42.5)

Data are presented as mean ± SD, median [interquartile range] or n (%)
Abbreviations: SD standard deviation, *CI* confidence interval
[a]Continuity correction

A significant difference was found in the interspace level of the puncture between the two groups ($P = 0.036$; Table 4). The T8 or T10 dermatome level could be reached in all cases, and no significant difference was found between the two groups ($P = 0.251$; Table 4). In terms of procedural adverse reactions and postoperative complications, no significant differences were found between the groups. There were no occurrences of paresthesia, backache, or post-dural puncture headache. No patients were converted to general anesthesia in either group. In the landmark group, two patients were converted to alternative techniques, however, the difference was not significant between the two groups ($P = 0.494$, Table 5). In terms of the quality of the ultrasound images, more images of good quality were obtained in PSO views than in TM views (Additional Table 1).

A subgroup analysis was conducted for 12 patients with scoliosis (Table 6). The first-pass success rate was 83.8% in the ultrasound group, and 0% in the landmark group ($P = 0.015$). Fewer attempts ($P = 0.022$) and needle passes ($P = 0.016$) were achieved in the ultrasound group. The locating time was longer in the ultrasound group ($P = 0.004$), while the puncture time was shorter ($P = 0.043$). The total time ($P = 0.659$) and patient satisfaction score ($P = 0.061$) were not significantly different between the two groups.

Table 3 Angulation information obtained by ultrasonography

	Number of views
Comparison between actual and maximum cephalad angle	
actual angle ≤ maximum angle	35 (87.5%)
actual angle > maximum angle	5 (12.5%)
Cephalad angle discrepancy	
accurate 0° ≤ Δ[a] ≤ 5° n (%)	28 (70%)
acceptable 5° < Δ ≤ 10° n (%)	7 (17.5%)
inaccurate Δ > 10° n (%)	5 (12.5%)
Medial angle discrepancy	
accurate 0° ≤ Δ ≤ 5° n (%)	32 (80%)
acceptable 5° < Δ ≤ 10° n (%)	6 (15%)
inaccurate Δ > 10° n (%)	2 (25%)

[a]Δ indicates the discrepancy between the suggested and actual angles

Discussion

The current study shows that in comparison with the landmark-guided technique, the ultrasound-assisted technique had a higher first-pass and first-attempt success rate, fewer needle passes and insertion attempts, and a shorter puncture time; this improved the efficacy of CSE anesthesia, as well as patient satisfaction.

CSE anesthesia was applied to reduce the dose of local anesthetic in spinal anesthesia; this lowered the risk of unstable hemodynamic conditions among the elderly patients, who had a high prevalence of underlying diseases. Epidural cathetering was applied to ensure an adequate block level during the surgery, and maintenance of postoperative analgesia [34]. Ultrasound scan was conducted

Table 4 Interspinous level of successful puncture and block level

	Landmark- guided group $n = 40$	Ultrasound- assisted group $n = 40$	*P* value
Interspace level of successful puncture n (%)			0.036
L2/L3	10 (25%)	19 (47.5%)	
L3/L4	30 (75%)	21 (52.5%)	
Peak dermatome level n (%)			0.251
T8	13 (32.5%)	18 (45%)	
T10	27 (67.5%)	22 (55%)	

Data are presented as n (%)

Table 5 Procedural adverse reactions and postoperative complications

	Landmark group (*n* = 40)	Ultrasound group (*n* = 40)	*P* value[a]
Radicular pain	2 (5.0%)	2 (5.0%)	1
Bloody tap	3 (7.5%)	1 (2.5%)	0.615
Unintentional dural puncture	2 (5.0%)	1 (2.5%)	1
Backache	0 (0%)	0 (0%)	–
Post-dural puncture headache	0 (0%)	0 (0%)	–
Paresthesia	0 (0%)	0 (0%)	–
Alternative technique	2 (5.0%)	0 (0%)	0.494
Conversion to general anesthesia	0 (0%)	0 (0%)	–

Data are presented as n (%)
[a]Fisher's exact test

in all patients for three reasons. Firstly, it is for safety concern, even the occurrence of L1-L2 is very unlikely, this procedure can ensure the needle insertion point is below L1-L2, which is endorsed by A. Chin et al. [23]. Secondly, the ultrasound scan can provide more data for evaluation of the ultrasound image quality. Lastly, since the patients were blinded to the procedure, ultrasound scan in both groups could reduce the procedural difference which may influence the patients' satisfaction rating.

Compared with previous studies [24, 25], the subjects in the current study had a higher mean age and lower lumbar curvature ability; furthermore, patients with scoliosis were also included. Thus, puncture was relatively more difficult in the present study. Additionally, although total duration of the procedure was significantly longer in the ultrasound group, more time was used in ultrasound scan which will not discomfort the patients. In landmark-guided group, more time was used for puncture or repositioning, which may reduce the patients' satisfaction. Overall, we believe at the sacrifice of certain effectiveness for a better patients' satisfaction is worthwhile.

The higher first-pass success rate in the ultrasound group can be attributed to several modifications to previous ultrasound-assisted technique. First, accurately measured personalized insertion angles provided a better needle trajectory. Then the anesthesiologist used an aseptic protractor to guide the puncture. Previous studies have suggested 10–15° medial and cephalad angles during the puncture [28]. However, in practice, these angulations are estimated based on personal judgment. The results (Table 3) showed that for most cases (70%), the actual cephalad angle discrepancies were within 5°. Indeed, the first pass was also achieved in these cases. For the medial angle, 80% of the cases showed a discrepancy within 5°. These results demonstrated that the suggested angles could provide reasonable guidance. Second, for elderly patients with hip fractures, limitations associated with patient positioning may have led to a narrow interlaminar space. The current study placed the upper edge of the inferior lamina at the center of the screen to obtain a lower needle insertion point and a larger cephalad angle, resulting in a wider operating space for the puncture (Fig. 3). Previous studies have often placed the posterior and anterior complex at the center of the screen, and identified the needle insertion point by skin-marking the midpoint of the probe at that time [24, 29], thereby resulting in a relatively limited operating space (Fig. 3). Similar studies involving elderly patients also indicated that the first-pass success rate in the ultrasound group was higher than that reported in a study conducted by Park et al. [24], and a higher first-attempt rate was achieved compared with that reported in a study conducted by Geng et al. [25]. These favorable results could also be contributed by the modifications to the previous ultrasound-assisted technique.

In the current study, a successful first pass was not always accomplished. In most circumstances, this was because of bony contact, most frequently with the inferior laminar. Therefore, needle redirection and more needle passes were needed for a successful puncture. In five cases, the actual cephalad angle exceeded the maximum

Table 6 Subgroup analysis for patients with scoliosis

	Landmark- guided group *n* = 6	Ultrasound- assisted group *n* = 6	*P* value	95% CI of differences (%)
First pass success, n (%)	0 (0.0%)	5 (83.3%)	0.015[a]	(71.7, 94.9)
Number of attempts	2 [1 to 5]	1 [1 to 1]	0.022	
Number of passes	3.5 [2.75 to 12.5]	1 [1 to 1.75]	0.016	
Locating time(s)	40.0 [33.75 to 45.75]	405.0 [256.75 to 466.25]	0.004	
Puncture Time(s)	535.33 ± 185.24	272.50 ± 206.80	0.043	
Total time(s)	576.33 ± 180.21	641.17 ± 298.78	0.659	
Satisfaction; 4–5	2 (33.3%)	6 (100.0%)	0.061[a]	(52.1, 81.3)

Data are presented as mean ± SD, median [interquartile range] or n (%)
Abbreviations: SD standard deviation, *CI* confidence interval
[a]Fisher's exact test

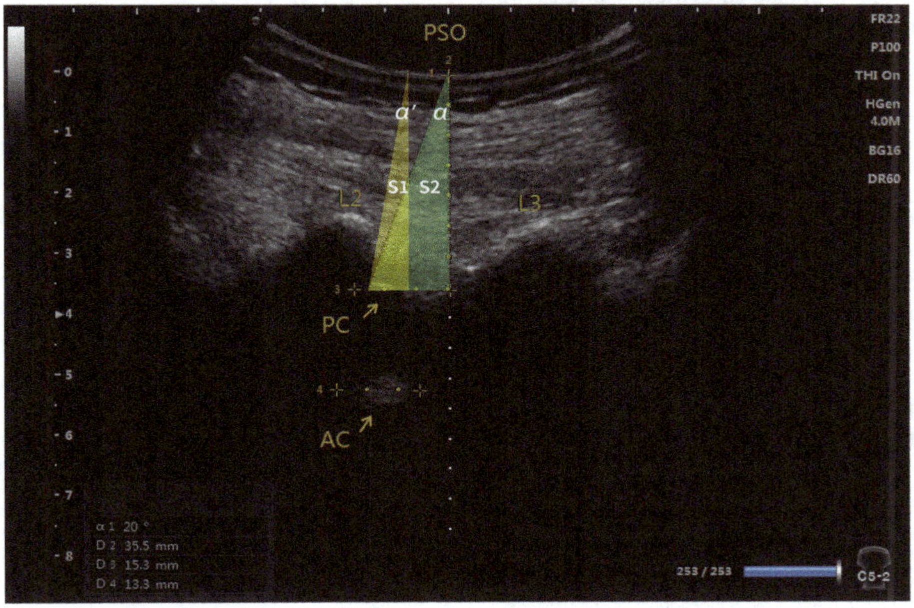

Fig. 3 Comparison of operating spaces. The ultrasound image shows the L2-L3 interlaminar space in the parasagittal oblique (PSO) view. The posterior complex (PC) and anterior complex (AC) are shown at the same time. The modified preprocedural ultrasound-guided technique placed the upper edge of the inferior laminar at the center of the ultrasound screen and suggested a lower needle insertion point, which provided a larger cephalad angle (∠α), and a wider operation space (S2) than the previous technique which placed the PC and AC at the center of the screen (∠α' and S1)

suggested angle (∠α) measured by the ultrasound image; this may have been explained by the deviation of the insertion point. If the marked needle insertion point was lower than the ideal point, the needle encountered the inferior laminar, and a larger cephalad angle was needed.

There is a difference in successful puncture interspace level between two groups. More patients achieved successful puncture at L2-L3 in landmark-guided group while L3-L4 in ultrasound-assisted group. The possible explanation is: in landmark-guided group, the anesthesiologist may not be absolutely sure about the identification of the intervertebral space. For safety concern, the anesthesiologist may intentionally choose a lower intervertebral space for needle insertion, resulted in a large proportion of L3-L4 level. In this case, the choice of the anesthesiologist is purely based on personal experiences and preferences. In the ultrasound-assisted group, the intervertebral space was identified by ultrasound scan, which is relatively more accurate. The ultrasound image indicated the L2-L3 level had better quality and were more suitable for needle insertion. In this case, this is not a choice but rather a more precise point derived from imaging results. When ultrasound scan showed the L3-L4 level had same image quality with L2-L3, the anesthesiologist would prefer L2-L3 for insertion according to surgery requirement.

Some procedural adverse reactions were observed in current study. Unintentional dural puncture occurred in three cases, possibly because the degenerative disc disease, ligament calcification, and stenosis of the spinal canal in elderly patients made it difficult to identify the tissue layer and control the force to perform the procedure [35]. Two cases in the landmark group required the use of alternative techniques, indicating that the variability of performance in the landmark group was relatively large compared with the ultrasound group. The differences in adverse reactions and postoperative complications were not statistically significant between the two groups. This might be attributed to the fact that the anesthesiologists in this study have ample experiences (> 15 years in average) in conducting CSE anesthesia.

Sub-group analysis for patients with scoliosis indicated that the modified ultrasound-assisted technique showed superiority in improving the first-pass success rate, reducing needle passes and attempts. The difference in total time was not statistically significant but longer time was consumed for puncture in the landmark-guided group which is invasive. In spite of patient satisfaction score was not statistically significant different in sub-group, which can be possibly explained by the limited number of cased for analysis, all patients in the ultrasound-assisted group scored 4–5.

However, we do acknowledge the limitations of this study. First, due to the nature of the study design, only the patients were blinded during the CSE anesthesia procedure. Second, measurement error was inevitable, even though the suggested cephalad and medial angles were measured by the same operator. Finally, in some cases, inaccuracy in the needle insertion point was unavoidable, as elderly patients often have loose and mobile skin.

Conclusion

In conclusion, the modified preprocedural ultrasound-assisted CSE anesthesia technique with suggested needle insertion angulations and a more caudad needle insertion point can increase the first-pass and first-attempt success rate, reduce the puncture time and elevate patients' satisfaction in elderly patients with hip fractures, especially in patients with scoliosis. We believe that it has clinical benefits for elderly patients with hip fractures.

Abbreviations

AC: Anterior complex; ASA: American Society of Anesthesiologists; BMI: Body Mass Index; CI: Confidence Interval; CSE: Combined spinal-epidural; PC: Posterior complex; PSO: Paramedian sagittal oblique; SD: Standard deviation; TM: Transverse midline

Acknowledgements

The authors thank the patients who participated in the study and Dr. Xiaohui Zheng (Department of Orthopedics, The First Affiliated Hospital of Guangzhou University of Chinese Medicine, Guangzhou City, Guangdong, China) for their help and support. Special thanks are also extended to Dr. Phei Er Saw and Dr. Zhengyuan Xia for their assistance in finalizing this manuscript. This work was supported by the Guangdong Medical Research Foundation (A2020221).

Authors' contributions

WM and YL designed the study and conducted the trial. BQ designed the study, analyzed the data, and wrote the manuscript. LC, YZ, and MJ collected and analyzed the data. CW conducted the trial and wrote the manuscript. All authors have read and approved the manuscript.

Author details

[1]Guangzhou University of Chinese Medicine, Guangzhou 510405, Guangdong, China. [2]Department of Anesthesiology, The First Affiliated Hospital of Guangzhou University of Chinese Medicine, Guangzhou 510405, Guangdong, China.

References

1. Chu CC, Weng SF, Chen KT, Chien CC, Shieh JP, Chen JY, Wang JJ. Propensity score-matched comparison of postoperative adverse outcomes between geriatric patients given a general or a Neuraxial anesthetic for hip surgery: a population-based study. Anesthesiology. 2015;123(1):136–47.
2. Kannus P, Parkkari J, Sievanen H, Heinonen A, Vuori I, Jarvinen M. Epidemiology of hip fractures. Bone. 1996;18(1 Suppl):57S–63S.
3. Holloway KL, Sajjad MA, Mohebbi M, Kotowicz MA, Livingston PM, Khasraw M, Hakkennes S, Dunning TL, Brumby S, Page RS, et al. The epidemiology of hip fractures across western Victoria, Australia. Bone. 2018;108:1–9.
4. Perlas A, Chan VW, Beattie S. Anesthesia technique and mortality after Total hip or knee Arthroplasty: a retrospective, Propensity Score-matched Cohort Study. Anesthesiology. 2016;125(4):724–31.
5. Mclsaac DI, Wijeysundera DN, Huang A, Bryson GL, van Walraven C. Association of Hospital-level Neuraxial Anesthesia use for hip fracture surgery with outcomes: a population-based cohort study. Anesthesiology. 2018;128(3):480–91.
6. Johnson RL, Kopp SL, Burkle CM, Duncan CM, Jacob AK, Erwin PJ, Murad MH, Mantilla CB. Neuraxial vs general anaesthesia for total hip and total knee arthroplasty: a systematic review of comparative-effectiveness research. Br J Anaesth. 2016;116(2):163–76.
7. Aylott CE, Puna R, Robertson PA, Walker C. Spinous process morphology: the effect of ageing through adulthood on spinous process size and relationship to sagittal alignment. Eur Spine J. 2012;21(5):1007–12.
8. Scapinelli R. Morphological and functional changes of the lumbar spinous processes in the elderly. Surg Radiol Anat. 1989;11(2):129–33.
9. Chin KJ, Perlas A, Chan V, Brown-Shreves D, Koshkin A, Vaishnav V. Ultrasound imaging facilitates spinal anesthesia in adults with difficult surface anatomic landmarks. Anesthesiology. 2011;115(1):94–101.
10. Kim H, Won D, Chang JE, Lee JM, Ryu JH, Min SW, Jun K, Row HS, Hwang JY. Ultrasound assessment of the anatomic landmarks for spinal anesthesia in elderly patients with hip fracture: a prospective observational study. Medicine (Baltimore). 2019;98(27):e16388.
11. Tessler MJ, Kardash K, Wahba RM, Kleiman SJ, Trihas ST, Rossignol M. The performance of spinal anesthesia is marginally more difficult in the elderly. Reg Anesth Pain Med. 1999;24(2):126–30.
12. Chin KJ, Perlas A, Singh M, Arzola C, Prasad A, Chan V, Brull R. An ultrasound-assisted approach facilitates spinal anesthesia for total joint arthroplasty. Can J Anaesth. 2009;56(9):643–50.
13. Perlas A, Chaparro LE, Chin KJ. Lumbar Neuraxial ultrasound for spinal and epidural anesthesia: a systematic review and meta-analysis. Reg Anesth Pain Med. 2016;41(2):251–60.
14. Elgueta MF, Duong S, Finlayson RJ, Tran DQ. Ultrasonography for neuraxial blocks: a review of the evidence. Minerva Anestesiol. 2017;83(5):512–23.
15. Chin KJ, Karmakar MK, Peng P. Ultrasonography of the adult thoracic and lumbar spine for central neuraxial blockade. Anesthesiology. 2011;114(6): 1459–85.
16. Ghosh S, Madjdpour C, Chin K. Ultrasound-guided lumbar central neuraxial block. BJA Education. 2015;16(7):213–20.
17. Oh TT, Ikhsan M, Tan KK, Rehena S, Han NR, Sia ATH, Sng BL. A novel approach to neuraxial anesthesia: application of an automated ultrasound spinal landmark identification. BMC Anesthesiol. 2019;19(1):57.
18. Morimoto Y, Ihara Y, Shimamoto Y, Shiramoto H. Use of ultrasound for spinal anesthesia in a super morbidly obese patient. J Clin Anesth. 2017;36: 88–9.
19. Chin KJ, Perlas A, Chan V. The ultrasound-assisted paraspinous approach to lumbar neuraxial blockade: a simplified technique in patients with difficult anatomy. Acta Anaesthesiol Scand. 2015;59(5):668–73.
20. Grau T, Leipold RW, Conradi R, Martin E, Motsch J. Efficacy of ultrasound imaging in obstetric epidural anesthesia. J Clin Anesth. 2002;14(3):169–75.
21. Ekinci M, Alici HA, Ahiskalioglu A, Ince I, Aksoy M, Celik EC, Dostbil A, Celik M, Baysal PK, Golboyu BE, et al. The use of ultrasound in planned cesarean delivery under spinal anesthesia for patients having nonprominent anatomic landmarks. J Clin Anesth. 2017;37:82–5.
22. Li M, Ni X, Xu Z, Shen F, Song Y, Li Q, Liu Z. Ultrasound-assisted technology versus the conventional landmark location method in spinal anesthesia for cesarean delivery in obese Parturients: a randomized controlled trial. Anesth Analg. 2019;129(1):155–61.
23. Chin A, Crooke B, Heywood L, Brijball R, Pelecanos AM, Abeypala W. A randomised controlled trial comparing needle movements during combined spinal-epidural anaesthesia with and without ultrasound assistance. Anaesthesia. 2018;73(4):466–73.
24. Park SK, Yoo S, Kim WH, Lim YJ, Bahk JH, Kim JT. Ultrasound-assisted vs. landmark-guided paramedian spinal anaesthesia in the elderly: a randomised controlled trial. Eur J Anaesthesiol. 2019;36:1–9.
25. Geng J, Chen X, Wang X, Guo X, Li M. Ultrasound imaging increases first-attempt success rate of neuraxial block in elderly patients. Natl Med J China. 2016;96(43):3459–63.
26. Park SK, Bae J, Yoo S, Kim WH, Lim YJ, Bahk JH, Kim JT. Ultrasound-assisted versus landmark-guided spinal anesthesia in patients with abnormal spinal anatomy: a randomized controlled trial. Anesth Analg. 2020;130(3):787–95.
27. Chin KJ. Recent developments in ultrasound imaging for neuraxial blockade. Curr Opin Anaesthesiol. 2018;31(5):608–13.
28. Rabinowitz A, Bourdet B, Minville V, Chassery C, Pianezza A, Colombani A, Eychenne B, Samii K, Fourcade O. The paramedian technique: a superior initial approach to continuous spinal anesthesia in the elderly. Anesth Analg. 2007;105(6):1855–7.
29. Kallidaikurichi Srinivasan K, Iohom G, Loughnane F, Lee PJ. Conventional landmark-guided midline versus Preprocedure ultrasound-guided Paramedian techniques in spinal anesthesia. Anesth Analg. 2015;121(4): 1089–96.

30. Rizk MS, Zeeni CA, Bouez JN, Bteich NJ, Sayyid SK, Alfahel WS, Siddik-Sayyid SM. Preprocedural ultrasound versus landmark techniques for spinal anesthesia performed by novice residents in elderly: a randomized controlled trial. BMC Anesthesiol. 2019;19(1):208.
31. Jones MR, Novitch MB, Hall OM, Bourgeois AP, Jeha GM, Kaye RJ, Orhurhu V, Orhurhu MS, Eng M, Cornett EM, et al. Fascia iliaca block, history, technique, and efficacy in clinical practice. Best Pract Res Clin Anaesthesiol. 2019;33(4): 407–13.
32. Kumar D, Hooda S, Kiran S, Devi J. Analgesic efficacy of ultrasound guided FICB in patients with hip fracture. J Clin Diagn Res. 2016;10(7):UC13–6.
33. Chin KJ, Ramlogan R, Arzola C, Singh M, Chan V. The utility of ultrasound imaging in predicting ease of performance of spinal anesthesia in an orthopedic patient population. Reg Anesth Pain Med. 2013;38(1):34–8.
34. Miller R, Cohen N, Eriksson L, Fleisher L, Wiener-Kronish J, Young W: Miller's anesthesia 8th ed. Philadelphia: Saunders; 2015.
35. Meyer-Bender A, Kern A, Pollwein B, Crispin A, Lang PM. Incidence and predictors of immediate complications following perioperative non-obstetric epidural punctures. BMC Anesthesiol. 2012;12:31.

7

Retroclavicular vs Infraclavicular block for brachial plexus anesthesia

Andrés Felipe Gil Blanco[1], Pascal Laferrière-Langlois[1], David Jessop[2], Frédérick D'Aragon[1], Yanick Sansoucy[1], Natalie Albert[2], Pascal Tétreault[3] and Pablo Echave[1*]

Abstract

Background: The coracoid approach is a simple method to perform ultrasound-guided brachial plexus regional anesthesia (RA) but its simplicity is counterbalanced by a difficult needle visualization. We hypothesized that the retroclavicular (RCB) approach is not longer to perform when compared to the coracoid (ICB) approach, and improves needle visualization.

Methods: This randomized, controlled, non-inferiority trial conducted in two hospitals, included patients undergoing distal upper limb surgery. Patients were randomly assigned to a brachial plexus block (ICB or RCB). The primary outcome was performance time (sum of visualization and needling time), and was analyzed with a non-inferiority test of averages. Depth of sensory and motor blockade, surgical success, total anesthesia time, needle visualization, number of needle passes and complications were also evaluated. Subgroup analysis restricted to patients with higher body mass index was completed.

Results: We included 109 patients between September 2016 and May 2017. Mean RCB performance time was 4.8 ± 2.0 min while ICB was 5.2 ± 2.3 min ($p = 0.06$) with a 95% CI reaching up to 5.8% longer. RCB conferred an ultrasound-needle angle closer to 0° and significantly improved needle visibility after the clavicle was cleared and before local anesthetic administration. No differences were found in the secondary outcomes. Similar results were found in the subgroup analysis.

Conclusion: RCB approach for brachial plexus anesthesia was similar to ICB approach in terms of time performance. Needle visibility, which represent an important clinical variable, was superior and angle between needle and ultrasound probe was close to 0° in the RCB group.

Keywords: Regional anesthesia, Brachial plexus, Upper extremity, Ambulatory, Anatomy

Background

Regional anesthesia (RA) offers several advantages over general anesthesia (GA) for upper limb orthopedic surgery. One of the advantages is the improvement in postoperative pain, which leads to decreased use of postoperative opioids needs and reduces the recovery time for patients [1, 2]. The infraclavicular (ICB) (coracoid) approach for brachial plexus anesthesia is recognized for its facility and simplicity to perform. However, an inevitable pitfall of this method is the steep angle between the needle and the ultrasound probe that makes needle visibility challenging [3–8]. Because of its different needle entry point, the retroclavicular (RCB) approach [9] offers an almost perpendicular needle-ultrasound (US) beam angle, but aims at the same goal as the ICB. This simple yet critical difference can theoretically improve block performance conditions [6]. Our group and others have provided evidence that this technique is efficient, rapid, safe and simple to perform [10–12].

* Correspondence: Pablo.Echave@USherbrooke.ca
[1]Department of Anesthesiology, Medicine and Health Sciences Faculty, Centre Hospitalier Universitaire de Sherbrooke (CHUS), 3001, 12e Avenue Nord, Sherbrooke, QC J1H 5N4, Canada

The purpose of this randomized controlled trial was to perform a systematic comparison between these two RA techniques for upper limb surgery. By providing better needle visibility, our main hypothesis is that the total time required to perform RCB will be non-inferior to the time required to perform ICB while providing at least identical block quality and success. To that extent, several secondary outcomes were collected and analyzed such as needle visibility, imaging and needling time, depth of sensory and motor blocks, total anesthesia time, block success, angle and number of passes, procedural pain and incidence of complications.

Methods

Design and setting

We conducted this non-inferiority randomized trial at Centre hospitalier universitaire de Sherbrooke (CHUS, performing over 200 RCB per year) and Centre Hospitalier de l'Université Laval (CHUL, where this method was recently implemented), Quebec, Canada between September 2016 and May 2017. The trial was approved by the research ethics board of *Centre intégré universitaire de santé et service sociaux de l'Estrie (*MP-31-2017-1298), which provided a provincial-wide approval. Clinical Trial Registration: ClinicalTrials.gov (NCT02913625). All study participants provided written informed consent before randomization. A detailed study protocol was previously published [10, 13]. This study fully adhere to CONSORT guidelines [14].

Study participants

All patients scheduled for elective or urgent surgery (mainly open reduction and internal fixation of arm and forearm, fasciectomy, epicondylitis, elbow and wrist arthroscopy and elbow arthroplasty) were eligible for the study if they were ≥ 18 years old; ASA (American Society of Anesthesiologists) class I-III; able to provide a valid written consent and weighed > 50 kg, regardless of body mass index (BMI). Patients with previous surgery or gross anatomical deformities of the clavicle, systemic or local infection at the needle entry point, coagulopathy, severe pulmonary disease, local anesthetic (LA) allergy, known neuropathy affecting the operated limb, pregnancy and for whom surgeon requested an indwelling catheter for postoperative analgesia were excluded.

Intervention

In the intervention group, an RCB was performed by inserting the needle at the supraclavicular fossa and aiming the posterior wall of the axillary artery, strictly in-plane with the US probe resting in the delto-pectoral groove [10]. For the control group, the ICB was performed by placing the US probe in the infraclavicular fossa, medially to the coracoid process and by directing the needle towards the posterior wall of the axillary artery. Local anesthetic bolus (20 ml of 0.5% ropivacaine and 20 ml of 1.5% mepivacaine) was deposited under the axillary artery for both approaches. As defined a priori, ICB and RCB feasibility needed to be confirmed by a pre-scan before the randomization envelope was opened, to avoid recruitment of patients with gross anatomical deformation. Objective evaluation of motor and sensory blockade was required for all patients.

Randomization and blinding process

Clinical and epidemiological research unit at the CHUS generated the random allocation sequence. Participants were randomly assigned to control or experimental group with a 1:1 allocation ratio and stratified by sites using permuted blocks of random sizes. To ensure concealment, block sizes will not be disclosed and sequentially numbered, opaque and sealed envelopes were used. Only the research assistant had access to the envelopes. A research assistant, resident or anesthesiology department staff member was responsible for assessing participant eligibility and recruitment. All anesthetic interventions were performed by an anesthesiology resident (minimally in its 2nd year of training) or an anesthesiologist of the recruiting centers. Before the study, all operators, including experienced attending anesthesiologists, had a minimum experience of three successful retroclavicular blocks, as well as a minimum overall experience of 20 regional blocks. Only the outcome assessor for the motor block and sensory block could be blinded since it was technically impossible to blind the person performing the block and the patient. To reinforce blinding of the motor and sensory block assessor, chlorhexidine and bandages were applied over the two theoretical needle entry points. Video assessors of needle visibility could not be blinded because needle position on the screen was evident, but the adjudication was made independently to minimize this bias.

Outcomes assessment

A research assistant recorded the different times needed using a standard chronometer. Imaging time was the interval between initial contact of US probe with the skin and acquisition of a satisfactory axillary artery image. Needling time was the interval between the skin wheal and block needle withdrawal. Total anesthesia time was the sum of performance time (imaging plus needling) and the time required to achieve a sensory loss score of 9/10 (further described). The primary outcome, performance time, was measured in minutes (min) and corresponded to the sum of imaging time and needling time.

Detailed methodology of the following outcomes can be found in our previously published protocol [13].

Briefly, depth of sensitive and motor blocks was evaluated every 10 min after complete LA injection. Sensory loss was assessed in the territory of the radial, median, ulnar, musculocutaneous, and medial cutaneous nerve of the forearm using a 3-point score. As previously described [10, 15], the sum of these five scores represents the final sensory loss score (minimum score of 9/10 required). Motor function was tested for the radial, median, ulnar, and musculocutaneous nerves. The sum of these four scores represents the motor block final score [10, 15]. An independent, blinded, research assistant completed the sensory and the motor assessment and noted the final scores up to 30 min after block was performed. Blocks were considered successful only if surgery was completed without additional LA infiltration or GA. Blocks were recorded on video and two blinded independent anesthesiologists evaluated needle visibility using a 5-point Likert scale and ImageJ software (version 1.50i, developed by the National Institutes of Health [NIH]). This evaluation was done twice and needle angle on the horizontal axis was measured and noted before LA injection.

Immediately after complete LA bolus injection, an independent and blind outcome assessor evaluated procedural pain using a 10 cm visual analogue scale. Following our detailed protocol [13], number of needle passes (defined as positive integer unit each time the block needle needs to be realigned on the skin) as well as early and 48 h complications (such as paresthesia, vascular puncture, Horner syndrome, dyspnea, etc.) were also documented. We considered the use of neurostimulator as positive when the purpose of its use was not only for safety sentinel stimulation (< 0.3 mA). Details of complications and follow-up assessments are presented in our protocol [13]. Briefly, early complications were assessed on the day of surgery, all patients were further contacted 48 h after surgery to query for any delayed complications (dyspnea, paresthesia, weaknesses, pain, at the puncture site or hematoma). If a complication was suspected, patients were immediately referred for medical assessment.

Statistical methods

The statistics software SPSS (version 24.0.0.0), SAS (version 9.4), R (version 3.5.1) and Graph Pad Prism (version 6.0 h) were used. Primary outcome was analyzed with the non-inferiority test of the averages. Data was not normally distributed and required a logarithmic transformation to perform pre-defined parametric tests. Primary outcome was interpreted based on the logarithmic transformation. Secondary outcomes were analyzed using superiority analysis. For continuous data or ordinal data with > 8 categories, data were compiled as averages and standard deviation. Student t test was used for parametric data and the Mann-Whitney test was used for non-parametric data. Chi square (data $n > 5$) or Fisher exact (data $n < 5$) test were used for dichotomous data. Finally, for ordinal parametric data the chi square test was used and the Mann-Whitney test was used for ordinal non-parametric data. Subgroup analysis were performed following the same criteria as the main group and was conducted to evaluate if BMI higher than our study population average was influencing the outcomes. For all analysis, the intention-to-treat principle was used for analysis of missing data. When required, results are reported as mean (SD). No interim analysis was performed.

Sample size

Sample size calculation for this study has been presented in detail previously [13]. Briefly, it was calculated on the basis of a recent study [16] where the performance time for coracoid ICB approach was 5.6 min, with 45 s of visualization time and using our feasibility study recently conducted [10] where the needling time for the RCB approach was 3 min 42 s. As we explained in our published protocol [13] and based on our clinical judgement and statistical convention, we deemed that a time superiority of 5% would be significant and therefore have set the non-inferiority margin at 5%. An initial sample size of 49 patients per group was required to provide a statistical power of 0.9 (0.05 one-sided type 1 error), but to account for dropouts and inadequate procedures, the final sample size was set to 55 patients per group.

Results

Between September 2016 and May 2017, 163 patients were screened, 110 patients were randomized in the trial, and 109 were available for analysis (Fig. 1). No patient was lost to follow up. Baseline characteristics are presented in Table 1.

Primary outcome

The RCB group was composed of 53 participants and the ICB group was composed of 56. The average time required to perform an RCB was 4.8 min (SD 2.0 min) and 5.2 min (SD 2.3 min) for an ICB. Natural logarithmic average for performance time was 5.6 (SD: 0.4; 95% Confidence Interval [CI] 5.5–5.7) and 5.7 (SD: 0.4; 95% CI 5.6–5.8) for RCB and ICB respectively. Difference between the logarithmic averages was 0.073 (95% IC diff: [− 5.8% - infinity]; $p = 0.06$) or 7.1% when expressed in percentage change of performance time and was therefore going over the pre-specified non-inferiority margin of 5.0% by 0.8% (Fig. 2).

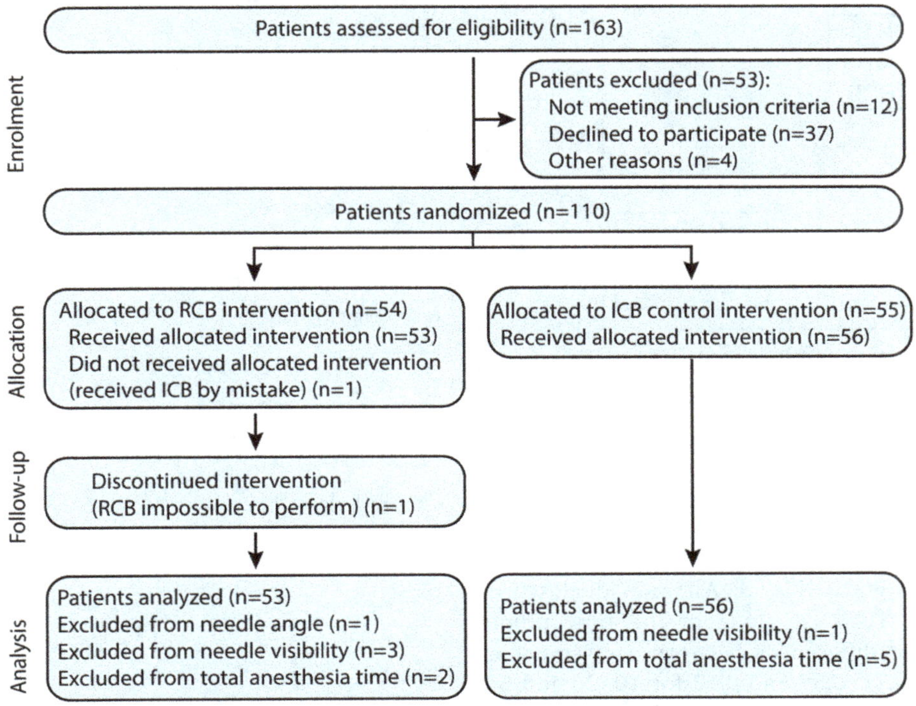

Fig. 1 Study flow chart summarizes overall experimental design. A total of 163 patients were originally assessed for eligibility, from which 109 were analyzed. Grouping and dropout causes are indicated. Reason of exclusion for needle angle and visibility: improper image quality; Reason of exclusion for total anesthesia time: minimal sensitive block not obtained at 30 min. RCB, retroclavicular and ICB, infraclavicular approach

Secondary outcomes

Imaging time did not show any differences between the two methods (35 ± 42 s for RCB vs 41 ± 52 s for ICB, $p = 0.725$). Similar results were observed for needling time, where no differences were present between groups (4.2 ± 1.7 min for RCB vs 4.5 ± 2.2 min for ICB, $p = 0.702$).

A minimal sensory block score of 9/10 was also used to compute the proportion of patients that were ready

Table 1 Demographics, ASA stratification and block repartition by center

	RCB ($n = 53$)	ICB ($n = 56$)
Age (years)	51 ± 16	52 ± 16
Female	16 (30%)	20 (36%)
BMI	26.6 ± 4.5	27.3 ± 5.1
ASA I	27 (51%)	22 (39%)
ASA II	24 (45%)	25 (45%)
ASA III	2 (4%)	9 (16%)
CHUL	38 (72%)	41 (73%)
CHUS	15 (28%)	15 (27%)

Data are given as number (%) or mean ± SD. Test of baseline characteristics were not performed [14]

ASA American Society of Anesthesiologists physical status classification score, *BMI* Body Mass Index, *CHUL* Centre Hospitalier Universitaire de l'Université Laval, *CHUS* Centre Hospitalier Universitaire de l'Université de Sherbrooke

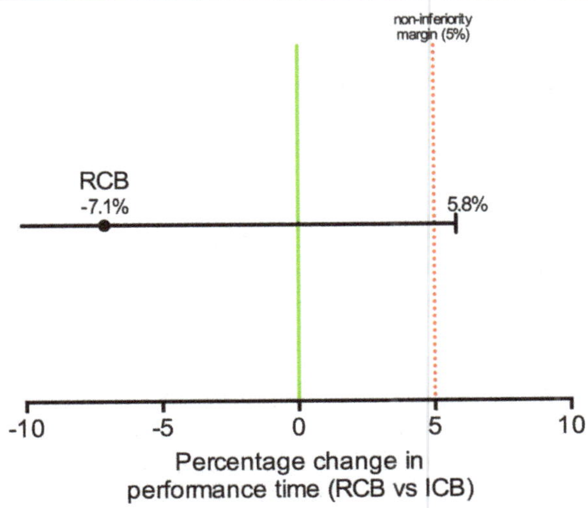

Fig. 2 Visual representation of non-inferiority margin for the change in percentage of the performance time when comparing RCB approach to the standard ICB. The RCB approach is 7.1% faster than the ICB approach while the one-sided 95%CI is going over the 5% margin by 0.8%

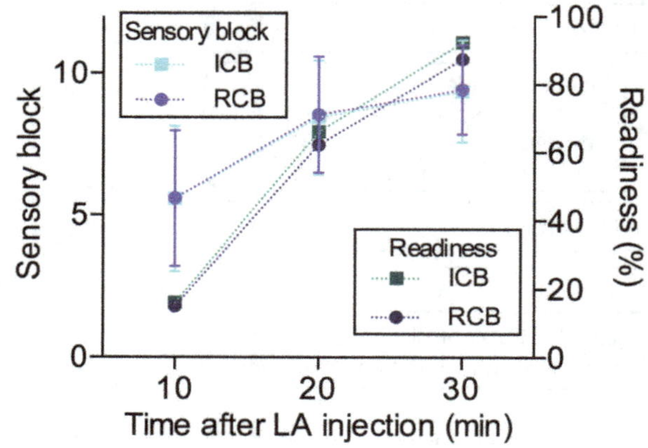

Fig. 3 Sensory block performance and readiness for surgery did not show any differences between the two regional anesthesia approaches, providing a similar proportion of participants that could undergo their respective surgical procedure at each time points

for surgery as shown in Fig. 3. All individual scores are presented in Table 2. None of the time points showed significant differences between assessment of sensory loss ($p = 0.71$, 0.59 and 0.12 for 10, 20 and 30 min respectively), motor block ($p = 0.75$, 0.46 and 0.11 for 10, 20 and 30 min respectively) and readiness for surgery ($p = 0.89$, 0.68 and 0.39 for 10, 20 and 30 min respectively).

For 7 (6%) patients, the time needed to obtain a 9/10 sensitive score was longer than the time allotted for evaluation. Thus, participants with missing data were imputed. RCB total anesthesia time ($n = 51$) was 27.3 min (SD 8.0 min) and ICB total anesthesia time ($n = 51$) was 26.4 min (SD 8.3 min) ($p = 0.433$). Success of plexus block was similar in both groups: 50/53 (94.3%) for RCB and 51/56 (91.1%) for ICB ($p = 0.717$).

Images from 4 patients (one in ICB group and three in RCB group) were excluded because of poor acquired images. First Likert evaluation score was 3.49/5 (SD 1.04) for RCB and 2.84/5 (SD 0.90) for ICB ($p < 0.001$); and second Likert evaluation score was 4.47/5 (SD 0.66) for RCB and 3.09/5 (SD 1.05) for ICB (p < 0.001). Average angle to horizontal axis was 7.8° (SD 6.4°) for RCB ($n = 52$) and 32.3° (SD 10.3°) for ICB ($n = 56$) (p < 0.001).

Immediate complications consisted of three paresthesias (5.7%) in RCB group and one (1.8%) in ICB group ($p = 0.35$); one arterial puncture (1.9%) in RCB group and four (7.1%) in ICB ($p = 0.364$); and one Horner's episode in each group ($p = 1$). Late complications consisted of two participants (3.8%) with pain at the injection site in RCB group and four (7.1%) in ICB group ($P = 0.679$); No significant difference was found between the groups. No patient developed permanent complications after follow-up (48 h).

Table 2 Descriptive information about procedures and outcomes

	RCB	ICB	*p*-value
Performance time	4.8 ± 2.0 min	5.2 ± 2.3 min	$p = 0.0608$
Imaging time	35 ± 42 s	41 ± 52 s	$p = 0.725$
Needle time	4.2 ± 1.7 min	4.5 ± 2.2 min	$p = 0.702$
Total anesthesia time	$n = 51$	$n = 51$	
	27.3 ± 8.0 min	26.4 ± 8.3 min	$p = 0.4331$
Number of needle passes	1.1 ± 0.4	1.2 ± 0.7	$p = 0.909$
Neurostimulation use	37/53 (67.9%)	38/56 (69.8%)	$p = 0.826$
Needle angle	7.8 ± 6.4°	32.3 ± 10.3°	**$p < 0.001$**
Procedural pain	2.9/10 ± 1.6	2.9/10 ± 1.9	$p = 1$
Needle visualization	$n = 51$	$n = 55$	
Likert evaluation time 1	3.49/5 ± 1.044	2.84/5 ± 0.9	**$p < 0.001$**
Likert evaluation time 2	4.47/5 ± 0.66	3.09/5 ± 1.05	**$p < 0.001$**
Person performing the block			
Residents	$n = 41$ (77.4%)	$n = 43$ (76.8%)	$p = 1$
Staff anesthesiologist	$n = 12$ (22.6%)	$n = 13$ (23.2%)	$p = 0.818$
Sensory loss at 10 min	5.6/10 ± 2.38	5.59/10 ± 2.55	$p = 0.706$
Sensory loss at 20 min	8.55/10 ± 2.05	8.45/10 ± 2.02	$p = 0.587$
Sensory loss at 30 min	9.43/10 ± 1.58	9.38/10 ± 1.80	$p = 0.121$
Ready for surgery at 10 min	$n = 8$ (15.1%)	$n = 9$ (16.1%)	$p = 0.888$
Ready for surgery at 20 min	$n = 33$ (62.3%)	$n = 37$ (66.1%)	$p = 0.679$
Ready for surgery at 30 min	$n = 49$ (87.5%)	$n = 49$ (92.5%)	$p = 0.391$
Motor block at 10 min	4.49/8 ± 1.77	4.25/8 ± 2.12	$p = 0.750$
Motor block at 20 min	6.70/8 ± 1.76	6.57/8 ± 1.99	$p = 0.462$
Motor block at 30 min	7.47/8 ± 1.50	7.13/8 ± 2.01	$p = 0.112$
Success of plexus block	50/53 (94.3%)	51/56 (91.1%)	$p = 0.717$
Sedation during surgery	$n = 14$	$n = 23$	$p = 0.106$
Rescue	$n = 5$	$n = 7$	$p = 0.609$
Local anesthesia	$n = 2$ (3.8%)	$n = 3$ (5.4%)	$p = 1$
Axillar block	$n = 0$	$n = 3$ (5.4%)	$p = 0.244$
Other block	$n = 2$ (3.8%)	$n = 1$ (1.8%)	$p = 0.611$
General anesthesia	n = 1 (1.9%)	$n = 0$	$p = 0.486$
Duration of surgery	49 ± 28 min	55 ± 29 min	$p = 0.230$
Immediate complications			
Paresthesia	$n = 3$ (5.7%)	$n = 1$ (1.8%)	$p = 0.354$
Arterial puncture	$n = 1$ (1.9%)	$n = 4$ (7.1%)	$p = 0.364$
Horner's	$n = 1$ (1.9%)	$n = 1$ (1.8%)	$p = 1$
Late complications			
Pain at injection site	$n = 2$ (3.8%)	$n = 4$ (7.1%)	$p = 0.679$

Data are given as number (%) or mean ± SD. RCB indicates retroclavicular block; ICB, infraclavicular block; *p*-values in bold represent significant differences between RCB and ICB method

Subgroup analysis

Mean BMI was 27.13 kg/m^2 (5.00 kg/m^2) and patients with a higher than mean BMI were included in the subgroup analysis. Groups were composed of 27 participants for ICB and 24 for RCB (Table 3). Performance time for ICB was 6.10 min (SD 2.92 min) and for RCB was 4.99 min (SD 2.09 min) ($p = 0.193$) (Table 4). Poor quality images were imputed (analyzed data: RCB $n = 22$ and ICB $n = 27$). First Likert evaluation score was 3.45/5 (SD 0.76) for RCB and 2.85/5 (SD 1.03) for ICB ($p < 0.05$). Second evaluation score was 4.33/5 (SD 0.75) for RCB and 2.7/5 (SD 0.99) for ICB ($p < 0.001$). Needle angle was 8.48° (SD 7.14°) for RCB and 36.26° (SD 9.94°) for ICB ($p < 0.001$). Number of needle passes was 1.17 (SD 0.48) for RCB and 1.22 (SD 0.97) ($p = 0.571$).

Discussion

For patients with a palpable supraclavicular fossa and no clavicle anatomical abnormalities, we were not able to prove complete statistical non-inferiority of the RCB in terms of performance time when compared to the ICB namely because both techniques were found to be efficient. However, when evaluating secondary outcomes, we found that total anesthesia time, needle and image time, blocks success and dynamics, complications incidence, procedural pain and number of needle passes were not different between approaches. These results therefore suggest that RCB is globally non-inferior when compared to ICB. Furthermore, these results were also found in the high BMI subgroup analysis.

Needle visibility is also an important clinical variable that can influence the choice of a method for brachial plexus anesthesia. As the needle approaches the plexus (Table 2, Likert evaluation time 2), RCB visibility score was > 1 point higher than ICB on Likert scale. This likely relates to the almost perpendicular angle (Table 2, needle angle) between US beam and needle. Good visibility provides a safer technique and a quicker needling time [6–8]. ICB and RCB actually confer an opposite gradient of visibility to sensitive structures. Improved needle visibility with RCB occurs near the neurovascular bundle as opposed to the limited visibility offered by ICB. The opposite occurs at or near the skin.

Table 3 Subgroups demographics, ASA stratification and block repartition by center participants

	RCB ($n = 24$)	ICB (n = 27)
Age	46.6 ± 15.8	51.5 ± 12.4
Female	4 (16.7%)	9 (33.3%)
BMI	30.7 ± 3.7	31.2 ± 4.2
ASA I	13 (54.2%)	10 (37%)
ASA II	10 (41.7%)	14 (51.9%)
ASA III	1 (4.2%)	3 (11.1%)
CHUL	19 (79.2%)	20 (74.1)
CHUS	5 (20.8%)	7 (25.9%)

Test of baseline characteristics were not performed. Data are given as number (%) or mean ± SD. *ASA* American Society of Anesthesiologists physical status classification score, *BMI* Body Mass Index, *CHUL* Centre Hospitalier Universitaire de l'Université Laval, *CHUS* Centre Hospitalier Universitaire de l'Université de Sherbrooke

Table 4 Descriptive information about procedures and outcomes for subgroups analysis

	RCB ($n = 24$)	ICB ($n = 27$)	p-value
Performance time	4.99 ± 2.09 min	6.10 ± 2.92 min	$p = 0.193$
Imaging time	33.04 ± 17.82 s.	51.37 ± 67.78 s.	$p = 0.713$
Needling time	4.44 ± 2.04 min	5.24 ± 2.62 min	$p = 0.238$
Total anesthesia time	28.95 ± 9.02 min	28.67 ± 8.36 min	$p = 0.982$
Number of passes	1.17 ± 0.48	1.22 ± 0.97	$p = 0.571$
Needle angle	8.48 ± 7.14	36.26 ± 9.94	$\mathbf{p < 0.001}$
Visibility score	$n = 22$	$n = 27$	
Likert 1st evaluation	3.45/5 ± 0.80	2.85/5 ± 1.03	$\mathbf{p < 0.05}$
Likert 2nd evaluation	4.32/5 ± 0.78	2.70/5 ± 0.99	$\mathbf{p < 0.001}$

Patients above average BMI (27.13) were grouped according to the type of block they received. RCB indicates retro-clavicular block, *ICB*; infraclavicular block; *p*-values in bold represent significant differences between RCB and ICB method

A recent anatomical study of RCB [17] highlights the potential risk of suprascapular nerve injury as the needle passes under the clavicle. No patients presented permanent neurologic complications during this study nor over the ~ 1000 RCB performed at the CHUS in recent years (albeit all of them were not performed within a research setting where this data is specifically recorded). Early and late incidence of paresthesia were also not considered statistically different between study groups, RCB paresthesia incidence was of 5.7% and is lower than reported by literature for ICB [8, 15, 18, 19]. A higher than usual arterial puncture rate for ICB can be linked to a lower needle visibility score inherent of the ICB method and possibly the primary nature of the study, performance time, which could lead clinicians to "beat the clock". Nonetheless, no complications were recorded at 48 h for both groups.

The high BMI subgroup analysis, comprising almost 50% of the total number of patients recruited, also suggests that needle visibility and needle angle improvements with RCB over ICB are still present and not affected by a higher BMI. Our clinical experience leads us to infer that if the supraclavicular fossa is palpable and depressible, RCB is likely to be feasible even with high BMI patients, until an arterial depth of 5 cm is reached. In a time where there is increased interest, controversies and discussion about the RCB method [19–22], our study represents one of the first that properly compare these two methods and confirms its safety and efficacy.

Limitations and Bias

Even if the majority of the blocks (> 75%) were performed by trainees in this study, success rate was comparable to more experienced clinicians (92.9% for resident and 92.0% for experience clinicians). Both procedures were still performed within a reasonable average time, but it is, however, likely that smaller standard deviation would be observed with experienced anesthesiologist only and therefore non-inferiority of the primary outcome could be statistically proven. It is important to mention that the RCB approach was newly introduced in the center where most patients were recruited but still present standard deviations similar to the ICB method, suggesting that this new regional anesthesia method appears to offer a fast learning curve. Likert scale was not validated previously in this context, but its use is becoming more popular [19, 23] and we deemed it appropriate to evaluate a secondary outcome of our trial. This is also one of the reasons we used performance time as our primary outcome even though needle visibility is clinically more important. We felt a pre-scan was necessary because needle travel under the clavicle can be impossible in case of unrepaired clavicle fracture. Pre-scan was done for both blocks and therefore did not limit internal validity although it did dilute imaging time. Despite these limitations, because randomization, blinding and adherence to protocol were strict and detection and experimental bias were limited we consider the internal validity to be good. We did not identify confounding factors.

Conclusion

In the context of clinical reality where each approach possesses pros and cons, proving the usefulness of RCB is valuable as it offers another option to the regionalist. The implications of our work can be summarized as an improved strategy to easily keep track of the tip of the needle as it nears the neurovascular bundle. The downside of RCB is the acoustic shadow of the clavicle but our clinical experience so far leads us to believe that with strict in-plane US guidance, needle angled parallel to US probe and never posteriorly together with the confirmation of distance A and B [10] the RCB is a safe method. As previously observed [10], operators also found in this study that the fullness of the supraclavicular fossa and its lack of compressibility is increasing technical difficulty. Recent studies suggest that RCB could be used in emergency room settings because of its simplicity, safety and efficacity [24]. Taken altogether, despite falling short statistically to prove the non-inferiority in performance time, we consider that the absence of differences in all the other relevant secondary outcomes suggests that retroclavicular approach (RCB) represents an interesting alternative to coracoid approach.

Abbreviations

ASA: American Society of Anesthesiologists; BMI: Body mass index; CHUL: Centre Hospitalier de l'Université Laval; CHUS: Centre hospitalier universitaire de Sherbrooke; GA: General anesthesia; ICB: coracoid; LA: Local anesthetic; NIH: National Institutes of Health; RA: Regional anesthesia; RCB: Retroclavicular; US: Ultrasound

Acknowledgments

We kindly acknowledge the excellent work done by Mrs. Veronique Gagnon and Dr. Joshua Fortin by recruiting patients for our trial. We are also thankful to Dr. Marie-Josée Loignon and Dr. Stéphanie Deziel Malouin for their precious contribution and expertise in this trial.

Author's contribution

PE conceived the original idea. AFGB, DJ, FDA, NA, PE, PLL and YS designed the study and helped with implementation. AFGB and PLL wrote the study protocol. AFGB drafted the manuscript. DJ, FDA, NA, PE and YS implemented through revision. FDA provided statistical expertise in clinical trial design. PT revised, proofread and wrote the manuscript to produce a final version. All authors contributed to the refinement of this article and approved the final manuscript.

Author details

[1]Department of Anesthesiology, Medicine and Health Sciences Faculty, Centre Hospitalier Universitaire de Sherbrooke (CHUS), 3001, 12e Avenue Nord, Sherbrooke, QC J1H 5N4, Canada. [2]Department of Anesthesiology, Medicine and Health Sciences Faculty, Centre Hospitalier Universitaire de Laval (CHUL), 2705 boul Laurier, Quebec G1V 4G2, QC, Canada. [3]Department of Biomedical Engineering, Faculty of medicine and Dentistry, University of Alberta, 1098 Research Transition Facility, Edmonton T6G 2V2, AB, Canada.

References

1. Hadzic A, Arliss J, Kerimoglu B, Karaca PE, Yufa M, Claudio RE, et al. A comparison of infraclavicular nerve block versus general anesthesia for hand and wrist day-case surgeries. Anesthesiology. 2004;101(1):127–32.
2. Bruce BG, Green A, Blaine TA, Wesner LV. Brachial plexus blocks for upper extremity orthopaedic surgery. J Am Acad Orthop Surg. 2012;20(1):38–47.
3. de Gusmao LC, Lima JS, Ramalho Jda R, Leite AL, da Silva AM. Evaluation of brachial plexus fascicles involvement on infraclavicular block: unfixed cadaver study. Braz J Anesthesiol (Elsevier). 2015;65(3):213–6.
4. Tsui BC-H. Atlas of ultrasound and nerve stimulation-guided regional anesthesia. New York: Springer; 2007.
5. Sites BD, Brull R, Chan VW, Spence BC, Gallagher J, Beach ML, et al. Artifacts and pitfall errors associated with ultrasound-guided regional anesthesia. Part I: understanding the basic principles of ultrasound physics and machine operations. Reg Anesth Pain Med. 2007;32(5):412–8.
6. Sites BD, Brull R, Chan VW, Spence BC, Gallagher J, Beach ML, et al. Artifacts and pitfall errors associated with ultrasound-guided regional anesthesia: part II: a pictorial approach to understanding and avoidance. Reg Anesth Pain Med. 2010;35(2 Suppl):S81–92.
7. Chin KJ, Perlas A, Chan VW, Brull R. Needle visualization in ultrasound-guided regional anesthesia: challenges and solutions. Reg Anesth Pain Med. 2008;33(6):532–44.
8. Chin KJ, Alakkad H, Adhikary SD, Singh M. Infraclavicular brachial plexus block for regional anaesthesia of the lower arm. Cochrane Database Syst Rev. 2013;8:Cd005487.
9. Hebbard P, Royse C. Ultrasound guided posterior approach to the infraclavicular brachial plexus. Anaesthesia. 2007;62(5):539.
10. Charbonneau J, Frechette Y, Sansoucy Y, Echave P. The ultrasound-guided Retroclavicular block: a prospective feasibility study. Reg Anesth Pain Med. 2015;40(5):605–9.
11. Grape S, Pawa A, Weber E, Albrecht E. Retroclavicular vs supraclavicular brachial plexus block for distal upper limb surgery: a randomised, controlled, single-blinded trial. British journal of anaesthesia. 2019;In Press.
12. Beh ZY, Hasan MS, Lai HY, Kassim NM, Md Zin SR, Chin KF. Posterior parasagittal in-plane ultrasound-guided infraclavicular brachial plexus block-a case series. BMC Anesthesiol. 2015;15:105.
13. Langlois PL, Gil-Blanco AF, Jessop D, Sansoucy Y, D'Aragon F, Albert N, et al. Retroclavicular approach vs infraclavicular approach for plexic bloc anesthesia of the upper limb: study protocol randomized controlled trial. Trials. 2017;18(1):346.
14. Moher D, Hopewell S, Schulz KF, Montori V, Gotzsche PC, Devereaux PJ, et al. CONSORT 2010 explanation and elaboration: updated guidelines for reporting parallel group randomised trials. BMJ (Clinical research ed). 2010;340:c869.

15. Tran DQ, Russo G, Munoz L, Zaouter C, Finlayson RJ. A prospective, randomized comparison between ultrasound-guided supraclavicular, infraclavicular, and axillary brachial plexus blocks. Reg Anesth Pain Med. 2009;34(4):366–71.
16. Yazer MS, Finlayson RJ, Tran DQ. A randomized comparison between infraclavicular block and targeted intracluster injection supraclavicular block. Reg Anesth Pain Med. 2015;40(1):11–5.
17. Sancheti SF, Uppal V, Sandeski R, Kwofie MK, Szerb JJ. A cadaver study investigating structures encountered by the needle during a Retroclavicular approach to Infraclavicular brachial plexus block. Reg Anesth Pain Med. 2018;43(7):752–5.
18. Frederiksen BS, Koscielniak-Nielsen ZJ, Jacobsen RB, Rasmussen H, Hesselbjerg L. Procedural pain of an ultrasound-guided brachial plexus block: a comparison of axillary and infraclavicular approaches. Acta Anaesthesiol Scand. 2010;54(4):408–13.
19. Kavrut Ozturk N, Kavakli AS. Comparison of the coracoid and retroclavicular approaches for ultrasound-guided infraclavicular brachial plexus block. J Anesth. 2017;31(4):572–8.
20. Uppal V, Sancheti SF, Kwofie MK, Szerb JJ. Novel approaches to the brachial plexus in the infraclavicular space: filling up the tool box. Reg Anesth Pain Med. 2019.
21. Leurcharusmee P, Layera S, Finlayson RJ, Tran Q. Retroclavicular approach to infraclavicular brachial plexus block: a logical conundrum. Reg Anesth Pain Med. 2019.
22. Uppal V, Kalagara HKP, Sondekoppam RV. Tips and tricks to improve the safety of the retroclavicular brachial plexus block. Am J Emerg Med. 2018; 36(6):1107–8.
23. Wiegel M, Moriggl B, Schwarzkopf P, Petroff D, Reske AW. Anterior Suprascapular nerve block versus Interscalene brachial plexus block for shoulder surgery in the outpatient setting: a randomized controlled patient- and Assessor-blinded trial. Reg Anesth Pain Med. 2017;42(3):310–8.
24. Luftig J, Mantuani D, Herring AA, Nagdev A. Ultrasound-guided retroclavicular approach infraclavicular brachial plexus block for upper extremity emergency procedures. Am J Emerg Med. 2017;35(5):773–7.

8

The efficacy and safety of intrathecal dexmedetomidine for parturients undergoing cesarean section

Xiao-xiao Li[1†], Yu-mei Li[2†], Xue-li Lv[1], Xing-he Wang[1] and Su Liu[1,3*]

Abstract

Background: The efficacy and safety of spinal anesthesia by intrathecal dexmedetomidine (DEX) for parturients undergoing cesarean section are still lack of evidence. This aim of our study was to evaluate the efficacy and safety of intrathecal DEX for parturients undergoing cesarean section to provide more data evidence for intrathecal applications.

Methods: Three hundred parturients undergoing cesarean section under spinal anesthesia were randomly assigned into three groups: group B: 9.0 mg (1.2 ml) of 0.75% bupivacaine with saline (1 ml); group FB: 9.0 mg (1.2 ml) of 0.75% bupivacaine with 20 μg of fentanyl (1 ml); group DB: 9.0 mg (1.2 ml) of 0.75% bupivacaine with 5 μg of DEX (1 ml). Intraoperative block characteristics, parturients' postoperative quality of recovery, maternal and neonatal outcomes and the plasma concentration of DEX were measured. All parturients were followed up for 30 days to determine whether nerve injury occurred.

Results: Compared with group B, the duration of sensory block in group FB and group DB were significantly prolonged (108.4 min [95% Confidence Interval (CI) = 104.6–112.3] in group B, and 122.0 min [95% CI = 116.8–127.3] in group FB, 148.2 min [95% CI = 145.3–151.1] in group DB). The overall score of quality recovery in group DB (71.6 [95% CI = 71.0–72.2]) was significantly higher than that in group FB (61.5 [95% CI = 60.8–62.2]) and group B (61.7 [95% CI = 61.0–62.4]). There was no statistically significant difference among the three groups for PH, PaO_2, and $PaCO_2$ of newborn. The plasma concentration of DEX in umbilical artery and umbilical vein was low and cannot be detected. The 30-days follow-up of parturients did not show any new onset of back, buttock or leg pain or paresthesia.

Conclusions: DEX is a potential local anesthetic adjuvant that the intrathecal combination of 5 μg DEX can safely exhibit a facilitatory block effect and improve parturients' recovery quality.

(Continued on next page)

* Correspondence: liusu112277@gmail.com
†Xiao-xiao Li and Yu-mei Li contributed equally to this work.
[1]Jiangsu Province Key Laboratory of Anesthesiology, Xuzhou Medical University, Xuzhou, Jiangsu, China
[3]Department of Anesthesiology, the Affiliated Hospital of Xuzhou Medical University, 99 Huaihai West Road, Xuzhou 221000, Jiangsu, China

(Continued from previous page)
Keywords: Intrathecal dexmedetomidine, Spinal anesthesia, Cesarean section

Background

Spinal anesthesia, with the advantage of easy-operating and avoiding the maternal risk of general anesthesia, including tracheal intubation failure, aspiration and lung infection, has been recommended as the preferred anesthesia for cesarean section [1–4]. However, some disadvantages caused by single-shot spinal anesthesia such us the limited duration of action and insufficient postoperative analgesia, which will lower the maternal postoperative recovery quality, and increasing local anesthetics doses is prone to cause maternal and neonatal adverse events [5, 6]. Therefore, several adjuvants [7, 8] in combination with local anesthetics have gradually been applied to further improve spinal anesthesia, of which dexmedetomidine (DEX) is a good choice.

DEX, a highly selective α-2 adrenergic receptor agonist, provides sedative, analgesic, anti-sympathetic effects and has no significant effect on respiration [9]. Several clinical trials [10–13] have shown that DEX can be applicated as an auxiliary for spinal anesthesia through enhancing the anesthetic effects, preventing and reducing adverse reactions caused by local anesthetics. However, there are only a few studies on intrathecal DEX for cesarean section and these studies were mostly single-center with a small sample size, and whether the parturients' recovery quality would be improved and whether DEX would adversely affect the fetus are still lack of plasma concentration evidence. Therefore, this two-centers, prospective, double-blind, randomized controlled trial was designed to evaluate the efficacy and safety of intrathecal DEX for parturients undergoing cesarean section to provide more data evidence for intrathecal applications.

Methods

Study participants

This trial was approved by the ethics committee of Feng Xian People's Hospital and the Affiliated Hospital of Xuzhou Medical University. Written informed consent was obtained from all enrolled participants. This manuscript adheres to the applicable CONSORT guidelines. This study was a two-centers, prospective, double-blind, randomized controlled trial, and the two centers are the Affiliated Hospital of Xuzhou Medical University and Feng Xian People's Hospital. Patient recruitment and data collection were started in April 2019 and ended in July 2019. The inclusion criteria of our study were: (1) Full-term pregnant women undergoing elective cesarean section under spinal anesthesia; (2) Age: 20 ~ 35 years; (3) ASA physical status II ~ III; The exclusion criteria were: (1) Multiple pregnancies; (2) Cardiovascular disease (e.g., pre-eclampsia and hypertension); (3) Serious hepatic dysfunction (Child-Pugh class C); (4) serious renal dysfunction (undergoing dialysis before surgery); (4) History of alcohol or opioid addiction; (5) Contraindication to spinal anesthesia; (7) Refusing to sign informed consent.

Randomization, blinding and allocation concealment

According to the random number generated by computer, parturients were randomly allocated into three equal groups to receive either DEX, fentanyl or normal saline in combination with bupivacaine. The randomization sequence was placed in serially numbered opaque envelopes. Before the start of spinal anesthesia, an anesthesiologist prepared relevant drugs according to the randomization sequence and the anesthesiologist would not participate in the data collection, follow-up, and analysis.

Study interventions

All parturients included in the study routinely fasted for 6–8 h before surgery, and none of them received premedication. When parturients were admitted into the operating room, standard monitoring for pulse oxygen saturation (SpO_2), heart rate (HR), electrocardiogram (ECG), and noninvasive blood pressure (NIBP) was carried out. All parturients were given a supplementation of 3 L/min O_2 through the nasal catheter. Then an intravenous 18-G cannula was inserted and patients were preloaded with ringer lactate 10 ml/kg 15–20 min before anesthesia.

With the parturients in the left lateral position, spinal anesthesia was performed at the L3-L4 interspace with a 25 G spinal Quincke-tip needle and study drugs were injected slowly within 15 s after the cerebrospinal fluid flowing out. The three groups were scheduled to receive drugs as follows: bupivacaine group (group B): 9 mg (1.2 ml) of 0.75% bupivacaine, with 1.0 ml of normal saline. Bupivacaine + fentanyl group: (group FB): 9 mg (1.2 ml) of 0.75% bupivacaine, with 20 μg of fentanyl in 1.0 ml of normal saline. Bupivacaine + DEX group (group DB): 9 mg (1.2 ml) of 0.75% bupivacaine, with 5 μg of DEX in 1.0 ml of normal saline. After removing the spinal needle, parturients were in the position with a 15-degree tilt to the left side immediately. All spinal anesthesia procedures were performed by experienced anesthesiologists. The sensory block level was tested by the pinprick method using a blunt 25-G needle. Assessment of the dermatomal level was done every 1 min until the peak sensory block level was achieved. Subsequently frequent testing every 10 min was performed until regression to S1 dermatome. The motor block was assessed by the modified Bromage scale (MBS, 0 = no paralysis,1 = inability to raise the leg, 2 = inability to flex the knee, and 3 = inability to flex the ankle) [14]. Surgery was allowed to commence once the sensory block level reached T6 [15]. Any patient showing moderate pain (visual analog score (VAS) ≥3) was administered intravenous 0.5 mg/kg ketamine. If hypotension (systolic blood pressure (SBP) < 90 mmHg or descending baseline values by 30%) persisted, intravenous 6 mg of ephedrine was administered; If bradycardia (HR < 50 bpm) occurs, intravenous 0.5 mg of atropine was administered. Repeat if necessary. Intraoperative ephedrine and atropine consumption were recorded. After surgery, all patients underwent patient-controlled intravenous analgesia (PCIA) with 2 μg/kg of sufentanil and 10 mg of tropisetron.

Outcomes

The primary outcome of our study was the duration of sensory block, which was defined as time taken from intrathecal injection to sensory regression to S1 dermatome. The secondary outcomes of our study were as follows: the onset time of sensory block, which was defined as time taken from intrathecal injection to the maternal feeling of lower extremities temperature increment or numbness [16]; the onset time of motor block, which was defined as time taken from intrathecal injection to MBS > 1; the duration of motor block, which was defined as time taken from intrathecal injection to MBS = 0; the peak sensory block level; the blood gas analysis for PH, PaO_2, and $PaCO_2$ of the umbilical artery (UA) and umbilical vein (UV) blood samples of the newborn, which was performed immediately after collection; the plasma concentration of DEX in the UA and UV, which was determined by High-Performance Liquid Chromatography Tandem Mass Spectrometry methods [17]; Apgar scores, which were assessed at 1st and 5th min by the obstetrician who was blinded to the study; the hemodynamic parameters of parturient including BP, HR, which were evaluated at: baseline values (T0), immediately after blockcade (T1), 5 min (T2), 10 min (T3), 15 min (T4) and 20 min (T5) after blockcade. BP and HR at T0 were defined as the average values measured for 3 consecutive times at rest after entering the operating room.

The recovery quality of parturients within 24 h after surgery was assessed by obstetric quality of recovery-11 score [18] (ObsQoR-11, score from 0 to 10 in each term, where 0 = strongly agree and 10 = strongly disagree, the higher of the score, the higher of recovery quality), which was designed for parturients and presented by Ciechanowicz S; intra-and postoperative adverse events including nausea, vomiting and shivering, time to the first analgesic request and total sufentanil comsumption at 24 h after surgery were also recorded. Parturients were contacted by telephone for a post-operative 30 days following discharge to determine whether nerve injury occurred, including any new onset of back, buttock or leg pain or paresthesia. All of these evaluations were performed by an anesthesiologist blind to any other aspect of the trial.

Statistical analysis

The sample size was calculated using PASS 15.0 software (NCSS, LLC, Kaysville, USA). The sample size calculation was based on the primary outcome, the duration of sensory block. According to our pilot trial results, the duration of sensory block was 114.3 ± 28.5 min for group B, 120.1 ± 29.4 min for group FB, 128.8 ± 29.5 min for group DB. A total of 80 patients were required to achieve 80% power with an alpha error of 5% based on the module of analysis of variance (ANOVA) in PASS. Considering a lost-to-follow-up rate of about 15%, 94 patients are required for each group. Finally, a total of 100 parturients were recruited in our study.

Statistical analysis was performed using IBM SPSS 22.0 software (SPSS Inc., IBM, Chicago, IL, USA). Numeric variables were analyzed for normality by the Kolmogorov-Smirnov test. Normally distributed continuous variables were expressed as mean with a standard deviation and compared using ANOVA with post hoc analysis using Bonferroni test. The categorical variables were presented as number (%) and compared using Chi-square test or Fischer exact test. Kaplan-Meier curve illustrated the time to first analgesic request and comparisons between groups were conducted with the log-rank test. Hemodynamic parameters were compared by repetitive measurement deviation analysis. $P < 0.05$ was considered statistically significant.

Results

Between April and July in 2019, 342 pregnant women at two centers were evaluated for study participation. Of these, eighteen women did not meet the inclusion criteria, twenty women refused to participate, and four women were excluded for other reasons (Fig. 1). Finally, three hundred patients were randomly 1:1:1 divided into

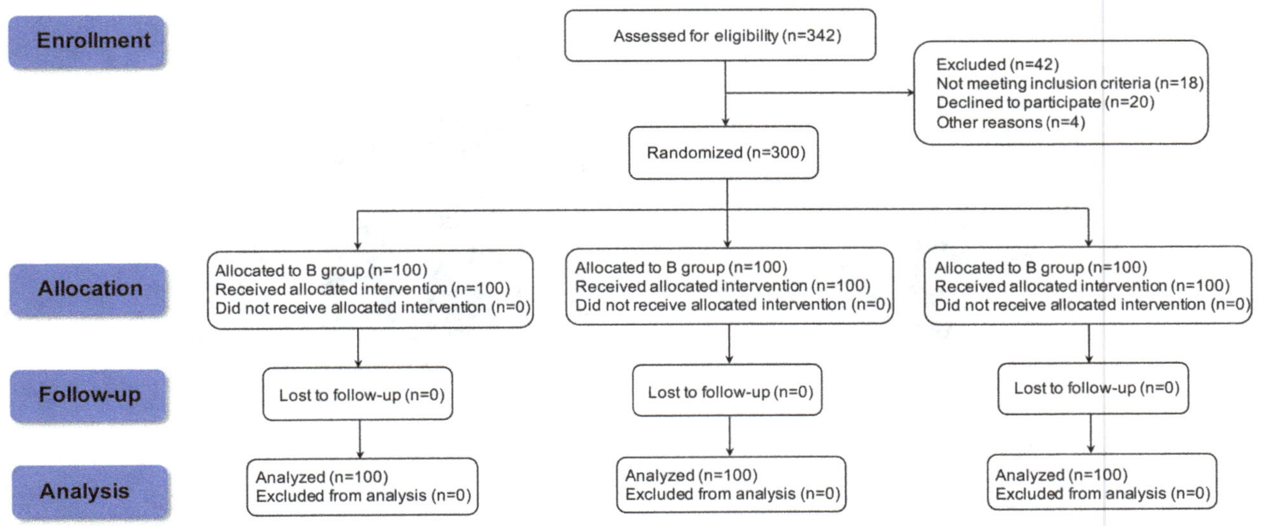

Fig. 1 Study population flow diagram

group B ($n = 100$), group FB ($n = 100$) and group DB ($n = 100$). All patients were well-blocked and no one needed additional analgesia during the surgery. In addition, all patients completed the assessment and received postoperative follow-up for 30 days.

The three groups were comparable with regard to baseline variables include age, height, weight, BMI, ASA physical status, gestational age. There were also no significant differences in perioperative variables including peak sensory level, duration of surgery, intraoperative fluid volume and blood loss (Table 1).

Compared with group B, the duration of sensory block in group FB and group DB were prolonged (108.4 min [95% Confidence Interval (CI) = 104.6–112.3] in group B, and 122.0 min [95% CI = 116.8–127.3] in group FB, 148.2 min [95% CI = 145.3–151.1] in group DB) with statistical significance ($P < 0.001$) (Fig. 2a). The duration of sensory block was significantly longer in group DB as compared with group FB ($P < 0.001$). Compared with group B, the onset time of sensory block (Fig. 2b) in group DB was significantly shorter (12.2 s [95% CI = 12.0–12.4]) in group DB, 14.5 s [95% CI = 14.0–15.1] in

Table 1 Baseline and perioperative characteristics of parturients

	Group B ($n = 100$)	Group FB ($n = 100$)	Group DB ($n = 100$)	*P*-Value
Age (yr.)	27 (26–29)	27 (25–30)	27 (25–29)	0.244
Height (cm)	161.5 (159.0–164.0)	162.0 (159.0–165.0)	160 (159.0–164.0)	0.284
Weight (kg)	72.3 ± 6.2	72.8 ± 5.3	72.6 ± 5.3	0.771
BMI (kg/m^2)	27.6 ± 2.5	27.6 ± 2.2	27.8 ± 2.3	0.865
ASA physical status, n (%)				0.394
II	78 (78)	74 (74)	82 (82)	
III	22 (22)	26 (26)	18 (18)	
Gestational week (Wk.)	39 (38–39)	39 (38–39)	39 (38–39)	0.379
Peak sensory level				0.846
T2	2 (2)	1 (1)	1 (1)	
T4	37 (37)	36 (36)	42 (42)	
T6	61 (61)	63 (63)	57 (57)	
Surgery duration (min)	41.0 (38.0–44.0)	41.0 (39.0–44.0)	41.0 (39.0–44.0)	0.746
Intraoperative fluid volume (ml)	1351.1 ± 115.4	1361.6 ± 97.8	1356.5 ± 98.7	0.775
Intraoperative blood loss (ml)	421.2 ± 36.0	424.5 ± 30.5	423.1 ± 30.7	0.773

Notes: Data are presented as n (%) or mean ± SD or median (range); There were no significant differences among the three groups ($P > 0.05$). Group B = bupivacaine group; Group FB = bupivacaine and fentanyl group; Group DB = bupivacaine and dexmedetomidine group
Abbreviations: *ASA* American Society of Anesthesiologists, *BMI* Body Mass Index

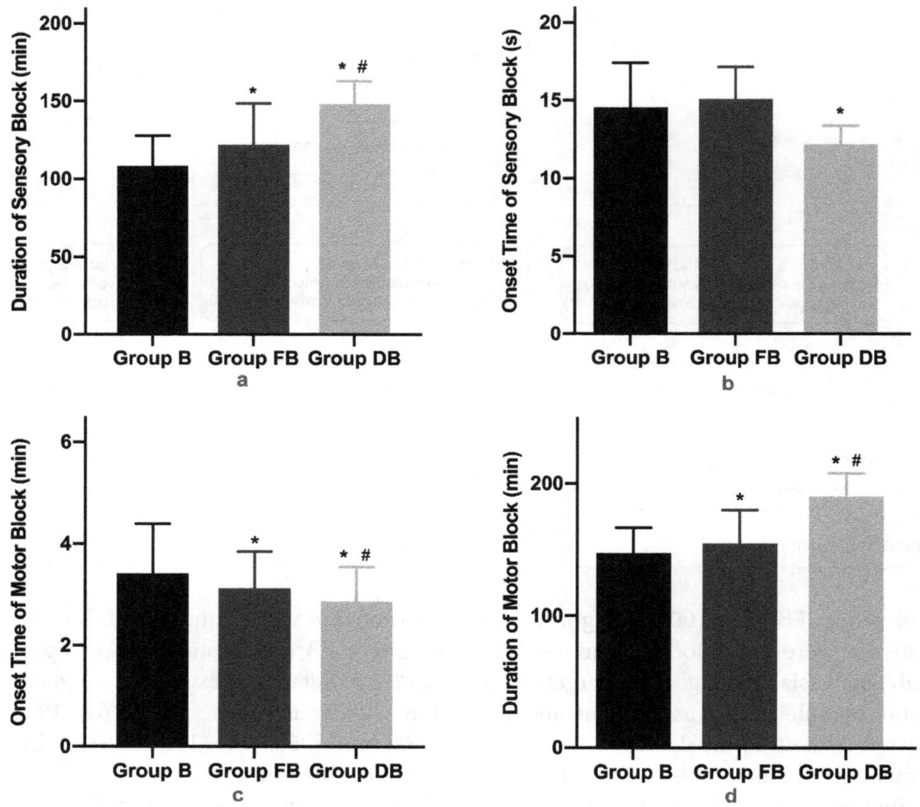

Fig. 2 Block characteristics of parturientsNotes: Group B = bupivacaine group; Group FB = bupivacaine and fentanyl group; Group DB = bupivacaine and dexmedetomidine group. * $P < 0.017$ Group DB or Group FB vs Group B; # $P < 0.017$ Group DB vs Group FB.

group B, $P < 0.001$). Besides, compared with group B and group FB (Fig. 2c), the onset time of motor block in group DB was statistically shorter (2.9 min [95% CI = 2.7–3.0] in group DB, 3.1 min [95% CI = 3.0–3.3] in group FB, 3.4 min [95% CI = 3.2–3.6], in group B, $P < 0.001$). However, compared with group B (147.5 min [95% CI = 143.7–151.3]), the duration of motor block (Fig. 2d) in group DB (190.3 min [95% CI = 186.9–193.8]) was prolonged by 43 min ($P < 0.001$), while that in group FB (154.9 min [95% CI = 150.0–160.0]) was prolonged by 7 min ($P = 0.038$).

There were 11 items in ObsQoR-11 score Table (Table 2) to reflect the quality of postoperative recovery. The overall score of group DB (71.6 [95% CI = 71.0–72.2]) was higher than that of group FB (61.5 [95% CI = 60.8–62.2], $P < 0.001$) and group B (61.7 [95% CI = 61.0–62.4], $P < 0.001$). All items showed recovery quality of group DB was significantly better than that of group B, except in terms of feeling dizzy ($P > 0.05$). Moreover, there was no statistical difference between group B and group FB about the ObsQoR-11 score.

Kaplan-Meier curve (Fig. 3) showed that time to first analgesic request in group DB was longer than that in group FB and group B (log-rank $P < 0.017$). However, the sufentanil dosage within postoperative 24 h was not statistically different among three groups ($P = 0.681$).

The maternal hemodynamic characteristics including HR and mean arterial pressure (MAP) were found significantly higher in group DB than that in group B (Fig. 4). The incidence of shivering (Table 3) was statistically lowered in group DB (3%) compared with group FB (18%) and group B (35%). The incidence of hypotension in group DB (33%) was higher than that in group FB (25%) and group B (28%) but with no statistical difference. There was no statistical difference for the dosage of ephedrine and atropine, intra-operative or post-operative nausea and vomiting among three groups.

For PH, PaO_2, and $PaCO_2$ in the umbilical artery and umbilical vein blood of newborn (Table 4), there were no statistically significant among the three groups. The concentration of DEX in umbilical artery and umbilical vein was too low to be detected by High-Performance Liquid Chromatography Tandem Mass Spectrometry. The mean values of Apgar scores at 1st and 5th min were all beyond 8, which also showed no statistical significance. Moreover, the 30-daysfollow-up did not show any new onset of back, buttock or leg pain or paresthesia.

Table 2 ObsQoR-11 of parturients

	Group B (n = 100)	Group FB (n = 100)	Group DB (n = 100)	P-Value
Moderate pain	3.6 ± 1.1	5.6 ± 0.9*	7.3 ± 1.2*#	< 0.001
Severe pain	4.4 ± 1.2	5.0 ± 2.1*	7.5 ± 1.6*#	< 0.001
Nausea or vomiting	5.2 ± 1.0	6.0 ± 0.9*	7.3 ± 1.2*#	< 0.001
Feeling dizzy	6.3 ± 1.2	5.0 ± 0.8*	6.3 ± 1.1#	< 0.001
Shivering	3.7 ± 0.8	5.3 ± 0.7*	7.2 ± 1.0*#	< 0.001
Have been comfortable	6.4 ± 1.0	6.4 ± 0.6	7.4 ± 1.8*#	< 0.001
Able to mobilize independently	6.0 ± 1.9	6.9 ± 1.5*	6.9 ± 1.1*	< 0.001
Can hold baby without assistance	6.9 ± 0.8	8.2 ± 0.7*	8.1 ± 0.8*	< 0.001
Can feed/nurse baby without assistance	6.6 ± 0.7	7.0 ± 1.0*	7.1 ± 0.7*	< 0.001
Can look after personal hygiene/toilet	5.6 ± 0.9	6.3 ± 0.6*	6.5 ± 0.9*	< 0.001
Feeling in control	7.0 ± 0.8	7.3 ± 1.0*	8.0 ± 0.8*#	< 0.001
Total	61.7 ± 3.3	61.5 ± 3.6	71.6 ± 3.1*#	< 0.001

Notes: Data are presented as mean ± SD; Group B = bupivacaine group; Group FB = bupivacaine and fentanyl group; Group DB = bupivacaine and dexmedetomidine group; ObsQoR-11 = obstetric quality of recovery-11 score, 0–10 in each term, where 0 = strongly agree and 10 = strongly disagree
* P < 0.017 Group DB or Group FB vs Group B; # P < 0.017 Group DB vs Group FB

Discussion

Our results showed that compared with 9 mg of bupivacaine alone, the combination of 5 μg of DEX for cesarean section could significantly prolong the duration of sensory block and improve paturients' recovery quality with no neonatal adverse effects or maternal neurotoxicity in the short term.

Spinal anesthesia, which is block-well, easy to operate, not as complicated as epidural anesthesia [19], and avoiding the maternal risk of general anesthesia, has become the preferred anesthesia type for cesarean section. However, in clinical practice, single-shot spinal anesthesia was often not sufficient to inhibit visceral pain, causing maternal discomfort during the surgery, which affect parturients' postoperative recovery quality [6]. While increasing the doses of local anesthetics to prolong the analgesic time could lead to adverse effects such as central nervous system problems and cardiotoxicity. In our study, compared with intrathecal 9 mg of bupivacaine alone, the onset time of sensory and motor block of parturients in combination of 9 mg of intrathecal bupivacaine with 5 μg of DEX was significantly

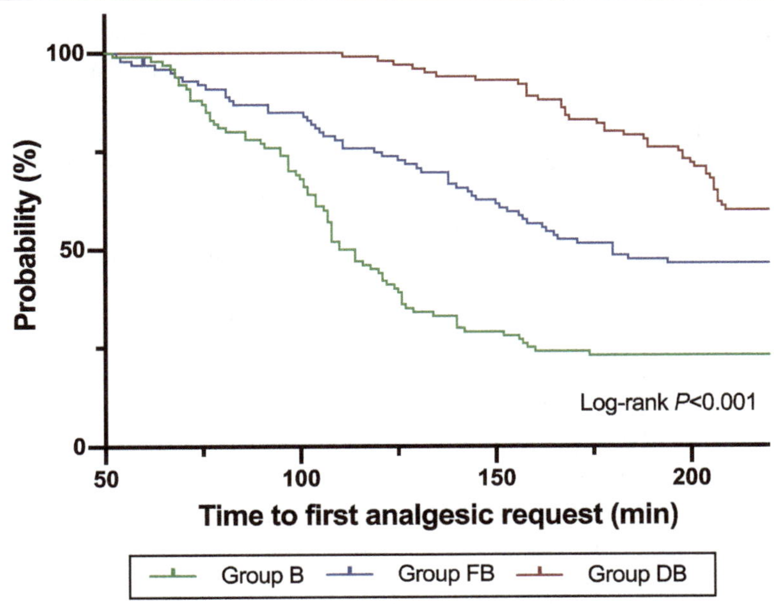

Fig. 3 Kaplan-Meier curves for time to first analgesic request. Notes: Group B = bupivacaine group; Group FB = bupivacaine and fentanyl group; Group DB = bupivacaine and dexmedetomidine group

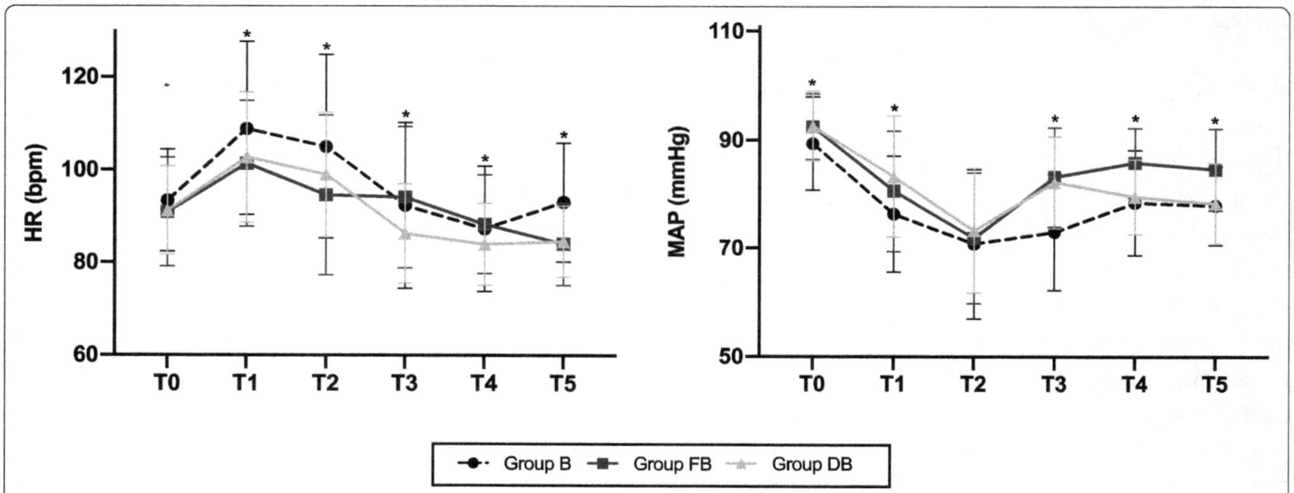

Fig. 4 Hemodynamic parameters. Notes: Group B = bupivacaine group; Group FB = bupivacaine and fentanyl group; Group DB = bupivacaine and dexmedetomidine group; T0 = before spinal anesthesia, T1, T2, T3, T4, T5 = 0, 5, 10, 15, 20 min after spinal anesthesia. HR = Heart Rate; MAP = Mean Arterial Pressure; *There were significant differences among the three groups ($P < 0.05$)

shortened, and the duration of sensory block was significantly prolonged by 40 min, which is consistent with the research results of Suthar's [20] and Sushruta's [10]. The mechanism may be as follows: DEX can activate the α-2 adrenergic receptor in the dorsal horn neurons, activate the spinal cord intermediate neurons by reducing the neurotransmitter released by the primary afferent end and G-protein-mediated potassium channel, and make the spinal cord intermediate neurons hyperpolarized, thus reducing the pain transmission. In addition, DEX can also block the internal flow of Na + and enhance the blocking effect of local anesthetics on the sodium channel of the cell membrane [21, 22]. However, consisted with the results of a meta-analysis [23] that included 9 RCTs, our study found that motor block duration of paturients with intrathecal DEX was also prolonged, which suggest that combination with DEX may increase the fall risk and delay the early rehabilitation of parturients.

Currently, the commonly used postoperative recovery quality scales were QoR-40 [24] and QoR-15 [25]. However, both of them are developed and verified in non-obstetric patients and day surgery population [26], so there are many items unrelated to cesarean section, and lack of critical elements to evaluate postoperative recovery after delivery such as the ability of caring babies [18]. The ObsQoR-11 scale has been proved to be reliable, clinically acceptable, feasible and effective in patients undergoing elective and emergency cesarean section [18, 27]. In our study, all questionnaire feedback had been received and the results showed that scores in group DB was higher than in both group FB and group B ($P < 0.017$), suggesting that parturients with intrathecal DEX had a better recovery quality.

Consistent with the findings of meta-analysis conducted by Miao [12], intrathecal DEX can significantly reduce the incidence of shivering in parturients undergoing spinal anesthesia. The mechanism of anti-shivering effect can be inferred that DEX could reduce central thermos-sensitivity by weakening the electrical conductivity of neurons through mediating the α-2 adrenergic receptors in the brain and spinal cord [28, 29]. Moreover, intrathecal DEX showed added advantages on block characteristics and ObsQoR-11 score compared with intrathecal fentanyl, suggesting a better clinical application prospect.

Table 3 Maternal outcomes

	Group B (*n* = 100)	Group FB (*n* = 100)	Group DB (*n* = 100)	*P*-Value
Shivering, n (%)	35 (35)	18 (82) *	3 (97) *#	< 0.001
Hypotension, n (%)	28 (28)	25 (25)	33 (33)	0.450
Dose of ephedrine (mg)	2.8 ± 3.9	2.1 ± 3.6	1.5 ± 3.0	0.029
Nausea and/or vomiting, n (%)	11 (11)	17 (17)	14 (14)	0.474
Sufentanil consumption (μg)	106.0 ± 9.2	105.5 ± 7.7	105.0 ± 7.8	0.681

Notes: Data are presented as n (%) or mean ± SD; Group B = bupivacaine group; Group FB = bupivacaine and fentanyl group; Group DB = bupivacaine and dexmedetomidine group

*$P < 0.017$ Group DB or Group FB vs Group B; #$P < 0.017$ Group DB vs Group FB

Table 4 Neonatal outcomes

	Group B ($n = 100$)	Group FB ($n = 100$)	Group DB ($n = 100$)	*P*-Value
Umbilical artery				
pH	7.3 ± 0.3	7.3 ± 0.2	7.3 ± 0.4	0.581
PaO_2 (mmHg)	15.6 ± 2.0	15.0 ± 2.3	15.4 ± 2.4	0.217
$PaCO_2$ (mmHg)	49.9 ± 3.4	49.8 ± 4.0	50.4 ± 4.6	0.545
Umbilical vein				
pH	7.4 ± 0.2	7.4 ± 0.1	7.4 ± 0.5	0.711
PaO_2 (mmHg)	30.0 ± 3.4	30.7 ± 4.4	30.80 ± 3.5	0.277
$PaCO_2$ (mmHg)	42.6 ± 3.2	41.6 ± 3.8	42.0 ± 3.2	0.111
Apgar score				
1 min	8.7 ± 0.5	8.7 ± 0.5	8.7 ± 0.5	0.752
5 min	9.7 ± 0.5	9.7 ± 0.4	9.7 ± 0.5	0.809

Notes: Data are presented as mean ± SD; Group B = bupivacaine group; Group FB = bupivacaine and fentanyl group; Group DB = bupivacaine and dexmedetomidine group
$^*P < 0.017$ Group DB or Group FB vs Group B; $^\#P < 0.017$ Group DB vs Group FB

When intrathecal DEX during cesarean section, one of the main concerns was the maternal neurotoxicity. Therefore, all participants were followed up for 30 days after surgery, and none of them showed neurological complications of lower limbs and buttocks, indicating that intrathecal DEX would not lead to nerve injury in the short term. Ozdamar [30] injected 10 rats with DEX 10 μg through the subarachnoid path and extracted spinal medulla for histological and electron microscopy examination after 7 days, and the results showed that compared with saline group, no signs of neuronal or axonal injury, gliosis, or myelin sheath damage was found. Another concern was the adverse effects on the fetus, which was excluded by the blood gas analysis and Apgar scores in our study. Li et al. [31] showed similar results, which further confirmed our conclusion. A placental perfusion study in vitro conducted by Ala-Kokko [32] found that the DEX fetal: maternal concentration ratio was 0.77, which meant DEX in maternal circulation was easy to pass through the placental barrier. Currently, there is no firm clinical data about whether DEX would be absorbed into the maternal circulation and transferred to the fetus via the placenta under the intrathecal administration. In our study, the plasma concentration of DEX in the UA and UV was measured and no DEX accumulation was detected, suggesting that intrathecal 5 μg of DEX caused a low or even no drug exposure on the fetus, which would not lead to adverse effects.

There were also some limitations in our study. Firstly, the adequacy of muscle relaxation during the surgery and the satisfaction of parturients and obstetricians were not measured, further studies should use more parameters to explore the efficacy of intrathecal DEX; Secondly, due to the invasive arterial blood pressure monitoring was not performed during the operation, the information concerning the placental transfer was not obtained with no maternal blood plasma sample collected; Thirdly, we did not investigate the dose-response reaction of DEX, and the optimal clinical dose was not determined. Furthermore, the postoperative follow-up period in this study was only 30 days, so it is unknown whether patients had delayed adverse neuron reactions.

Conclusion

DEX is a potential local anesthetic adjuvant that the intrathecal combination of 5 μg DEX can safely exhibit a facilitatory block effect and improve parturients' recovery quality. However, large sample clinical studies to support the safety of intrathecal DEX use in the clinical setting are still needed.

Abbreviations

DEX: Dexmedetomidine; CI: Confidence Interval;; SpO2: Pulse Oxygen Saturation; HR: Heart Rate; ECG: Electrocardiogram; NIBP: Noninvasive Blood Pressure; SBP: Systolic Blood Pressure; MBS: Modified Bromage scale; ObsQoR-11: Obstetric Quality of Recovery-11 Score; MAP: Mean Arterial Pressure; RR: Relative Risk; ASA: American Society of Anesthesiologists; BMI: Body Mass Index

Acknowledgments

This study thanked Ph.D. Yuan and his team for offering help in plasma concentration measurement of dexmedetomidine.

Authors' contributions

LXX contributed to study design, interpretation of data, and drafted the manuscript. LS contributed to study design, and interpretation of the data, revised the manuscript, and approved the final version. LYM was primarily responsible for the processing and analysis of blood samples. LXL contributed to analysis, and approved the final version. WXH was responsible for the follow up. All authors have read and approved the final manuscript.

Author details

[1]Jiangsu Province Key Laboratory of Anesthesiology, Xuzhou Medical University, Xuzhou, Jiangsu, China. [2]Feng Xian People's Hospital of Jiangsu Province, Xuzhou, Jiangsu, China. [3]Department of Anesthesiology, the Affiliated Hospital of Xuzhou Medical University, 99 Huaihai West Road, Xuzhou 221000, Jiangsu, China.

References

1. Juang J, Gabriel RA, Dutton RP, et al. Choice of anesthesia for cesarean delivery: an analysis of the national anesthesia clinical outcomes registry. Anesth Analg. 2017;124:1914–7.
2. Kim WH, Hur M, Park SK, et al. Comparison between general, spinal, epidural, and combined spinal-epidural anesthesia for cesarean delivery: a network meta-analysis. Int J Obstet Anesth. 2019;37:5–15.
3. Ghaffari S, Dehghanpisheh L, Tavakkoli F, et al. The effect of spinal versus general anesthesia on quality of life in women undergoing cesarean delivery on maternal request. Cureus. 2018;11(12):e3715.
4. Riley ET. Regional anesthesia for cesarean section. Tech Reg Anesth Pain Manage. 2003;7:204–12.
5. Wu CL, Rowlingson AJ, Partin AW, et al. Correlation of postoperative pain to quality of recovery in the immediate postoperative period. Reg Anesth Pain Med. 2005;30(6):516–22.
6. Catro A, Lucas S, De A, et al. The effect of Neuraxial versus general anesthesia techniques on postoperative quality of recovery and analgesia after abdominal hysterectomy: a prospective randomized controlled trial. Anesth Analg. 2011;113(6):1480–6.
7. Fernandes HS, Bliacheriene F, Vago TM, et al. Clonidine effect on pain after cesarean delivery: a randomized controlled trial of different routes of administration. Anesth Analg. 2018;127(1):165–70.
8. Uppal V, Retter S, Casey M, et al. Efficacy of intrathecal fentanyl for cesarean delivery: a systematic review and meta-analysis of randomized controlled trials with trial sequential analysis. Anesth Analg. 2019;130(1):111.
9. Hall JE, Uhrich TD, Barney JA, et al. Sedative, amnestic, and analgesic properties of small-dose Dexmedetomidine infusions. Anesth Analg. 2000; 90(3):699–705.
10. Sushruth MR, Rao DG. Effect of adding intrathecal dexmedetomidine as an adjuvant to hyperbaric bupivacaine for elective cesarean section. Anaesth Pain Intensive Care. 2018;22(3):348–54.
11. Gupta M, Gupta P, Singh DK. Effect of 3 different doses of intrathecal dexmedetomidine (2.5mg, 5mg, and 10 mg) on subarachnoid block characteristics: a prospective randomized double-blind dose-response trial. Pain Physician. 2016;19(3):e411–20.
12. Miao S, Shi M, Zou L, et al. Effect of intrathecal dexmedetomidine on preventing shivering in cesarean section after spinal anesthesia: a meta-analysis and trial sequential analysis. Drug Des Devel Ther. 2018;12:3775–83.
13. Singh AP, Chawla S, Bajwa SJS, et al. Efficacy and safety of dexmedetomidine as an intrathecal agent: a dose finding clinical study. Anaesth Pain Intensive Care. 2017;21(1):13–8.
14. Axelsson K, Widman GB. A comparison of bupivacaine and tetracaine in spinal anaesthesia with special reference to motor block. Acta Anaesthesiol Scand. 1985;29:79–86.
15. Russell IF. Assessing the block for caesarean section. Int J Obstet Anesth. 2001;10(2):83–5.
16. Wang X, Fang F, Zhu XG. Clinical application of combined spinal-epidural anesthesia with fentanyl and ropivacaine in cesarean section. J Southeast Univ (Med Sci Edi). 2014;33(2):170–3.
17. Pais de Barros JP, Gautier T, Sali W, et al. Quantitative lipopolysaccharide analysis using HPLC/MS/MS and its combination with the limulus Amebocyte lysate assay. J Lipid Res. 2015;56(7):1363–9.
18. Ciechanowicz S, Setty T, Robson E, et al. Development and evaluation of an obstetric quality-of-recovery score (ObsQoR-11) after elective caesarean delivery. Br J Anaesth. 2019;122(1):69–78.
19. Heesen M, Klöhr S, Rossaint R, et al. Insertion of an intrathecal catheter following accidental dural puncture: a meta-analysis. Int J Obstet Anesth. 2013;22(1):26–30.
20. Suthar O, Sethi P, Sharma UD. A comparison of intrathecal dexmedetomidine, clonidine, and fentanyl as adjuvants to hyperbaric bupivacaine for lower limb surgery: a double-blind controlled study. J Anaesthesiol Clin Pharmacol. 2013;29(4):496–502.
21. Khan ZP, Ferguson CN, Jones RM. Alpha-2 and imidazoline receptor agonists. Their pharmacology and therapeutic role. Anaesthesia. 1999;54(2): 146–65.
22. Oda A, Iida H, Tanahashi S, et al. Effects of alpha2-adrenoceptor agonists on tetrodotoxin-resistant Na+ channels in rat dorsal root ganglion neurons. Eur J Anaesthesiol. 2007;24(11):934–41.
23. Abdallah FW, Brull R. Facilitatory effects of perineural dexmedetomidine on neuraxial and peripheral nerve block: a systematic review and meta-analysis. Br J Anaesth. 2013;110(6):915–25.
24. Myles PS, Weitkamp B, Jones K, et al. Validity and reliability of a postoperative quality of recovery score: the QoR-40. Br J Anaesth. 2000;84: 11e5.
25. Stark PA, Myles PS, Burke JA. Development and psychometric evaluation of a postoperative quality of recovery score: the QoR-15. Anesthesiology. 2013; 118:1332e40.
26. Chazapis M, Walker EM, Rooms MA, et al. Measuring quality of recovery-15 after day-case surgery. Br J Anaesth. 2016;116:241e8.
27. Ciechanowicz S, Howle R, Heppolette C, et al. Evaluation of the obstetric quality-of-recovery score (ObsQoR-11) following non-elective caesarean delivery. Int J Obstet Anesth. 2019;39:51–9.
28. Nasseri K, Ghadami N, Nouri B. Effects of intrathecal dexmedetomidine on shivering after spinal anesthesia for cesarean section: a double-blind randomized clinical trial. Drug Des Devel Ther. 2017;11:1107–13.
29. Mittal G, Gupta K, Katyal S, et al. Randomised double-blind comparative study of dexmedetomidine and tramadol for post-spinal anaesthesia shivering. Indian J Anaesth. 2014;58:257–62.
30. Ozdamar D, Dayioglu H, Anik I, et al. Evaluation of the neurotoxicity of intrathecal dexmedetomidine on rat spinal cord (electro microscopic observations). Saudi J Anaesth. 2018;12(1):10–5.
31. Li Z, Tian M, Zhang CY, et al. A randomized controlled trial to evaluate the effectiveness of intrathecal bupivacaine combined with different adjuvants (fentanyl, clonidine and Dexmedetomidine) in caesarean section. Drug Res. 2015;65(11):581–6.
32. Ala-Kokko TI, Pienimäki P, Lampela E, Hollmén AI, Pelkonen O, Vähäkangas K. Transfer of clonidine and dexmedetomidine across the isolated perfused human placenta. Acta Anaesthesiol Scand. 1997;41(2):313–9.

Comparative study between intrathecal dexmedetomidine and intrathecal magnesium sulfate for the prevention of post-spinal anaesthesia shivering in uroscopic surgery

Heba Omar[1], Wessam Adel Aboella[2], Mohammed Mahmoud Hassan[3], Amany Hassan[1], Passaint Hassan[1], Ahmed Elshall[1], Dalia Khaled[1], Maha Mostafa[1], Pierre Zarif Tawadros[1], Mona Hossam Eldin[1], Mai Wedad[1] and Bassant Mohamed Abdelhamid[1*]

Abstract

Background: Hypothermia and shivering are common complications after spinal anaesthesia, especially after uroscopic procedures in which large amounts of cold intraluminal irrigation fluids are used. Magnesium sulfate and dexmedetomidine are the most effective adjuvants with the least side effects. The aim of this study was to compare the effects of intrathecal dexmedetomidine versus intrathecal magnesium sulfate on the prevention of post-spinal anaesthesia shivering.

Methods: This prospective randomized, double-blinded controlled study included 105 patients who were scheduled for uroscopic surgery at the Kasr El-Aini Hospital. The patients were randomly allocated into three groups. **Group C (*n* = 35) received** 2.5 ml of hyperbaric bupivacaine 0.5% (12.5 mg) + 0.5 ml of normal saline, **Group M (*n* = 35)** received 2.5 ml of hyperbaric bupivacaine 0.5% (12.5 mg) + 25 mg of magnesium sulfate in 0.5 ml saline, and **Group D (*n* = 35)** received 2.5 ml of hyperbaric bupivacaine 0.5% (12.5 mg) + 5 μg of dexmedetomidine in 0.5 ml saline. The primary outcomes were the incidence and intensity of shivering. The secondary outcomes were the incidence of hypothermia, sedation, the use of meperidine to control shivering and complications.

Results: Group C had significantly higher proportions of patients who developed shivering (21), developed grade IV shivering (20) and required meperidine (21) to treat shivering than group M (8,5,5) and group D (5,3,6), which were comparable to each other.

The time between block administration and meperidine administration was similar among the three groups. Hypothermia did not occur in any of the patients.

The three groups were comparable regarding the occurrence of nausea, vomiting, bradycardia and hypotension. All the patients in group C, 32 patients in group M and 33 patients in group D had a sedation score of 2. Three patients in group M and 2 patients in group D had a sedation score of 3.

Conclusions: Intrathecal injections of both dexmedetomidine and magnesium sulfate were effective in reducing the incidence of post-spinal anaesthesia shivering. Therefore, we encourage the use of magnesium sulfate, as it is more physiologically available, more readily available in most operating theatres and much less expensive than dexmedetomidine.

(Continued on next page)

* Correspondence: bassantmohamed197@yahoo.com
[1]Anesthesia Department, Faculty of Medicine, Cairo University, Cairo, Egypt

(Continued from previous page)

Keywords: Dexmedetomidine, Magnesium, Spinal, Shivering

Background

For short procedures such as uroscopic surgeries, spinal anaesthesia (SA) is a very reliable and convenient technique, especially for procedures in which patient consciousness must be maintained to detect intraoperative complications, such as transurethral resection of the prostate (TURP) syndrome [1]. However, hypothermia and shivering are common complications after SA, especially when large amounts of cold intraluminal irrigating fluids are used [2]. SA impairs thermoregulation, inhibits tonic vasoconstriction, and causes the redistribution of core heat from the trunk to the peripheral tissue [3]. Shivering interferes with proper monitoring and is associated with several adverse effects, as it increases the circulating catecholamine, heart rate, cardiac output, minute ventilation, patient oxygen consumption, metabolic CO_2 production, lactic acid level, intraocular and intracranial pressure, and postoperative pain from surgical incision stretching [4].

Various opioid and non-opioid agents, such as meperidine, ketamine, tramadol, and clonidine, have been used to prevent shivering, but they have many side effects, and their results have not been conclusive [5].

Dexmedetomidine is a highly selective alpha-2- adrenoreceptor agonist with potent effects on the central nervous system, decreasing the sympathetic tone [5]. It has been effectively used intravenously for the treatment [6–10] and prevention [11–14] of shivering following SA without any major adverse effects in several studies. Few trials have examined intrathecal dexmedetomidine for the prevention of post-SA shivering [5, 15].

Magnesium sulfate ($MgSO_4$), which is an inorganic salt, has been shown to suppress postoperative shivering, indicating that the agent reduces the shivering threshold [16]. It has a good safety profile, as there are no side effects related to the intrathecal use of the drug and no significant changes in haemodynamic parameters have been reported [17]. Intravenous (IV) $MgSO_4$ has been effectively examined in many trials [2, 18–20], but few trials involving intrathecal $MgSO_4$ [3] to control shivering have been conducted.

The aim of this study was to evaluate and compare the effects of intrathecal dexmedetomidine versus intrathecal $MgSO_4$ on the prevention of post-SA shivering.

The primary outcomes were the incidence and intensity of shivering. The secondary outcomes were the incidence of pethidine use, haemodynamic parameters and incidence of complications, including hypotension, bradycardia and sedation.

Methods

After approval from the Ethics Committee of Cairo University Hospital (12015006), protocol registration in the Pan African Clinical Trial Registry (PACTR) (clinical trial registration ID: PACTR201801003001727, -retrospectively registered-) and obtaining informed written consent from each patient, this prospective randomized, double-blinded randomized controlled study was conducted at Kasr El-Aini Hospital in the urosurgical operating theatre following the Consolidated Standards for Reporting Trials (CONSORT) guidelines. A total of 105 patients scheduled for uroscopic surgery were enrolled. The **inclusion criteria** were as follows: patients aged between 20 and 60 years and patients with American Society of Anesthesiologists (ASA) class I or class II physical status. **The exclusion criteria** were as follows: patients who refused patients with coagulopathy, patients with a history of allergic reactions to local anaesthetics or patients with severe cardiac, respiratory, hepatic or renal diseases.

In the operating room, after lidocaine 2% was applied to the skin, venous puncture was performed with an 18 gauge cannula, and a preload of 500 ml of lactated Ringer's solution was infused; no premedication was given. Five-lead electrocardiogram (ECG), pulse oximetry and non-invasive arterial blood pressure (NABP) monitoring was performed. The baseline systolic and diastolic arterial blood pressures (SBP and DBP), heart rate (HR) and arterial oxygen saturation (PSO_2) were recorded. A spinal block was performed at the L3-L4 or L4-L5 interspace with a 22-gauge spinal needle after sterilization by povidone iodine while the patient was sitting and leaning forward; 2 cm of lidocaine 1% was applied to the skin at the site of lumbar puncture.

The patients were randomly allocated into three equal groups using computer-generated randomization tables. **Group C (n = 35) received** 2.5 ml of hyperbaric bupivacaine 0.5% (12.5 mg) + 0.5 ml of normal saline, **Group M (n = 35)** received 2.5 ml of hyperbaric bupivacaine 0.5% (12.5 mg) + 25 mg $MgSO_4$ in 0.5 ml saline, and **Group D (n = 35)** received 2.5 ml of hyperbaric bupivacaine 0.5% (12.5 mg) + 5 μg dexmedetomidine in 0.5 ml saline. Patients' assigned numbers and treatments were concealed in closed opaque envelopes that were retained by two members on the authors' team who had no interaction with the patients. The specific intrathecal drug solutions were prepared and injected by an anaesthesiologist who was not involved in the study. The anaesthesiologists involved in patient observation and data collection were blinded to the treatment group, as were the patients.

The onset and durations of the motor and sensory blocks were assessed by the Bromage scale and pinprick test, respectively. The level of the block was assessed to ensure that it was between T10-T8; blocks higher than T8 and failed blocks were excluded. A surgical drape was placed over the patient, the room temperature was maintained at 24 °C, and all the irrigation and IV fluids were pre-warmed. No warming device was used. The incidence and intensity of shivering were assessed by a blinded observer immediately after the block was administered, every 5 min for the first 15 min, and then every 10 min for 2 h after the block using the Crossley and Mahajan scale [21] (0 = no shivering, 1 = piloerection or peripheral vasoconstriction but no visible shivering, 2 = muscular activity in only one muscle group, 3 = muscular activity in more than one muscle group but not generalized shivering, 4 = shivering involving the whole body). Twenty-five milligrams of IV meperidine was given when a patient presented grade 3 shivering. The core temperature was monitored using a tympanic probe before the block, immediately after the block and every 15 min for 2 h after the block. Hypothermia and active warming were considered if the core temperature reached 36 °C. The patient's HR, BP and SPO_2 were recorded every 5 min for the first 15 min and then every 10 min for 2 h after the block.

The sedation level was observed and recorded every 30 min for 2 h or until the administration of IV pethidine using the Ramsay sedation scale [22] (1 = the patient was anxious, agitated or restless; 2 = the patient was cooperative, oriented, and tranquil; 3 = the patient only responded to commands; 4 = the patient exhibited an immediate response to light glabellar tap or loud auditory stimulus; 5 = the patient exhibited a sluggish response to a light glabellar tap or loud auditory stimulus; and 6 = the patient exhibited no response).

The patients were monitored for complications. Hypotension (20% decrease in the SBP from baseline) was treated with incremental administration of 3 mg of ephedrine and 200 ml of lactated Ringer's solution, and bradycardia (HR < 50) was treated with a bolus of 0.01–0.02 mg/kg of atropine. Nausea and vomiting were treated with 10 mg of metoclopramide.

Postoperatively, patients were transferred to the postanaesthesia care unit (PACU), monitored and covered with a cotton sheet. The PACU temperature was maintained at 25 °C.

The primary outcomes were the incidence and intensity of shivering. The secondary outcomes were incidence of hypothermia, sedation, the use of pethidine to control shivering and complications including hypotension, bradycardia, nausea and vomiting.

Statistical analysis

Sample size

A power analysis using the chi-square test for independent samples was performed to analyse the frequency of patients complaining of intraoperative and early postoperative shivering because it was the main outcome variable in the present study. Previous studies showed that the frequency of patients with perioperative shivering was approximately 50% in patients who underwent elective minor lower abdominal operations under SA and 20% in patients who received dexmedetomidine [15]. Considering a power of 0.8 and an alpha error of 0.025, a minimum sample size of 35 patients was required for each group.

Method of analysis

The data were entered into the "Microsoft Office Excel" software program (2010) for Windows. The data were then entered into the Statistical Package for the Social Sciences software program, version 20 (IBM SPSS Statistics for Windows, Version 20.0. Armonk, NY: IBM Corp.), for statistical analysis.

The quantitative variables were presented as ranges and means plus standard deviations, and the qualitative variables were presented as frequencies and percentages.

Sex and ASA grade were presented as numbers and percentages. Age, height, weight, and sensory and motor block onset and duration were presented as means and standard deviations. Shivering incidence, ASA grades, the need for meperidine and complications were presented as numbers and percentages.

The Kolmogorov-Smirnov test was used to verify the normality of the distribution of the quantitative data described using means and standard deviations. Significance was considered at the 5% level. **Chi-square tests** were used to compare the categorical variables between the different groups. **F-tests (ANOVA)** were used to compare the normally distributed quantitative variables between the three groups, and post hoc tests (Tukey's tests) were used for the pairwise comparisons.

Results

One hundred eighteen patients scheduled for uroscopic surgery were enrolled in this study; 8 patients did not meet the inclusion criteria, and 5 patients were excluded from the study due to failure to achieve spinal block within 15 min (Fig. 1). The types of the performed surgeries included cystoscopy (41 patients), TURP (17

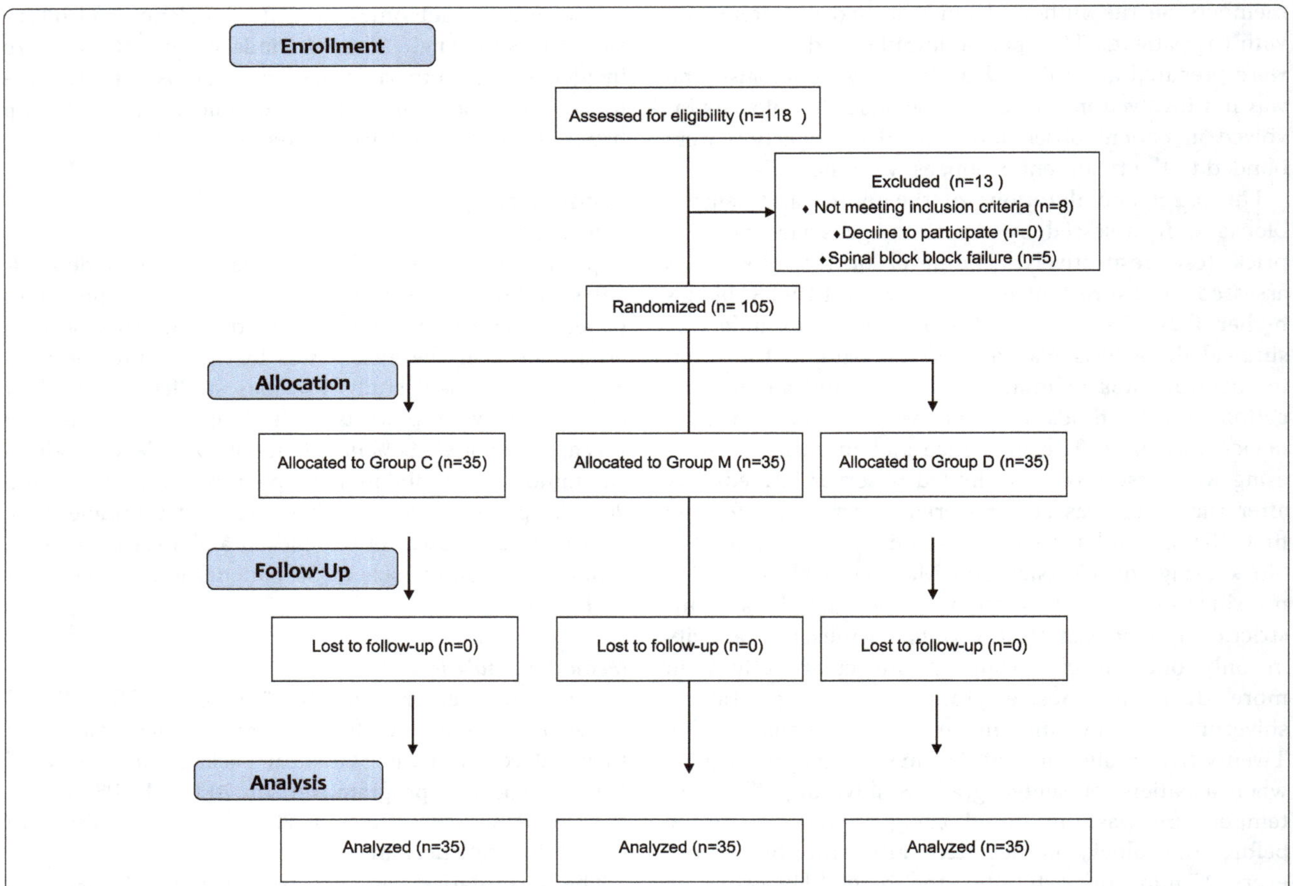

Fig. 1 Consort flow chart

patients), ureteroscopy (27 patients) and urethroscopy (20 patients); the proportions of patients according to the surgery types were comparable among the three groups.

All the patients were comparable regarding their demographic data, including age, weight, height, sex, duration of surgery and ASA classification (Table 1).

All the patients were comparable regarding their SBP and DBP (Fig. 2), HR and SpO_2 (Fig. 3) throughout the study.

The onset times and durations of the sensory and motor blocks were statistically different between the three groups. Group D presented the shortest onset, and group M presented the longest onset ($p < 0.001$). All the patients were comparable regarding their block levels (Table 1).

The tympanic temperature remained above 36 °C in all the patients at all times, and no patient required active warming (Fig. 4).

Group C had a significantly higher number of patients who developed shivering, who developed grade IV shivering and who needed meperidine to treat shivering than groups M and D, which were comparable to each other (Tables 2 and 3).

The time between block administration and meperidine administration was similar among the three groups.

The three groups were comparable regarding the occurrence of nausea, vomiting, bradycardia and hypotension. All the patients in group C, 32 patients in group M and 33 patients in group D had a sedation score of 2. Three patients in group M and 2 patients in group D had a sedation score of 3 (Table 4).

Discussion

In addition to its well-known advantages, SA has an additional advantage in uroscopic surgeries, especially procedures that require intraluminal fluid irrigation such as TURP, as it allows the early detection of complications such as TURP syndrome in conscious patients [1]. However, SA is not a complication-free technique; shivering is a common complication of SA, with an incidence of 40–60% in patients who undergo SA [5]. Though shivering is a protective mechanism to preserve body heat, it causes patient discomfort and pain and may be dangerous in patients with impaired cardiovascular reserves or limited respiratory capacity, as shivering increases the circulating catecholamine, HR, cardiac output, minute

Table 1 Demographic data

	C Group ($n = 35$)	M Group ($n = 35$)	D Group ($n = 35$)	*P*	P1	P2	P3
Gender (No &%)							
Male	28 (80.0)	26 (74.3)	29 (82.9)	0.669	0.569	0.759	0.382
Female	7 (20)	9 (25.7)	6 (17.1)				
Age (years)	50.29 ± 8.87	49.03 ± 8.83	49.23 ± 10.51	0.836	0.579	0.640	0.930
Height (cm)	173.71 ± 5.60	174.29 ± 5.02	173.86 ± 5.83	0.903	0.644	0.914	0.745
Weight (kg)	83.43 ± 7.93	82.29 ± 9.34	82.71 ± 10.24	0.872	0.605	0.747	0.846
ASA classif1cation							
I	17 (48.6)	17 (48.6)	15 (42.9)	0.858	0.858	0.631	0.631
II	18 (51.4)	18 (51.4)	20 (57.1)				
Duration of surgery (min)	105.03 ± 11.59	103.17 ± 7.83	101.60 ± 9.01	0.331	0.420	0.138	0.495
Sensory Block onset (time to reach T10)	4.20 ± 0.63	6.69 ± 0.90	3.40 ± 0.50	< 0.001*	< 0.001*	< 0.001*	< 0.001*
motor block onset (time to reach bromage 4)	4.97 ± 0.71	8.03 ± 0.79	3.80 ± 0.76	< 0.001*	< 0.001*	< 0.001*	< 0.001*
Block level Median (IQR)	9 (8–10)	9 (8–10)	9 (8–10)	0.921	0.08	0.954	0.084
Motor block duration	157.00 ± 13.07	193.71 ± 17.63	206.57 ± 22.06	< 0.001*	< 0.001*	< 0.001*	0.003*
Sensory block duration	198.14 ± 18.67	243.43 ± 23.22	301.57 ± 39.44	< 0.001*	< 0.001*	< 0.001*	< 0.001*
Intraoperative venous fluids	971.43 ± 161.01	997.14 ± 168.45	1002.86 ± 263.45	0.652	0.448	0.503	.0.914
No of patients had cystoscopy (41)	15	13	13				
No of patients had uretroscopy (27)	8	10	9				
No of patients had urethroscopy (20)	7	6	7				
No of patients had TURP (17)	5	6	6				

p1: *p* value for comparing between Control and MgSO4
p2: *p* value for comparing between Control and Dex
p3: *p* value for comparing between MgSO4and Dex
IQR Interquartile range, *TURP* Transurethral resection of prostate
*: Statistically significant at $p \leq 0.05$

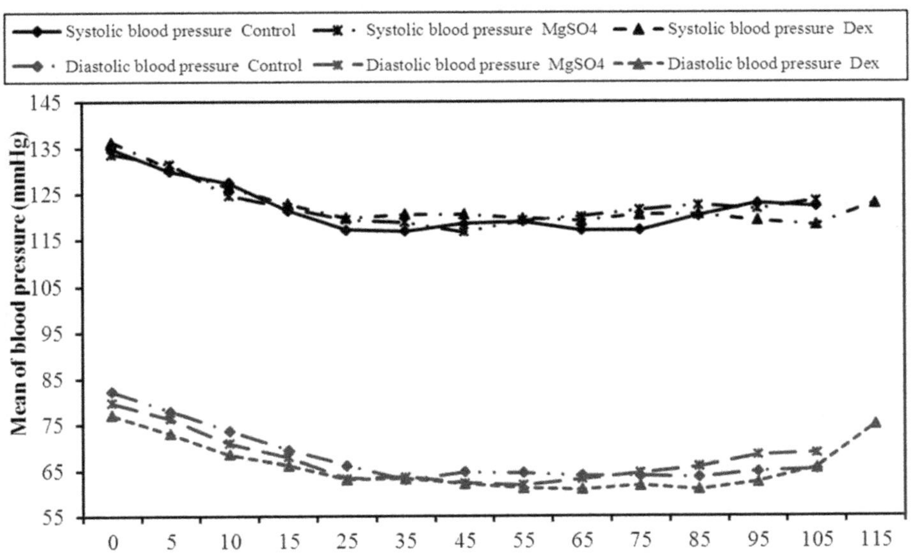

Fig. 2 Comparison between the three studied groups according to Systolic blood pressure and diastolic blood pressure (mmHg)

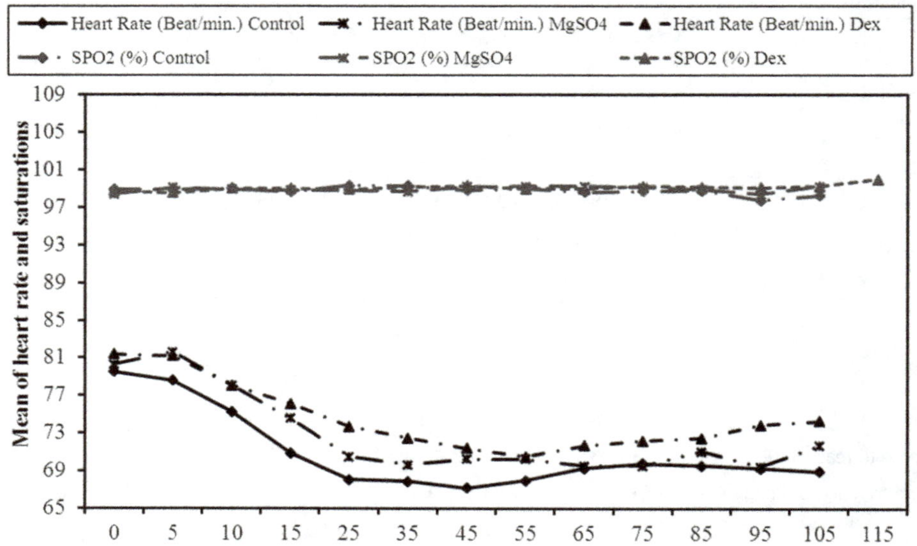

Fig. 3 Comparison between the three studied groups according to Heart Rate (Beat/min.) and SPO_2 (%)

ventilation, oxygen consumption, metabolic CO_2 production and lactic acid level. It also increases intraocular and intracranial pressure and postoperative pain due to surgical incision stretching. Shivering may also interfere with the monitoring of patients by causing artefacts on the ECG or disrupting BP and pulse oximetry readings [4]. Additionally, shivering in patients with ASA grades III and IV may cause challenges for the surgeon and increase the operative time.

Hypothermia is a major risk for shivering, but there is no definite linear relationship between body temperature and the occurrence of shivering. Other major risk factors include age, sensory block level, temperature of the operating room and temperatures of the IV solutions [23].

The exact mechanisms to explain the occurrence of shivering during SA have not yet been elucidated. Possible mechanisms include central thermoregulation disturbance, internal body heat redistribution, and body heat loss to the environment [24]. Regional and general anaesthesia are known to impair the efficiency of the hypothalamic thermoregulatory centre, causing different grades of hypothermia [25]. Under regional

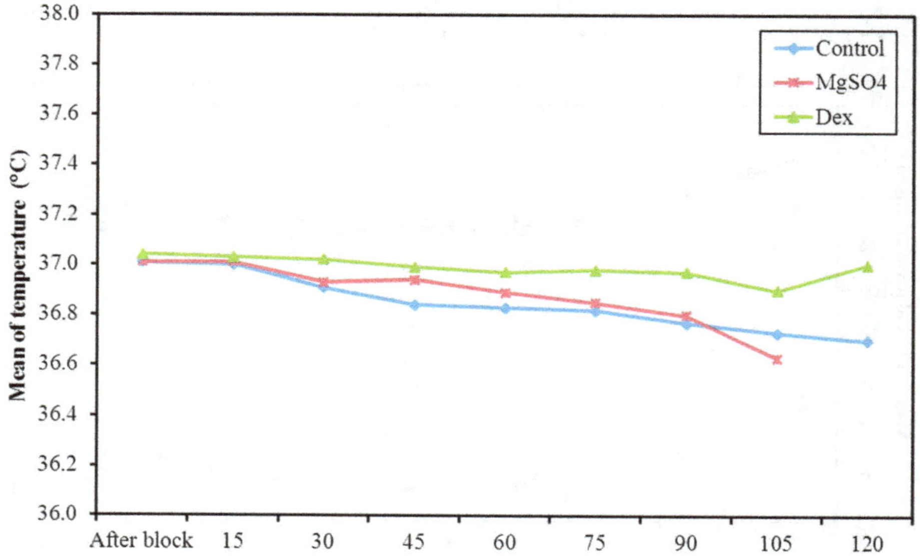

Fig. 4 Comparison between the three studied groups according to temperature (°C)

Table 2 Shivering incidence and grades

	C Group ($n = 35$)		M Group ($n = 35$)		D Group ($n = 35$)		P	p_1	p_2	p_3
	No.	%	No.	%	No.	%				
Grades										
No shivering	14	40.0	24	68.6	30	85.7	< 0.001*	0.016*	< 0.001*	0.088
I	0	0.0	0	0.0	0	0.0	–	–	–	–
II	0	0.0	2	5.7	0	0.0	0.331	0.493	–	0.493
III	1	2.9	1	2.9	2	5.7	1.000	1.000	1.000	1.000
IV	20	57.1	5	14.3	3	8.6	< 0.001*	< 0.001*	< 0.001*	0.716

p1: *p* value for comparing between Control and MgSO4
p2: *p* value for comparing between Control and Dex
p3: *p* value for comparing between MgSO4and Dex
*: Statistically significant at $p \leq 0.05$

anaesthesia, vasodilatation and redistribution of the core temperature are restricted to the lower body below the block, while vasoconstriction and shivering are restricted to the upper body, as they are inhibited below the level of the block due to sympathetic and somatic nerve blocks [26].

The neurotransmitter pathways responsible for shivering are complex, and different receptors patients, such as opioid, α-2 adrenergic, serotonergic, and anti-cholinergic receptors, are involved patients. Different drugs that act on these receptors have been examined in different trials for the prevention or treatment of shivering after SA [4]. The studied drugs include meperidine, fentanyl, clonidine, ketamine, and tramadol; they have resulted in different degrees of efficacy and many associated side effects, such as haemodynamic instability, respiratory depression, nausea and vomiting [27].

Dexmedetomidine [5–15] and magnesium sulfate [2, 3, 17–20] have been demonstrated to be effective and safe for the prevention and treatment of shivering following SA; their efficacy and safety are equal or superior to other adjuvants, with fewer adverse effects. Few trials [3, 5, 15, 17] have examined intrathecal administration to prevent SA-related shivering.

Dexmedetomidine is a highly selective alpha-2 adrenergic agonist, known for its sedative effect in anaesthesia and intensive care practice; its affinity for alpha-2 adrenoreceptors is ten times higher than that of clonidine [28]. The response to activation of these alpha-2- receptors includes a decreased sympathetic tone, resulting in a decreased BP and HR. Dexmedetomidine has been effectively examined in several studies for the prevention and treatment of shivering following general anaesthesia or SA at a dose that does not induce major sedation or haemodynamic instability, respiratory depression, nausea or vomiting [11]. The exact mechanism of dexmedetomidine in the control of shivering is unclear and complex. One suggested mechanism is as follows: dexmedetomidine and other alpha-2 agonists reduce shivering by inhibiting central thermoregulatory control by restraining neuronal conductance and suppressing vasoconstriction and shivering thresholds. Drugs that inhibit thermoregulatory vasoconstriction prevent shivering [29].

Magnesium (Mg^{+2}) is a naturally occurring non-competitive antagonist of N-methyl-D aspartate (NMDA) receptors with a good safety profile and neuroprotective properties under the condition of hypothermia [30]. There are many theories regarding the anti-shivering effect of $MgSO_4$; it has been reported to reduce shivering through a central effect by reducing the shivering threshold [16, 31]. Additionally, it blocks NMDA receptors and decreases norepinephrine and 5-HT, which both play a role in thermoregulation [32]. As a calcium antagonist, Mg^{+2} has a peripheral mild muscle relaxation effect that may reduce the intensity of

Table 3 Need of meperdine

	C Groupo		M Group		D Group		P	p_1	p_2	p_3
	No.	%	No.	%	No.	%				
No. of patients needed meperdine	21	60.0	6	17.4	5	14.3	< 0.001*	< 0.001*	< 0.001*	0.743
Timing after block/min.	39.52 ± 8.05		44.50 ± 11.17		52.0 ± 14.40		0.175	0.586	0.058	0.268
Recurrence of shivering	6	17.1	2	5.7	1	2.8	0.136	< 0.001*	< 0.001*	0.002*

p1: *p* value for comparing between Control and MgSO4
p2: *p* value for comparing between Control and Dex
p3: *p* value for comparing between MgSO4and Dex
*: Statistically significant at $p \leq 0.05$

Table 4 Complications

Complication	C Group ($n = 35$)		M Group ($n = 35$)		D Group ($n = 35$)		P	p_1	p_2	p_3
	No.	%	No.	%	No.	%				
Nausea	3	8.6	2	5.7	2	5.7	1.000	1.000	1.000	1.000
Vomiting	0	0.0	0	0.0	0	0.0	–	–	–	–
Bradycardia	4	11.4	4	11.4	3	8.6	1.000	1.000	1.000	1.000
Hypotension	7	20.0	6	17.1	7	20.0	0.940	0.759	1.000	0.759
Sedation (maximum score)										
1	0	0.0	0	0.0	0	0.0	0.364	0.239	0.493	1.000
2	35	100.0	32	91.4	33	94.3				
3	0	0.0	3	8.6	2	5.7				
4	0	0.0	0	0.0	0	0.0				
5	0	0.0	0	0.0	0	0.0				
6	0	0.0	0	0.0	0	0.0				

p1: *p* value for comparing between Control and MgSO4
p2: *p* value for comparing between Control and Dex
p3: *p* value for comparing between MgSO4and Dex

shivering (incremental shivering intensity with progressing hypothermia) [33]. Mg^{+2} also cause peripheral vasodilation, which increases cutaneous circulation, leading to a decrease in the incidence of shivering [34, 35].

Based on previous studies, we compared the effect of subarachnoid injections of dexmedetomidine and $MgSO_4$ on the prevention of shivering after SA in patients who underwent uroscopic surgery. The current study demonstrated that post-SA injection of both dexmedetomidine (5 μg) and $MgSO_4$ (25 mg) significantly reduced the incidence of post-SA shivering. Five patients (14.3%) in group D, 8 patients (22.8%) in group M, and 21 patients (60%) in group C developed shivering. The number of patients who developed shivering and required meperidine administration in group D group was 5 (14.3%), in group M was 6 (17.4%), and in group C was 21 (60.0%).

Similar to our study, Ellakany et al. [15] administered the same intrathecal dexmedetomidine dose (5 μg) and concluded that both intrathecal dexmedetomidine and meperidine effectively lowered the incidence of shivering following SA in patients who underwent lower abdominal surgery, but meperidine was associated with more side effects, such as pruritus, nausea and vomiting, than dexmedetomidine. In sixty patients who underwent lower abdominal surgery, Abdel Hamid et al. [36] concluded that adding 5 μg of dexmedetomidine to intrathecal bupivacaine improved the characteristics of the spinal block, with less postoperative analgesic requirements and a lower incidence of shivering than the placebo with no sedation or other complications.

Moawad et al. [5] studied the effect of adding dexmedetomidine to intrathecal bupivacaine at a higher dose (10 μg) than that in our study (5 μg). They found that it significantly decreased the incidence and degree of shivering in patients undergoing TURP.

Usta et al. [12] and Bajwa et al. [23] studied the prophylactic effect of IV dexmedetomidine on shivering in patients who received SA and general anaesthesia, respectively. They found that perioperative dexmedetomidine infusion significantly decreased the incidence and intensity of shivering, with no major adverse effects.

Botros et al. [14] compared the prophylactic effects of an intravenously infused placebo, 1 μg/kg of dexmedetomidine and 8 mg of ondansetron on the prevention of post-SA shivering in 120 patients undergoing different lower body surgeries and found that IV dexmedetomidine and ondansetron were equally as effective in reducing the incidence of post-SA shivering as the placebo.

Abdel-Ghaffar et al. [6] compared the clinical efficacy and side effects of three different doses of IV dexmedetomidine (0.5, 0.3 and 0.2 μg/kg) and IV meperidine 0.4 mg/kg for the treatment of post-SA shivering in 120 patients. They found that 0.3 μg/kg of dexmedetomidine was the most appropriate dose for the effective treatment of shivering after SA, with modest effects on haemodynamic characteristics and sedation.

Faiz et al. [3] concluded that an intrathecal injection of $MgSO_4$ (25 mg) improved perioperative shivering in female patients who underwent an elective caesarean section.

Ibrahim et al. [19] studied the prophylactic and therapeutic effects of IV $MgSO_4$ on SA-induced shivering and proved that it was effective.

Gozdemir et al. [2] found that following SA, an IV infusion of 80 kg/mg of $MgSO_4$ over 30 min, followed by

IV infusion at a rate of 2 g/hr. until the end of surgery had a significant effect on preventing post-SA shivering in patients undergoing TURP.

In a study by Sachidananda et al. [20], a prophylactic IV infusion of $MgSO_4$ and tramadol effectively reduced shivering during caesarean section under SA and the shivering intensity.

There was no difference between the three groups in terms of intraoperative haemodynamics. Regarding the sensory and motor block onset times, group D had the fastest sensory and motor blocks onset times, while group M had delayed sensory and motor block onset times compared to group D. This may be due to changes in the pH and baricity of bupivacaine due to the addition of $MgSO_4$. The durations of both the sensory and motor blocks in group D were longer than those in group M, which were longer than those in group C. Similar results were observed in two studies [37, 38] that compared the effects of 10 μg of intrathecal dexmedetomidine and 50 mg of intrathecal $MgSO_4$ when added to bupivacaine, considering the characteristics of the spinal block as the primary outcomes.

Limitations and recommendations

The limitation to this study was that we did not estimate the mean volumes of the irrigating fluids in each group. We recommend conducting further studies on both drugs with increased sample sizes and different doses.

Conclusion

We concluded that intrathecal injection of both dexmedetomidine and $MgSO_4$ with bupivacaine were effective in reducing the incidence of post-SA shivering. Therefore, we encourage the use of $MgSO_4$,as is it more physiologically available, more readily available in most operating theatres and much less expensive than dexmedetomidine.

Abbreviations

ASA: American Society of Anesthesiologists; °C: Degrees Celsius; CO_2: Carbon dioxide; DBP: Diastolic arterial blood pressure; ECG: Electrocardiogram; HR: Heart rate; IV: Intravenous; Mg^{+2}: Magnesium; $MgSO_4$: Magnesium sulfate; NABP: Non-invasive arterial blood pressure; NMDA: N-methyl-D-aspartate; PACU: Postanaesthesia care unit; PSO_2: Arterial oxygen saturation; SA: Spinal anaesthesia; SBP: Systolic arterial blood pressure; TURP: Transurethral resection of the prostate; μg: Microgram

Acknowledgements

We would like to thank our professors and colleagues in the anaesthesia department of Cairo University for their help and support.

Authors' contributions

MW, HO and BM were responsible for the conception of the study. HO, BA and MH contributed to the design of the study, analysis of the data, and writing of the manuscript. WA, BA, and HO contributed to the data collection. BA, MMH, HO, WA, PH, MH, AE, DK, MM, AH, PZ and MW contributed to the writing and revising of the manuscript. All the authors have read, revised and approved the final manuscript.

Author details

[1]Anesthesia Department, Faculty of Medicine, Cairo University, Cairo, Egypt. [2]El Sahel Teaching Hospital, Cairo, Egypt. [3]Anesthesia Department, National Cancer Institute, Cairo University, Cairo, Egypt.

References

1. Moeen SM, Moeen AM. Intrathecal dexamethasone vs. meperidine for prevention of shivering during transurethral prostatectomy: a randomized controlled trial. Acta Anaethesiol Scand. 2017;61:749–57.
2. Gozdemir M, Usta B, Demircioglu RI, Muslu B, Sert H, Karatas OF. Magnesium sulfate infusion prevents shivering during transurethral prostatectomy with spinal anesthesia: a randomized, double-blinded, controlled study. J Clin Anesth. 2010;22(3):184–93.
3. Faiz SH, Rahimzadeh P, Imani F, Bakhtiari A. Intrathecal injection of magnesium sulfate: shivering prevention during cesarean section: a randomized, double blinded, controlled study. Korean J Anaesth. 2013; 65(4):293–8.
4. De Witte J, Sessler DI. Perioperative shivering: physiology and pharmacology. Anesthesiology. 2002;96(2):467–84.
5. Moawad HES, Elawdy MM. Efficacy of intrathecal dexmedetomidine in prevention of shivering in patients undergoing transurethral prostatectomy: a randomized controlled trial. Egypt J Anaesth. 2015;31(2):178–81.
6. Abdel-Ghaffar HS, Mohamed SA, Fares KM, Osman MA. Safety and efficacy of dexmedetomidine in treating post spinal anesthesia shivering: a randomized clinically controlled dose-finding trial. Pain Physician. 2016;19: 243–53.
7. Kundra TS, Kuthiala G, Shrivastava A, Kaur P. A comparative study on the efficacy of dexmedetomidine and tramadol on post-spinal anesthesia shivering. Saudi J Anaesth. 2017;11:2–8.
8. Kranke P, Eberhart LH, Roewer N, Tramèr MR. Postoperative shivering in children: a review on pharmacologic prevention and treatment. Paediatr Drugs. 2003;5:373–83.
9. Lamontagne C, Lesage S, Villeneuve E, Lidzborski E, Derstenfeld A, Crochetière C. Intravenous dexmedetomidine for the treatment of shivering during cesarean delivery under neuraxial anesthesia: a randomized-controlled trial. Can J Anesth/J Can Anesth. 2019;66:762–11.
10. Megalla SA, Mansour HS. Dexmedetomidine versus Nalbuphine for treatment of postspinal shivering in patients undergoing vaginal hysterectomy: a randomized, double blind, controlled study. Egypt J Anaesth. 2017;3:47–52.
11. Mittal G, Gupta K, Katyal S, Kausal S. Randomized double blind comparative study of Dexmedetomidine and tramadol for post spinal anesthesia shivering. Indian J Anesth. 2014;58(3):257–62.
12. Usta B, Gozdemir M, Demircioglu RI, Muslu B, Sert H, Yaldiz A. Dexmedetomidine for prevention of shivering during spinal anesthesia. Clinics. 2011;66(7):1187–96.
13. Bozgeyik S, Mizrak A, Kiliç E, Yendi F, Ugur BK. The effects of preemptive tramadol and dexmedetomidineon shivering during arthroscopy. Saudi J Anaesth. 2014;8:238–43.
14. Botros JM, Mahmoud AMS, Ragab SG, Ahmed MAA, Roushdy HMS, Yassin HM, et al. Comparative study between dexmedetomidine and ondansteron for prevention of post spinal shivering, a randomized controlled trial. BMC Anesthesiol. 2018;18:179.
15. Ellakany M, Abdelhamid SA, Girgis M. Intrathecal dexmedetomidine or meperidine for post spinal shivering. Int J Anesth Anesth. 2014;1(2):1:004.
16. Wadhwa A, Senguta P, Durrani J, Akca O, Lenhardl R, Sessler DI, Doufas AG. Magnesium sulfate only slightly reduces the shivering threshold in humans. Br J Anesth. 2005;94(6):756–62.
17. Nath MP, Garg R, Talukdar T, Choudhary D, Chkrabarty A. To evaluate the efficacy of intrathecal magnesium sulfate for hysterectomy under subarachnoid block with bupivacaine and fentanyl: a prospective randomized double blind clinical trial. Saudi J Anaesth. 2012;6(3):254–8.
18. Elsonbaty M, Elsonbaty A, Saad D. Is this the time for magnesium sulfate to replace meperidine as an antishivering agent in spinal anesthesia? Egypt J Anaesth. 2013;29:213–7.
19. Ibrahim IT, Megalla SA, Khalifa OS, Salah El Deen HM. Prophylactic vs therapeutic magnesium sulfate for shivering during spinal anesthesia. Egypt J Anaesth. 2014;30:31–7.
20. Sachidananda R, Basavaraj K, Shaikh SI, Umesh G, Bhat T, Arpitha B. Comparison of prophylactic intravenous magnesium sulfate with tramadol for postspinal shivering in elective cesarean section: a placebo

controlled randomized double-blind pilot study. Anesth Essays Res. 2018;12:130–4.

21. Crossley AW, Mahajan RP. The intensity of postoperative shivering is unrelated to axillary temperature. Anesthesia. 1994;49:205–12.
22. Ramsay MA, Savege TM, Simpson BR, Goodwin R. Controlled sedation with alphaxolone-alphadalone. Br Med J. 1974;2:656–65.
23. Bajwa SJ, Gupta S, Kaur J, Singh A, Parmar S. Reduction in the incidence of shivering with perioperative dexmedetomidine. A randomized prospective study. J Anesthesiol Clin Pharmacol. 2012;28:86–91.
24. Kurz A, Sessler I, Schroeder M, Kurz M. Thermoregulatory response thresholds during spinal anaesthesia. Anesth Analg. 1993;77:721–6.
25. Joris J, Ozaki N, Sessler D, et al. Epidural anesthesia impairs both central and peripheral thermoregulatory control during general anesthesia. Anesthesiol. 1994;80:268–77.
26. Berti M, Fanelli G, Casati A, et al. Hypothermia prevention and treatment. Anaesthesia. 1998;53(2):46–7.
27. Park SM, Mangat HS, Berger K, Rosengart AJ. Efficacy spectrum of anti-shivering medications: meta-analysis of randomized controlled trials. Crit Care Med. 2012;40:3070–82.
28. Asano T, Dohi S, Ohta S, Shimonaka H, Iida H. Antinociception by epidural and systemic alpha 2 adrenoreceptor agonists and their binding affinity in rat spinal cord and brain. Anesth Analg. 2000;90:400–7.
29. Talke P, Tayefeh F, Sessler DI, Jeffrey R, Noursalehi M, Richardson C. Dexmedetomidine does not alter the sweating threshold, but comparably and linearly decreases the vasoconstriction and shivering thresholds. Anesthesiol. 1997;87:835–41.
30. Nowak L, Bregestovski P, Ascher P, Herbet A, Prochiantz A. Magnesium gates glutamate-activated channels in mouse central neurones. Nature. 1984;307(5950):462–7.
31. Cotton DB, Hallak M, Janusz C, Irtenkauf SM, Berman RF. Central anticonvulsant effects of magnesium sulfate on N-methyl-D-aspartate-induced seizures. Am J Obstet Gynecol. 1993;198:974–8.
32. Kizilirmak S, Karakaş SE, Akça O, Ozkan T, Yavru A, Pembeci K, et al. Magnesium sulfate stops postanesthetic shivering. Ann N Y Acad Sci. 1997; 813:799–806.
33. Lee C, Zhang X, Kwan WF. Electromyographic and mechanomyographic characteristics of neuromuscular block by magnesium sulphate in the pig. Br J Anaesth. 1996;76:278–83.
34. Kizihrmak S, Telci L, Akca O, et al. Magnesium sulphate in the treatment of post anesthetic shivering. Acta Anaethesiol Scand. 1996;40(109):250.
35. Miyakawa H, Matsumoto K, Matsumoto S, Mori M, Yoshitake S, Noguchi T, et al. A comparison of three drugs (pethidine, magnesium sulfate and droperidol) in patients with post-anesthesia shivering. Masui. 1991;40:1503–6.
36. Abdelhamid SA, El-lakany MH. Intrathecal dexmedetomidine: useful or not? J Anesth Clin Res. 2013;4:351.
37. Sunil BV, Sahana KS. Comparison of dexmedetomidine and magnesium sulfate as adjuvants with hyperbaric bupivacaine for spinal anesthesia. A double blind controlled study. J Med Sci Clin Res. 2013;1(3):117–41.
38. Shukla D, Verma A, Agarwal A, Pandey HD, Tyagic C. Comparative study of intrathecal dexmedetomidine with intrathecal magnesium sulfate used as adjuvant to bupivacaine. Anesthesiol Clin Pharmacy. 2011;27(4):495–9.

10

Prospective randomized comparison of cerebrospinal fluid aspiration and conventional popping methods using 27-gauge spinal needles in patients undergoing spinal anaesthesia

J. U. Han, B. G. Kim, C. Yang, W. H. Choi, J. Jeong, K. J. Lee and H. Kim*

Abstract

Background: Performing spinal anaesthesia using the conventional popping method with a 27-gauge (27G) spinal needle is technically difficult. In this study, we compared the aspiration and conventional popping method for spinal anaesthesia using 27G Quincke-type needles.

Methods: This prospective, randomized study enrolled 90 patients, aged 19 to 65 years, with American Society of Anesthesiologists physical status I-III, who were undergoing spinal anaesthesia. Patients were randomly assigned to one of two groups using a computer-generated random number table: patients receiving spinal anaesthesia using the aspiration method, in which the needle is advanced with continuous aspiration, or the conventional popping method. The primary outcome measure was the success rate of the first attempt to perform dural puncture. Number of attempts and passages, withdrawal cases, successful attempt time, total procedure time, and actual depth of dural puncture were recorded.

Results: Eighty-eight patients were included in the study. In the aspiration group, the success rate of first attempt for dural puncture was 93.3%, compared with 72.1% in the popping group ($P = 0.019$). Success involving needle withdrawal was recorded in 4 (8.9%) patients in the aspiration group and 13 (30.2%) in the popping group ($P = 0.024$). In the popping group, the number of attempts was significantly higher ($P = 0.044$), and total procedure time was significantly longer ($P = 0.023$). Actual depths of dural puncture were deeper in the popping group than in the aspiration group ($P = 0.019$).

Conclusions: The aspiration method using a 27G Quincke-type needle offers clinical benefits for dural puncture compared with the conventional popping method for spinal anaesthesia.

Keywords: Aspiration, Cerebrospinal fluid, Lumbar puncture, Spinal anaesthesia

* Correspondence: aneshyunzu@gmail.com
Department of Anesthesiology and Pain Medicine, Inha University College of Medicine, 27, Inhang-ro, Jung-gu, Incheon, Republic of Korea

Background

Spinal anaesthesia has various advantages and has been widely used for anaesthesia of the lower abdomen, genitourinary organs, and lower extremity. However, technique-related adverse effects have been reported due to spinal anaesthesia, such as backache, post-dural puncture headache (PDPH), and transient neurological symptoms. The appropriate external diameter of the spinal anaesthesia needle is important to prevent these mechanical complications. Notably, PDPH is a common and troublesome complication; however, it is less likely to occur when using a thinner spinal needle [1, 2]. Therefore, efforts have been made to use thinner needles, with punctures largely being performed with a 27-gauge (27G) needle in most patients.

Using a thinner needle for spinal anaesthesia has several advantages. However, this procedure is more difficult to perform and prolonged [3–5]. A thinner needle is more flexible, which restricts advancement of the needle in the intended direction [6–8]. Additionally, the practitioner cannot feel the dural puncture (known as the dural click or popping sensation), which can lead to a higher failure rate when performing spinal anesthesia [9]. In addition, nerve damage or vascular injury may be caused by inserting the spinal needle too deep, due to uncertainty as to whether the dural puncture occurred.

In our institute, a new method has been used in > 10, 000 cases over the past 10 years to advance the spinal needle with continuous aspiration into the syringe, by using a 27G needle. Here, we hypothesized that the aspiration method will provide more effective and safer spinal anaesthesia, compared with the conventional method. Therefore, the aim of this study was to compare the success rate, procedure time, depth of dural puncture, and complications between the aspiration method and the conventional popping method, using a 27G Quincke-type needle in adult patients undergoing spinal anaesthesia.

Methods

This study adheres to CONSORT guidelines and was registered with the Clinical Research Information Service (identifier: KCT0002815) after the protocol was approved by the Institutional Review Board of Inha University Hospital (Incheon, Republic of Korea). Written informed consent was obtained from adults undergoing elective or emergency lower abdominal or lower limb surgery under spinal anaesthesia. Ninety patients, 19 to 65 years of age, with of American Society of Anesthesiologists physical status I-III, and who fulfilled the study inclusion criteria were recruited. Patients with any contraindications to spinal anaesthesia (increased intracranial pressure, infection on injection site, coagulation disorder, severe hypovolemia, and aortic and/or mitral stenosis), body mass index $> 40\ kg{\cdot}(m^2)^{-1}$, history of spinal surgery, or congenital spinal deformity, were excluded. The patients were randomly assigned to one of two groups using a computer-generated random number table: patients in the popping group underwent spinal anaesthesia using the conventional popping method; those in the aspiration group received spinal anaesthesia using the novel aspiration method.

On entering the operating room, patients were monitored using electrocardiogram, pulse oximetry, and non-invasive blood pressure monitoring, measured every 5 min. After preloading with $5\ ml{\cdot}kg^{-1}$ of crystalloid, the patients were placed in the lateral decubitus position, on their side with their knees flexed and pulled high against the abdomen or chest, assuming a foetal position. All procedures were performed by a single expert anaesthesiologist. The operator had 3 years of experience in both the conventional popping and aspiration methods for spinal anaesthesia.

When lumbar spine X-rays were taken of the patients, the expected depth was measured as follows. We defined the junction of the inferior vertebral notch and inferior articular facet of the L3 vertebrate as the point of intersection with the posterior dura complex. The operator draws a line connecting the posterior dura complex and the nearest skin point, then extends the line to the L3 vertebral body on the lumbar spine lateral view. We defined the contact point of the line and the L3 vertebral body as the anterior dura complex. Before spinal anaesthesia, the operator measured distances from the skin to posterior dura complex, and from the skin to anterior dura complex.

After disinfection of the patient's back and skin, injection of local anaesthetic (2 ml lidocaine 2%) at L3-L4 was performed; spinal anaesthesia was performed using the 27G Quincke-type needle (spinal needle with Quinke bevel, Tachang Industrial co., Gongju, South Korea) and a 22G introducer needle attached to a 5 ml syringe (BD Emerald™ Syringe Luer Slip, Becton Dickinson India Pvt. Ltd., Rewari, India). The needle was inserted horizontally using the midline approach in all cases. In the aspiration group, cued by the sensation that the needle passed through the ligamentum flavum and subcutaneous tissue at the discretion of the operator, the stylet was removed. A 3-ml syringe (BD Emerald™ Syringe Luer Slip, Becton Dickinson India Pvt. Ltd.) was then connected to the needle and advanced while continuing aspiration with slight negative pressure till the cerebrospinal fluid (CSF) reached the syringe hub. In the popping group, the operator performed the conventional method, advancing the needle until the dural click was recognized. CSF was confirmed after the stylet was removed when CSF flowed out of the spinal needle. If the operator decided that the needle was too deep, considering the lumbar spine lateral view, or was contacting the bone, the needle was withdrawn until the subcutaneous tissue while checked the flow of CSF without the stylet without the stylet in the both groups. If CSF was present while withdrawing the needle, it was defined as a withdrawal case. This process of moving the spinal needle forward and backward movement was defined as a passage. If the operator could not confirm CSF flow during needle withdrawal, the needle was advanced repeatedly while changing its direction. If the operator could not confirm CSF flow during passages after 5 times, the attempt was regarded to be a failure. The needle was then completely removed and reinserted. If the operator could not confirm CSF flow even after 3 attempts, it was considered to be a failed case and the patient was excluded from the study. After confirming CSF flow, hyperbaric bupivacaine (Marcaine 0.5% Spinal Heavy®, AstraZeneca AB, Sodertalje, Sweden) was injected according to the patient's height and surgical indication. Before removing the needle after injection of the drug, the operator placed sterile tape on the needle at the point where it met the skin. Sensory block was determined using an alcohol stick 10 min after administration of the local anaesthetics.

Another anaesthesiologist recorded the number of attempts, number of passages, withdrawal cases, successful attempt time, total procedure time, and complications. The primary outcome measure was the success rate of the first attempt on the dural puncture procedure. The successful attempt time was defined as the time from insertion of the spinal needle into the introducing needle to identification of CSF during the successful attempt. The total procedure time was defined as the time from the initial spinal needle insertion into the introducing needle to identification of the CSF. The distances from skin to anterior or posterior dura mater from the lumbar spine lateral view were recorded. The actual depth of dural puncture was defined as the needle depth into the back of the patient at time of CSF identification. Doses of hyperbaric bupivacaine and levels of spinal anaesthesia used in both groups were recorded. Complications, including paraesthesia, and bloody tap were also recorded. The enrolled patients were followed up until discharge to assess the occurrence of PDPH.

Statistical analysis

The sample size estimations were performed in accordance with data from a pilot study, in which the success rate of first attempt was compared between the conventional popping method (45%) and aspiration method (82%) in 22 patients. We estimated that 90 subjects would be required to provide 95% power at a 5% significance level, which accounts for a 15% loss of study participants. Statistical analyses were performed using SPSS 19.0 (SPSS Inc., Chicago, IL, USA). All data are expressed as mean (standard deviation), number (%), or median (interquartile range [IQR]), as indicated. After testing for normally distributed data using the Kolmogorov-Smirnov test and Shapiro-Wilk test, continuous and categorical variables were analysed using a two-sample t-test and a chi-squared test, respectively. The variables that did not show normal distribution were analysed using a Mann-Whitney U test. Statistical significance was defined as $P < 0.05$.

Results

Fig. 1 illustrates patient enrolment and flow in the study. Of the 90 patients enrolled in the present study, two patients in the popping group were excluded because dural puncture failed. Therefore, 88 patients were included in the final analysis. There were no statistically significant differences in patient characteristics between the two groups (Table 1). The distances from skin to anterior or posterior dura mater in lumbar spine lateral view were comparable in both groups.

Data related to dural puncture between the two groups are summarized in Table 2. Figure 2 shows the number of attempts for successful dural puncture in both groups. In the aspiration group, the success rate of the first attempt for dural puncture was 93.3% compared to 72.1% in the popping group ($P = 0.019$). The success rate of the first passage was 55.6% in the aspiration group and 34.9% in the popping group ($P = 0.085$). In the popping group, the number of attempts was significantly higher than in the aspiration group ($P = 0.044$). There was no difference in the number of needle passages between the two groups ($P = 0.056$). Figure 3 shows that withdrawal cases included four (8.9%) patients in the aspiration group and 13 (30.2%) in the popping group ($P = 0.024$). There was no difference in the successful attempt time between the two groups. In the popping group, the total procedure time was significantly longer ($P = 0.023$). Figure 4 shows the depths for actual dura puncture in the two groups. The actual depths of dural puncture were deeper in the popping group than in the aspiration group ($P = 0.047$).

The median (IQR) hyperbaric bupivacaine dose was 10.5 (1.88) mg in the popping group and 11 (1.25) mg in aspiration group ($P = 0.071$). The median anaesthesia level was T10 in both groups and was not significantly different ($P = 0.364$). No complications occurred in either group. The participants' length of hospital stay was between 2 and 7 days; no patients presented with PDPH until discharge.

Discussion

This prospective randomized study revealed that the aspiration method yields a significantly higher success rate during the first attempt, lower incidence of withdrawal,

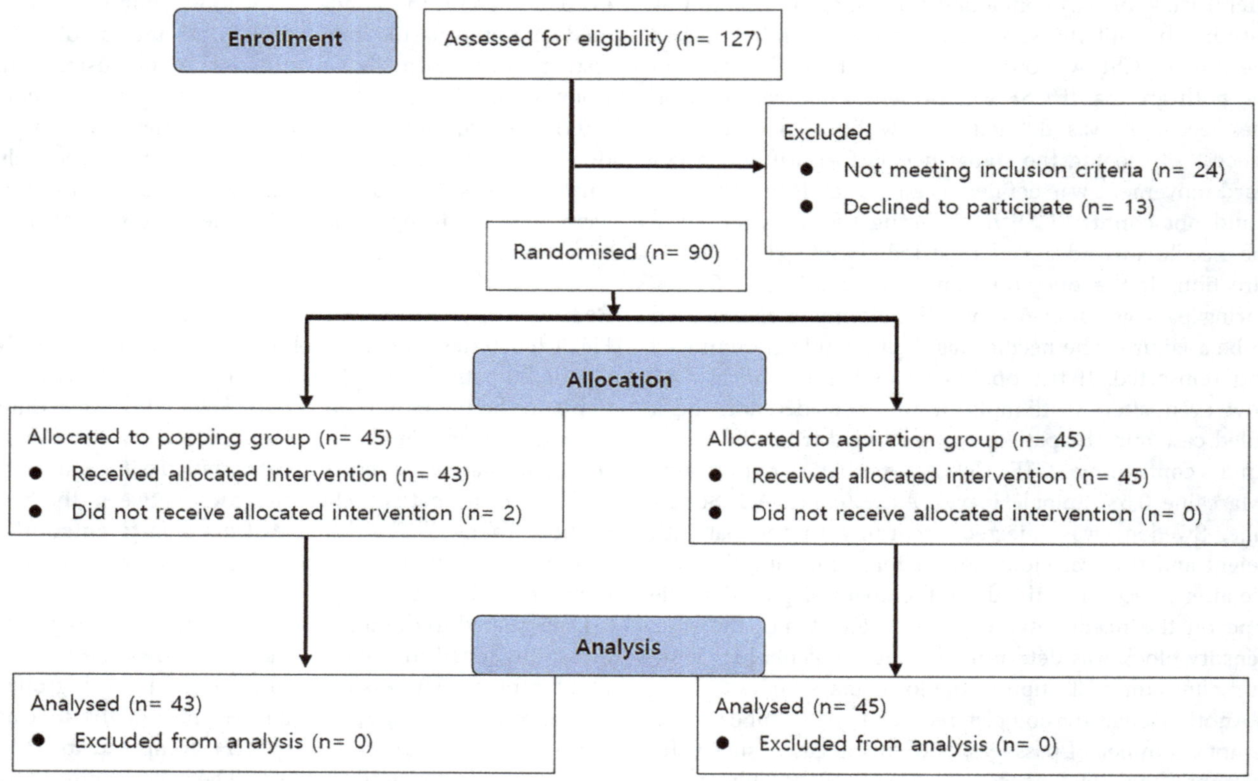

Fig. 1 Enrollment and allocation of patients in the study

and lower number of attempts, along with shorter total procedure time, compared with the conventional popping method for spinal anaesthesia.

Performing spinal anaesthesia using a 27G Quincke needle may be difficult because the CSF pressure varies from 9 to 28 cmH_2O, even in normal adults [10]. Even if a dural click is observed, CSF flow may be insufficient in a spinal needle with a thin diameter of 27G in situations involving low pressure. The dural puncture can be repeated without confirming the subarachnoid space only after spontaneous CSF flow is confirmed [11]. In this study, a higher first attempt success rate was noted in the aspiration group. The use of the aspiration method can help the operator detect the precise time of the dural puncture.

The number of attempts and total procedure time were significantly lower in the aspiration group. These favourable results suggest that the aspiration method can reduce complications arising from repeated manipulation of the spinal needle. Repeated attempts can directly damage the spinal cord or nerves of the central nervous system. Irritation of the filum terminale of the spinal cord causes paraesthesia, and in severe cases, nerve damage [12, 13]. There have been reports of damage to the conus medullaris [14] or discitis [15] after spinal anaesthesia. Considering the possibility of these

Table 1 Demographic data of participants undergoing aspiration or conventional popping for spinal anesthesia

Characteristic	Dural puncture		*P* value
	Popping group (*n* = 43)	Aspiration group (*n* = 45)	
Age (years)	44.3 ± 12.8	42.9 ± 14.0	0.623
Sex, male/female (n/n)	26/17	33/12	0.293
Height (cm)	165.5 ± 9.9	167.2 ± 7.3	0.369
Weight (kg)	68.9 ± 11.8	67.9 ± 11.2	0.672
Body mass index (kg/m^2)	25.1 ± 3.8	24.2 ± 3.5	0.291
Distance to posterior dura mater (mm)	6.5 ± 1.3	6.4 ± 1.5	0.409
Distance to anterior dura mater (mm)	7.7 ± 1.2	7.6 ± 1.3	0.533

Data are presented as mean ± standard deviation unless otherwise indicated

Table 2 Profiles related to dural puncture between patients undergoing aspiration or conventional popping for spinal anesthesia

Variable	Dural puncture		*P* value
	Popping group (n = 43)	Aspiration group (n = 45)	
First attempt, success/failure cases, (n/n)	31/12	42/3	0.019*
First passage, success/failure cases, (n/n)	15/28	25/20	0.085
Number of passage (n)	2 (3)	1 (2)	0.064
Successful attempt time (s)	25 (52)	22 (19)	0.254
Total procedure time (s)	43 (109)	22 (20)	0.023*

Data are presented as raw count or median (interquartile range) unless otherwise indicated

complications, it may be inappropriate to perform spinal anaesthesia using the conventional popping method for advancing a spinal needle based on subjective feeling of the anaesthesiologist.

The aspiration method group showed favourable results in terms of success rate, likely because the operator easily identified the moment of dural puncture and CSF flow based on the results of withdrawal and puncture depth. In the conventional popping group, there were more withdrawal cases, in which the CSF flow was identified during backward movement of the needle. We speculate that this difference was because the anaesthesiologist using the conventional popping method overlooked the point of dural puncture during advancement of the needle, as there is no objective clue for dural puncture. The actual depth of the dural puncture was significantly deeper using the conventional popping method. The aspiration method may reduce the side effects caused by unnecessary deep penetration of the spinal needle.

This study compared the two methods for using the 27G Quincke spinal needle, which has a sharp cutting edge. While thinner spinal needles have previously been used, the thinnest needle currently used in clinical practice is 27G. The aim of using a thinner spinal needle is to reduce the incidence of PDPH or back pain. However, if the dural click is not identified, repeated dural punctures are required, and the procedure time is prolonged. This leads to an increased risk of patient discomfort, PDPH, back pain, mechanical damage of the nerve, and infection [16, 17]. Therefore, the use of an aspiration method is appropriate when performing spinal anaesthesia with a thin needle.

The depth of dural puncture was significantly deeper in the popping group. The depth difference was only 3 mm; thus, its value could be underestimated. However,

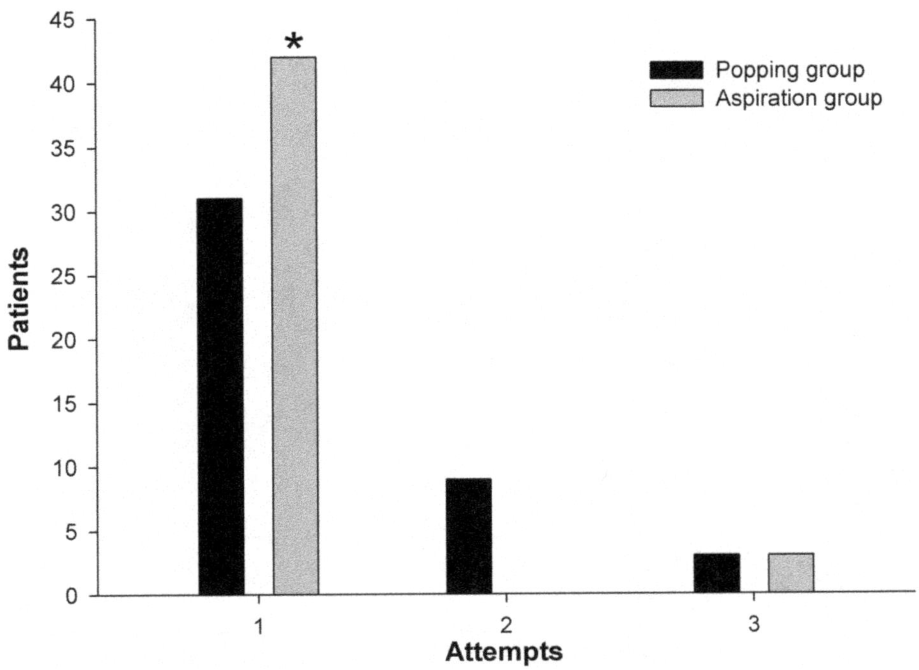

Fig. 2 Number of attempts to achieve successful dural puncture in both groups. *Statistically significant ($P \leq 0.05$)

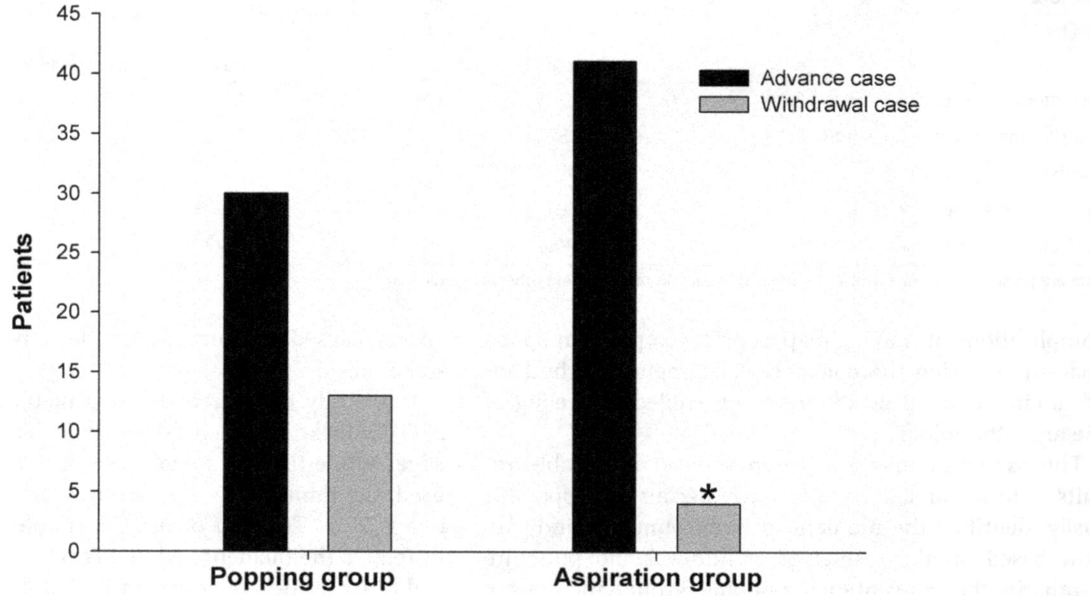

Fig. 3 Withdrawal cases where cerebrospinal fluid was identified while withdrawing the needle in both groups. *Statistically significant ($P \leq 0.05$)

it corresponded to 30% of the total subarachnoid space; the distance between anterior and posterior dura in this study was approximately 10 mm, a difference that should not be ignored. Spinal needles that are further advanced by 3 mm can penetrate the anterior dural mater through the subarachnoid space, increasing the possibility of damage to surrounding tissues. In addition, because the length of the needle bevel is 1.5 mm, the theoretical maximum difference between the two groups is 13 mm. In this study, a 3-mm difference in dural puncture is clinically relevant.

In this study, the measured distances from skin to the posterior and anterior dura complex were obtained from the lumbar spine lateral view. There were no differences in distances from the skin to the posterior and anterior dura complex on lumbar lateral X-ray film, as there were in other demographic characteristics of the patients. The distances from skin to the posterior and anterior dura

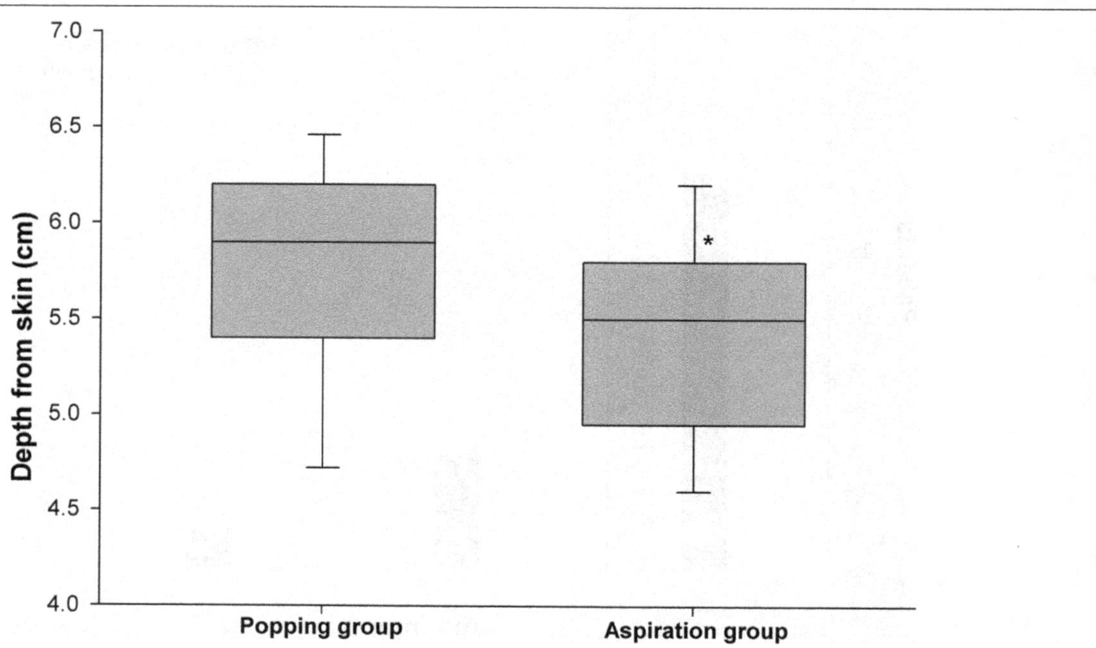

Fig. 4 Actual depths of dural puncture in both groups. *Statistically significant ($P \leq 0.05$)

complex are longer when compared to the actual depth of dural puncture. As the discrepancy is due to the patient's position, this comparison would be desirable if distances were measured in the foetal posture. This can serve as a guide to avoid advancing deeper than the depth when using the lumbar spine lateral view. Further studies are needed to provide reliable guidelines for safe spinal anaesthesia.

Notably, if a pencil-point needle is available, the results of this study may not be useful. Regarding the type of needle, a 25G pencil-point spinal needle causes PDPH similar to a cutting type spinal needle of less than 27G [18]. Furthermore, when using the pencil-point needle, dural clicks are easy to recognize [19]. Based on the actual cost of medical care, clinicians should use 27G Quincke-type spinal needles in most situations. In order to avoid the challenges faced using the 27G needle that are described above, we have attempted the aspiration method; the results of this study reveal that the aspiration method can be more effective and safer than the conventional popping method.

Limitations

There were some limitations to this study. First, there may be a concern about advancing the spinal needle without the stylet. If the needle passes the tissue without the stylet, a blood clot or tissue debris can occlude the needle. To minimize this problem, the operator used an introducing needle of 22G and removed the stylet when the needle entered the ligamentum flavum and proceeded with aspiration using the syringe. However, the stylet is not usually inserted when using the 27G needle in other procedure such as injection into the tissue. Second, the operator and investigator who watched the operator's procedure and evaluated and recorded the data were not blinded to the patient groups. Finally, all subjects were aged < 65 years and had no spinal disorders or history of spinal surgery. Thus, our results may not necessarily be applicable to different patient populations, particularly those of an older age with degenerative changes, obesity, or spinal diseases such as scoliosis.

Conclusions

The aspiration method has several clinical benefits for dural puncture compared with the conventional popping method for spinal anaesthesia that uses 27G Quincke-type needles.

Abbreviations

27G: 27-gauge; CSF: Cerebrospinal fluid; IQR: Interquartile range; PDPH: Post-dural puncture headache

Acknowledgements

Not applicable.

Authors' contributions

Study design: JUH, HK; Data collection: CY, WHC, KJL; Data analysis: BGK, JJ, HK; Manuscript writing: JUH, HK; all authors read and approved the final version of the manuscript.

References

1. Choi PT, Galinski SE, Takeuchi L, Lucas S, Tamayo C, Jadad AR. PDPH is a common complication of neuraxial blockade in parturients: a meta-analysis of obstetrical studies. Can J Anaesthesiol. 2003;50:460–9.
2. Gunaydin B, Karaca G. Prevention strategy for post dural puncture headache. Acta Anaesthesiol Belg. 2006;57:163–5.
3. Dahl JB, Schultz P, Anker-Møller E, Christensen EF, Staunstrup HG, Carlsson P. Spinal anaesthesia in young patients using a 29-gauge needle: technical considerations and an evaluation of postoperative complaints compared with general anaesthesia. Br J Anaesth. 1990;64:178–82.
4. Lyons G, Macdonald R. 29-gauge spinal needles. Br J Anaesth. 1991;67:222.
5. Smith EA, Thorburn J, Duckworth RA, Reid JA. A comparison of 25 G and 27 G Whitacre needles for caesarean section. Anaesthesia. 1994;49:859–62.
6. Sitzman BT, Uncles DR. The effects of needle type, gauge, and tip bend on spinal needle deflection. Anesth Analg. 1996;82:297–301.
7. Ahn WS, Bahk JH, Lim YJ, Kim YC. The effect of introducer gauge, design and bevel direction on the deflection of spinal needles. Anaesthesia. 2002; 57:1007–11.
8. Fama' F, Linard C, Bierlaire D, Gioffre'-Florio M, Fusciardi J, Laffon M. Influence of needle diameter on spinal anaesthesia puncture failures for caesarean section: A prospective, randomised, experimental study. Anaesth Crit Care Pain Med. 2015;34:277–80.
9. Shutt LE, Valentine SJ, Wee MY, Page RJ, Prosser A, Thomas TA. Spinal anaesthesia for caesarean section: comparison of 22-gauge and 25-gauge Whitacre needles with 26-gauge Quincke needles. Br J Anaesth. 1992;69: 589–94.
10. Whiteley W, Al-Shahi R, Warlow CP, Zeidler M, Lueck CJ. CSF opening pressure: reference interval and the effect of body mass index. Neurology. 2006;67:1690–1.
11. Ramachandran K, Ponnusamy N. Dry tap and spinal anesthesia. Can J Anaesth. 2005;52:1104–5.
12. Horlocker TT, McGregor DG, Matsushige DK, Schroeder DR, Besse JA. A retrospective review of 4767 consecutive spinal anesthetics: central nervous system complications. Perioperative Outcomes Group. Anesth Analg. 1997; 84:578–84.
13. Auroy Y, Narchi P, Messiah A, Litt L, Rouvier B, Samii K. Serious complications related to regional anesthesia: results of a prospective survey in France. Anesthesiology. 1997;87:479–86.
14. Reynolds F. Damage to the conus medullaris following spinal anaesthesia. Anaesthesia. 2001;56:238–47.
15. Bajwa ZH, Ho C, Grush A, Kleefield J, Warfield CA. Discitis associated with pregnancy and spinal anesthesia. Anesth Analg. 2002;94:415–6.
16. Tarkkila P. Complications associated with spinal anesthesia. In: Finucane BT, editor. editor Complications of regional Anaesthesia. New York: Springer Science; 2007. p. 149–66.
17. Krommendijk EJ, Verheijen R, van Dijk B, Spoelder EM, Gielen MJ, de Lange JJ. The PENCAN 25-gauge needle: a new pencil-point needle for spinal anesthesia tested in 1,193 patients. Reg Anesth Pain Med. 1999;24:43–50.
18. Zhang D, Chen L, Chen X, Wang X, Li Y, Ning G, et al. Lower incidence of postdural puncture headache using whitacre spinal needles after spinal anesthesia: a meta-analysis. Headache. 2016;56:501–10.
19. Kokki H, Hendolin H, Turunen M. Postdural puncture headache and transient neurologic symptoms in children after spinal anaesthesia using cutting and pencil point paediatric spinal needles. Acta Anaesthesiol Scand. 1998;42:1076–82.

11

Successful use of ultrasound-assisted spinal anesthesia for urgent cesarean section in a patient with implanted spinal cord stimulation system for giant chest wall arteriovenous malformation

Bruno Antonio Zanfini[*], Salvatore De Martino, Luciano Frassanito, Stefano Catarci, Francesco Vitale di Maio, Pietro Paolo Giuri, Gian Luigi Gonnella and Gaetano Draisci

Abstract

Background: The use of Spinal Cord Stimulation (SCS) system to treat medically refractory neuropathic pain is increasing. Severe neuropathic pain can be found in giant chest wall arteriovenous malformations (AVMs), exceedingly rare and debilitating abnormalities, rarely reported during pregnancy.

Case presentation: We present a report of a pregnant patient with implanted Spinal Cord Stimulation (SCS) system because of painful thoracic AVM scheduled for an urgent cesarean section in which we used lumbar ultrasound (US) to rule out the possibility to damage SCS electrodes and to find a safe site to perform spinal anesthesia.

Conclusions: The use of lumbar US to find a safe site for a lumbar puncture in presence of SCS system in a patient affected by painful thoracic AVM makes this case a particularly unique operative challenge and offers a new possible use of ultrasound to detect a safe space in patients with SCS implant.

Keywords: Spinal cord stimulation (SCS) system, Chest wall arteriovenous malformations, Cesarean section, Ultrasound

Background

The use of Spinal Cord Stimulation (SCS) system to treat medically refractory neuropathic pain is increasing [1]. Severe neuropathic pain can be found in giant chest wall arteriovenous malformations.

Arteriovenous malformations (AVMs) are rare abnormalities, associated with other congenital syndromes (Rendu-Osler-Weber Syndrome) or consequence of trauma, infection, cancer. Congenital AVMs can be found usually in the central nervous system but can be reported in abdominal organs (liver and gastrointestinal tract), thoracic organs (lung and heart) and lower limb. Congenital chest wall AVMs are rare, with few case reports available in the literature [2–6], but extremely debilitating: if no treatment is performed thoracic AVMs can cause severe bleeding, cardiac failure associated with arteriovenous shunting and severe neuropathic thoracic pain.

We report a case of a 29 years old pregnant patient with a giant, congenital, painful AVM of the left chest

* Correspondence: brunoantonio.zanfini@policlinicogemelli.it
Fondazione Policlinico Universitario Agostino Gemelli IRCCS, Università Cattolica del Sacro Cuore, Scienze dell'Emergenza, Anestesiologiche e della Rianimazione, Largo A. Gemelli 8, 00168 Rome, Italy

wall, treated with implanted Spinal Cord Stimulation (SCS) system, admitted to our obstetric emergency room for an urgent cesarean section.

The presence of SCS system in pregnant patients with congenital AVM and the use of lumbar ultrasound (US) to perform a safe spinal anesthesia made this case a particularly unique operative challenge.

Case presentation

A 29 years old pregnant patient with singleton pregnancy at 38th gestational week (GW) was admitted to our obstetric emergency room for membrane rupture. She referred to be affected by a giant, congenital AVM of the left chest wall, extending from the third to the seventh thoracic interspace, involving the overlying thoracic muscles and the correspondent thoracic nerves, the rib cage, the parietal pleura, the transverse process of seventh thoracic vertebra and the scapular girdle, with severe neuropathic pain and reduced mobility in her left arm. She underwent to multiple embolizations to treat the lesion, with no or mild improvement of her pain despite she was taking 60 mg Oral Morphine Equivalents (OME) per day and pregabalin 300 mg twice daily. To treat her medically refractory neuropathic pain she was therefore referred for SCS system implant. A Model SC-1200 Precision™ Montage™ Magnetic Resonance Imaging (Boston Scientific) was successfully implanted, with electrodes at thoracic level and Implantable Pulse Generator (IPG) in the left buttock. The procedure led to a dramatic improvement of the symptoms and withdrawal of opioids and antiepileptic drugs in 8 weeks. One year later she obtained a spontaneous pregnancy. During pregnancy her pain control improved, leading to SCS deactivation through the period. Despite the absence of stimulation she reported her neuropathic pain "go into remission". So she needed no other medications. Her pregnancy progressed normally until 38th GW. At admission just a pre-SCS implant Magnetic Resonance Imaging (MRI) was available (Fig. 1, axial view; Fig. 2, coronal view) thus making unpredictable the location of her SCS leads, extensions, and IPG. An urgent cesarean section was planned because of the membrane rupture and the risk of severe bleeding due to a possible AVM rupture in case of vaginal birth, due to the increasing of thoracic pressure during pushing (urgent CS type 3 according to NICE classification) [7]. To rule out a possible lesion to SCS system and to identify a safe lumbar interspace, a US assisted spinal anesthesia has been performed. No drugs have been administered before surgery. During anesthesiologic and surgical procedure standard hemodynamic monitoring has been provided for pregnant [Continuous Electrocardiographic monitoring (ECG), Pulse oximetry (SpO2), Non-invasive Blood Pressure (NIBP)]; fetal wellbeing has been registered by cardiotocographic monitoring. Supplemental oxygen has been provided by Venturi mask. In sitting position, after skin disinfection with surgical solution (ChloraPrep®, Carefusion, 244 LTD, UK) and using a broadband (5–8 MHz) convex probe, a left US paramedian sagittal

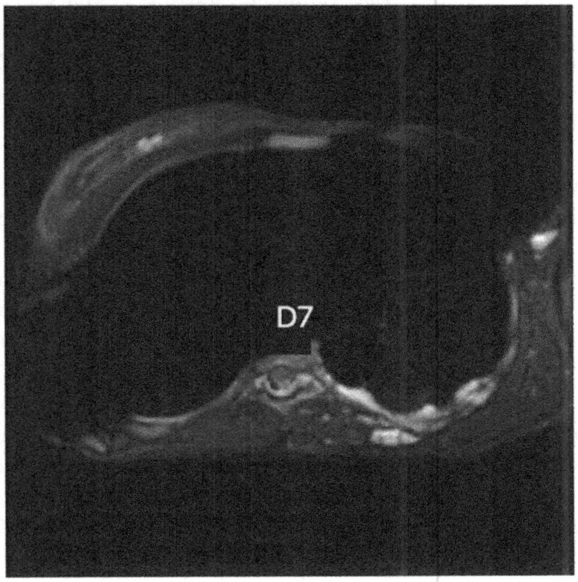

Fig. 1 MRI axial view

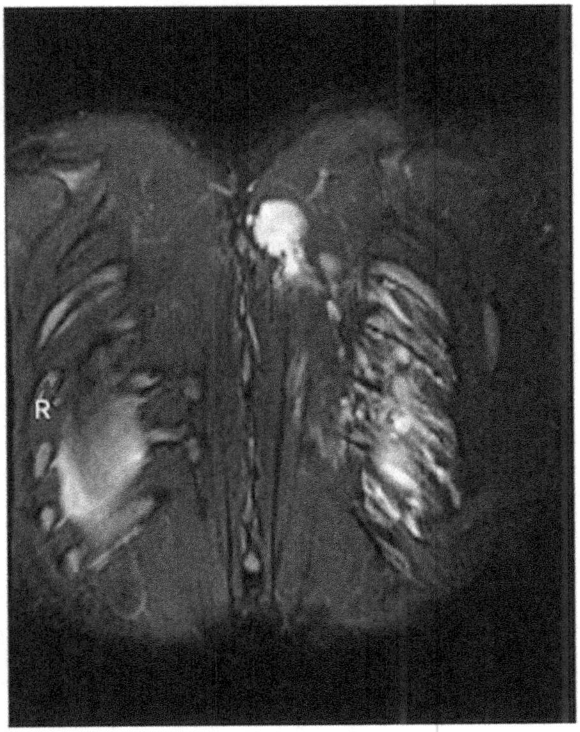

Fig. 2 MRI coronal view

oblique view has been obtained, starting at the sacrum and moving cephalad, to identify the L4-L5 lumbar interspaces (Fig. 3, paramedian sagittal oblique view). To identify the neuraxial midline, after rotating the probe 90° into a transverse orientation, a transverse interlaminar view has been obtained (Fig. 4, transverse interlaminar view). No electrodes have been reported in that interspace. After local anesthesia with lidocaine 2% (5 mL) a 25-gauge Whitacre spinal needle has been used to perform a spinal anesthesia using hyperbaric bupivacaine 0.5% 10 mg plus sufentanil 5 mcg and morphine 100 mcg intrathecally administered. Surgical procedure started when T4 level has been reached. An uneventful cesarean section has been performed. A healthy 3395-g female baby was born (Apgar scores of 9–10 at both 1 and 5 min). A postoperative thoracic X-Ray confirmed the right placement of thoracic electrodes but with entry point of SCS leads at L2-L3 interspace (Fig. 5, antero-posterior X ray; Fig. 6, lateral X ray). At postoperative day 3 patient has been discharged home.

Discussion and conclusions

Our case presents the successful use of lumbar US to detect a safe space for intrathecal injection in a patient with SCS implant because of thoracic AVM. Current data suggest that landmark identification using a pre-procedure ultrasound (US) is a useful adjunct to neuraxial anesthesia [8–10] that facilitates technical performance in obstetric [11–13] and pediatric patients. In adult patients with difficult spinal anatomy [14, 15] a pre-procedure US reduces the number of attempts [16] and the number of needle passes necessary for successful spinal anesthesia [16] and can predict technical difficulty [14, 17]; notably, compared to fluoroscopy, sonography

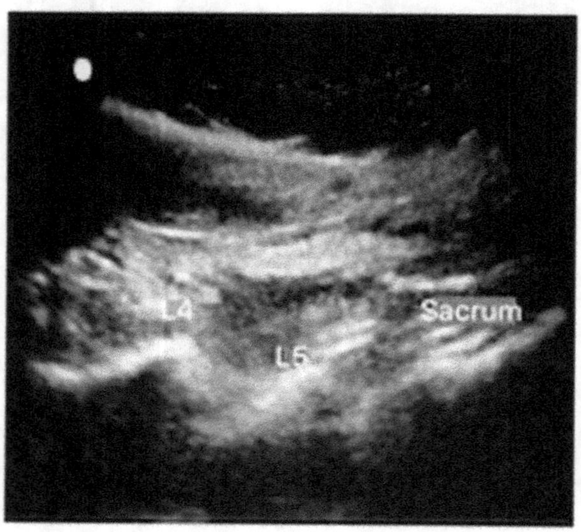

Fig. 3 Parasagittal oblique view of lumbar spine

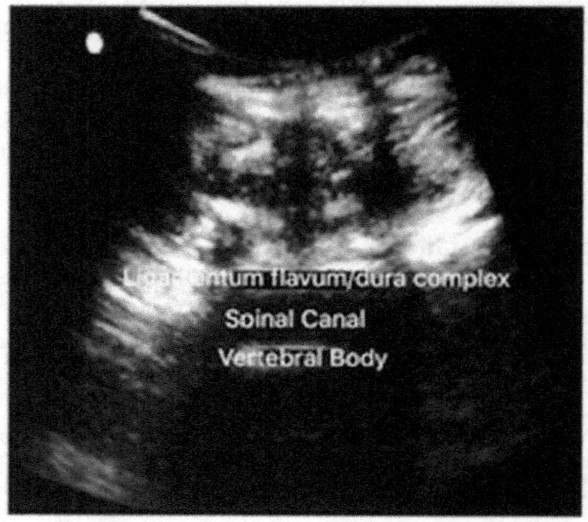

Fig. 4 Transverse interlaminar view at L4-L5 interspace

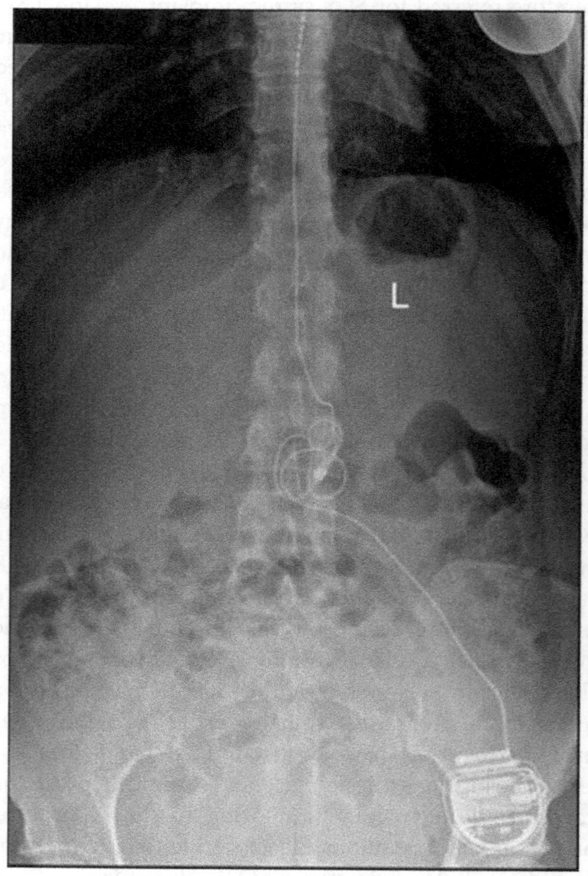

Fig. 5 Antero-posterior X ray of lumbar and thoracic spine

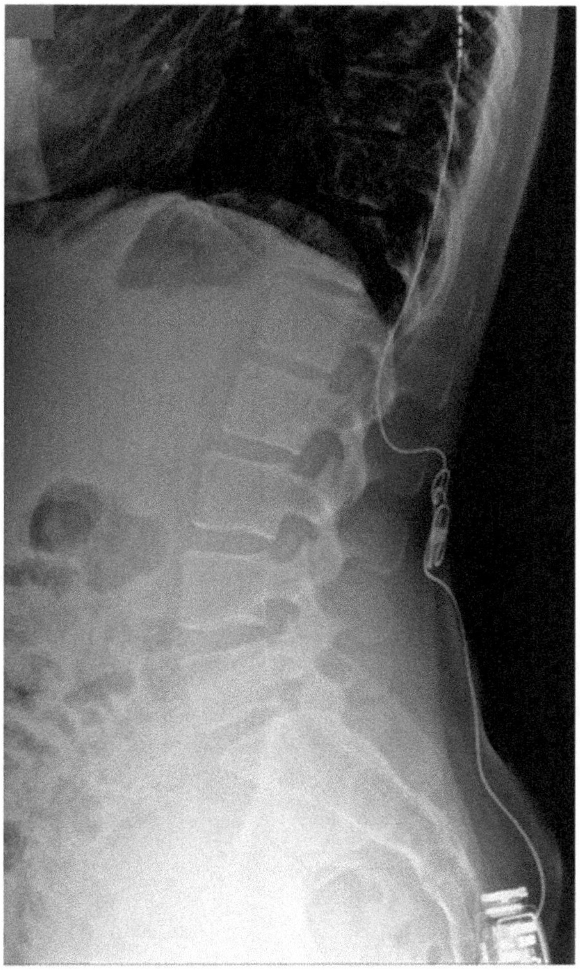

Fig. 6 Lateral X ray of lumbar and thoracic spine

allows for the elimination of radiation exposure for physician and for patient, mostly when, as in our case during a urgent admission to obstetric emergency room, a X-ray scan to identify the location of SCS leads, extensions, and IPG cannot be performed. Even though the first description of a SCS implant for pain in pregnant patients occurred only in 1999 [18] the number of pregnant patients with SCS is increasing. Mostly of these pregnants are affected by Complex Regional Pain Syndrome (CPRS) or Failed Back surgery Syndrome (FBSS) [19–24] with a SCS system implanted before pregnancy occurred. Because leads migration is one of the most common complications occurring in from 2.1 to 27% out of 5000 patients undergoing SCS [25], we performed a lumbar ultrasound scan to identify a safe interspace where perform a spinal anesthesia. The safest choice of anesthesia for cesarean section in pregnant patients with a vascular malformation requires careful consideration. No data have been reported about thoracic AVMs to pregnancy; most of data can be derived from AVMs of Central Nervous System (CNS). Ong discussed the relative risks of different anesthetic choices for cesarean for a patient with a known cervical (C3) AVM that was stable throughout pregnancy [26]. Although general anesthesia can provide good hemodynamic stability, airway manipulation may lead to coughing and bucking with attendant increases in intrathoracic and venous pressures on waking from the anesthesia. This has potential to precipitate rupture of the cervical AVM. We supposed the same for thoracic AVMs and this is the reason why we choose a spinal anesthesia.

A critical decision for anesthetic management of patients with implanted SCS system for painful thoracic AVM scheduled for urgent cesarean section is the feasibility of providing a safe neuraxial anesthesia. Potential risks include damage to electrodes with the spinal or epidural needle, introducer, or catheter. Ultrasound examination may be useful to rule out these risks.

Abbreviations

AVMs: Arteriovenous malformations; SCS: Spinal Cord Stimulation; US: Ultrasound; OME: Oral Morphine Equivalents; IPG: Implantable Pulse Generator; ECG: Continuous Electrocardiographic monitoring; SpO2: Pulse oximetry; NIBP: Non-invasive Blood Pressure; MHz: MegaHertz; CPRS: Complex Regional Pain Syndrome; EMF: Electromagnetic force; CNS: Central Nervous System

Acknowledgements

We thank Rosellina Russo MD for editorial assistance.

Authors' contributions

BAZ planned and conducted the case and drafted the manuscript. SDM conducted the case and revised the manuscript. LF acquired data and helped to write the manuscript. SC participated in the design of the case and helped in the draft of the manuscript. FVdiM studied the patient and planned anesthesiologic procedure. PPG acquired data and participated to planning of anesthesiologic procedure. GLG helped in the performing lumbar ultrasound. GD revised data, approved anesthesiologic procedure and revised the manuscript. All authors read and approved the final manuscript.

References

1. Camporeze B, Simm RF, Estevão IA, Mathias-Junior LR, Aguiar PH, Carrondo-Cottin S. Spinal cord stimulation in the treatment of neuropathic pain: current perspectives of indications, cost-effectiveness, complications and results. J Health Sci. 2017;1:1–35. https://doi.org/10.17532/jhsci.2017.399.
2. Ulku R, Onat S, Avci A, et al. Resection of intercostal hemangioma with involved chest wall and ribs in an 11-year- old girl. Texas Heart Inst J. 2010; 37(4):486–9 PMID:20844630.
3. Yilmaz S, Atinkaya C, Aktas A, et al. Giant arteriovenous malformation located on the chest wall—diagnosis and endovascular treatment: report of a case. Surg Today. 2010;40(12):1164–8. https://doi.org/10.1007/s00595-009-4249-5.
4. Rivera PP, Kole MK, Pelz DM, et al. Congenital intercostal arteriovenous malformation. AJR Am J Roentgenol. 2006;187(5):W503–6. https://doi.org/10.2214/AJR.05.0367.
5. Coulter TD, Maurer JR, Miller MT, et al. Chest wall arteriovenous fistula: an unusual complication after chest tube placement. Ann Thorac Surg. 1999; 67(3):849–50 PMID:10215249.
6. Urschel JD, Broad RW. Giant chest wall arteriovenous malformation with spinal cord compression. Postgrad Med J. 1995;71(834):252 PMID:7784298.
7. Caesarean section. NICE Clinical Guidelines, No. 132. National Collaborating Center for Women's and Children's Health (UK). London: RCOG Press; 2011. Accessed March 2020.

8. Sahin T, Balaban O, Sahin L, et al. A randomized controlled trial of preinsertion ultrasound guidance for spinal anaesthesia in pregnancy: outcomes among obese and lean parturients: ultrasound for spinal anesthesia in pregnancy. J Anesth. 2014;28:413–9. https://doi.org/10.1007/s00540-013-1726-1.
9. Scapinelli R. Morphological and functional changes of the lumbar spinous processes in the elderly. Surg Radiol Anat. 1989;11:129–33 PMID:2763004.
10. Angle P, Tang SL, Thompson D, et al. Expectant management of postdural puncture headache increases hospital length of stay and emergency room visits. Can J Anaesth. 2005;52:397–402 PMID: 15814755.
11. Vallejo MC, Phelps AL, Singh S, et al. Ultrasound decreases the failed labor epidural rate in resident trainees. Int J Obstet Anesth. 2010;19:373–8. https://doi.org/10.1016/j.ijoa.2010.04.002.
12. Grau T, Leipold RW, Conradi R, et al. Efficacy of ultrasound imaging in obstetric epidural anesthesia. J Clin Anesth. 2002;14:169–75 PMID:12031746.
13. Grau T, Leipold RW, Fatehi S, et al. Real time ultrasonic observation of combined spinal-epidural anaesthesia. Eur J Anaesthesiol. 2004;21(1):25–31 PMID:14768920.
14. Chin KJ, Perlas A, Chan V, et al. Ultrasound imaging facilitates spinal anesthesia in adults with difficult surface anatomic landmarks. Anesthesiology. 2011;115:94–10. https://doi.org/10.1097/ALN.0b013e31821a8ad4.
15. Willschke H, Bosenberg A, Marhofer P, et al. Epidural catheter placement in neonates: Sonoanatomy and feasibility of ultrasonographic guidance in term and preterm neonates. Reg Anesth Pain Med. 2007;32:34–40 PMID: 17449890.
16. Kallidaikurichi Srinivasan K, Iohom G, Loughnane F, et al. Conventional landmark-guided midline versus Preprocedure ultrasound-guided paramedian techniques in spinal anesthesia. Anesth Analg. 2015;121:1089–96. https://doi.org/10.1213/ANE.0000000000000911.
17. Chin KJ, Ramlogan R, Arzola C, et al. The utility of ultrasound imaging in predicting ease of performance of spinal anesthesia in an orthopedic patient population. Reg Anesth Pain Med. 2013;38:34–8. https://doi.org/10.1097/AAP.0b013e3182734927.
18. Segal R. Spinal cord stimulation, conception, pregnancy, and labor: case study in a complex regional pain syndrome patient. Neuromodulation. 1999;2:41–5. https://doi.org/10.1046/j.1525-1403.1999.00041.x.
19. Sommerfield D, Hu P, O'Keeffe D, et al. Caesarean section in a parturient with a spinal cord stimulator. Int J Obstet Anesth. 2010;19:114–7. https://doi.org/10.1016/j.ijoa.2009.08.006.
20. Bernardini DJ, Pratt SD, Takoudes TC, et al. Spinal cord stimulation and the pregnant patient-specific considerations for management: a case series and review of the literature. Neuromodulation. 2010;13:270–4. https://doi.org/10.1111/j.1525-1403.2010.00288.x.
21. Domínguez Suárez E, Camblor Suárez E, Vázquez Del Valle S, et al. Epidural analgesia in a woman with spinal neurostimulation for complex regional pain syndrome type 1. A clinical case and literature review. Rev Esp Anestesiol Reanim. 2012;59(9):515–6. https://doi.org/10.1016/j.redar.2012.05.041.
22. Fedoroff IC, Blackwell E, Malysh L, et al. Spinal cord stimulation in pregnancy: a literature review. Neuromodulation. 2012;15:537–41. https://doi.org/10.1111/j.1525-1403.2012.00448.
23. Ito S, Sugiura T, Azami T, et al. Spinal cord stimulation for a woman with complex regional pain syndrome who wished to get pregnant. J Anesth. 2013;27:124–7. https://doi.org/10.1007/s00540-012-1462-y.
24. Das B, McCrory C. Spinal cord stimulation in pregnancy with failed back surgery syndrome. Ir Med J. 2014;107(4):117–8 PMID: 24834587.
25. Eldabe S, Buchser E, Duarte RV. Complications of spinal cord stimulation and peripheral nerve stimulation techniques: a review of the literature. Pain Med. 2016;17:325–36 PMID: 26814260.
26. Ong BY, Littleford J, Segstro R, et al. Spinal anaesthesia for Caesarean section in a patient with cervical arteriovenous malformation. Can J Anaesth. 1996;43(10):1052–8 PMID: 8896858.

12

Lateral femoral cutaneous nerve block with different volumes of Ropivacaine

Frederik Vilhelmsen[1,2*], Mariam Nersesjan[1,2], Jakob Hessel Andersen[2], Jakob Klim Danker[2], Leif Broeng[3], Daniel Hägi-Pedersen[1], Ole Mathiesen[2] and Kasper Højgaard Thybo[1]

Abstract

Background: Nerve block of the lateral femoral cutaneous nerve (LFCN) is a predominantly sensory block. It reduces pain following total hip arthroplasty (THA), but the non-responder rate is high. We hypothesized, that an increased volume of ropivacaine, would result in greater coverage of incisions used for THA.

Methods: We conducted a randomized, blinded trial in 20 healthy volunteers. Participants were randomized to receive bilateral LFCN-blocks with 8 mL ropivacaine 0.75% on the left side and 16 mL ropivacaine 0.75% on the right side, or vice versa. Allocation was blinded to both participants and outcome assessors. Before nerve block performance, incision lines for posterior and lateral THA approaches were depicted with invisible ultraviolet-paint, thereby securing sufficient blinding during outcome assessment. The blocked area was mapped using temperature and mechanical discrimination tests. Quadriceps muscle strength was monitored. Primary outcome was coverage of the posterior incision line assessed by temperature discrimination test.

Results: We found no difference in coverage of the posterior or lateral incision lines when comparing LFCN-blocks with 8 mL versus 16 mL of ropivacaine. The blocked area was significantly larger in the 16 mL group, assessed by both temperature discrimination test ($p = 0.012$) and mechanical discrimination test ($p = 0.034$). We observed no difference between groups regarding quadriceps muscle strength ($p = 1.0$).

Conclusions: A LFCN-block with increased volume of ropivacaine from 8 mL to 16 mL did not result in a greater coverage of posterior or lateral incision lines used for THA, but in a larger blocked sensory area.

Keywords: Regional anesthetics, Lateral femoral cutaneous nerve block, Total hip arthroplasty, Ropivacaine, Anatomy, Clinical trial

Background

Total hip arthroplasty (THA) is often associated with moderate to severe postoperative pain [1] and peripheral nerve blocks have been used as part of a multimodal analgesic strategy [2–5]. The use of peripheral nerve blocks may be hindered by an accompanying motor blockade, which may lead to increased risk of falling [6].

* Correspondence: frederik.vilhelmsen@hotmail.com
[1]Department of Anesthesiology, Naestved Hospital, Naestved, Denmark
[2]CAR, Department of Anesthesiology, Centre of Anaesthesiological Research –ZealandUniversity Hospital, Koege, Denmark

The lateral femoral cutaneous nerve (LFCN) block is a predominantly sensory block and has been suggested to mitigate pain after hip surgery [7–9]. A clinical trial from 2016 showed that LFCN-blocks with 8 mL ropivacaine 0.75% reduced moderate to severe movement related pain after THA surgery using the posterior approach, but the non-responder rate was high (42%) [8]. Recently, several other studies have investigated the anatomical sensory distribution of a LFCN-block and consistently revealed a limited coverage of THA incisions using 5 to 10 mL of local anesthetics [10–12].

The LFCN most commonly originates from L2 and L3 spinal nerves and travels across the iliac muscle towards the anterior superior iliac spine (ASIS) as one single nerve, before passing beneath the inguinal ligament (IL). In most cases it divides immediately into two branches distal to the IL and continues superficially to supply the lateral aspect of the thigh. However various branching patterns and points of exit from the pelvis have been reported. Variations include, but are not limited to, bifurcation or even trifurcation within the pelvis, exits point through the IL, lateral to the ASIS, or through the ASIS. [13–15]. The LFCN has recently been described as being placed in its own fascial canal in the thigh, named the LFCN-canal [16] or fat-filled flat tunnel [10], created by a splitting of the fascia latae forming a lumen in which the nerve lies.

We hypothesized that injection of a larger volume of local anesthetic could migrate both proximally and distally within the above-described canal, spreading to additional lesser, local cutaneous branches arising from LFCN, thereby giving rise to a greater blocked distribution area. In this trial, we investigate if LFCN-blocks with 16 mL ropivacaine results in a greater coverage of the incision line for the posterior THA approach compared with LFCN-blocks with 8 mL ropivacaine, assessed by temperature discrimination test (primary outcome).

Methods

We conducted a randomized, blinded trial in healthy volunteers at the Department of Anesthesiology, Zealand University Hospital Koege, Denmark from the 19th of May 2017 to the 9th of June 2017.

Participants

Inclusion criteria were: ≥ 18 years of age, American Society of Anesthesiologists physical status classification (ASA) score of I or II, Body Mass Index between 18 and 30. Exclusion criteria were inability to understand or speak Danish, inability to cooperate, allergies to ropivacaine, alcohol or drug abuse (investigators judgement), consumption of prescription-required analgesic drugs within four weeks before the trial date or over-the-counter analgesic drugs within 48 h of trial date, neuromuscular defects, former surgery in lower extremity, large tattoos or trauma on the thigh or hip, and diabetes mellitus. Women had to use hormonal contraception and give a negative urine Human Chorionic Gonadotropine test prior to inclusion.

Each participant was screened for the above criteria on the day of the trial and gave their written informed consent before trial inclusion.

Incision lines

Before block performance, two hypothetical incisions were drawn on each side of the participants' hips, corresponding to the posterior [17] and lateral [18] approaches for THA. It should be noted that the lateral approach for any practical conditions corresponds to the anterolateral approach with respect to skin incision. The lines were approximately 9–13 cm in length. This was done by author LB, who is an orthopedic surgeon specialized in THA surgery. The incisions were drawn with ultraviolet (UV) paint (SkinSafe UV12 blue reflection, J & Maya, Denmark), only visible when exposed to UV light. To ensure that only the orthopedic surgeon knew the exact placement of the incision lines, drawing of the incision lines took place behind a curtain and with blindfolding of the participants.

Randomization and blinding

Participants were enrolled and allocated at random into two groups. Group A received a LFCN-block with 8 mL ropivacaine 0.75% on their right side and a LFCN-block containing 16 mL ropivacaine 0.75% on the left side. Group B received 16 mL ropivacaine 0.75% on the right side and 8 mL ropivacaine 0.75% on their left side.

The pharmacy of The Capital Region (Herlev, Denmark) prepared a computer-generated simple randomization list (1:1 ratio) of identification (ID) numbers and cognate allocation group, and packed the trial medicine in accordance, one medicine package for each ID number. The ID numbers were assigned consecutively. Each medicine package included two identical ampoules containing 20 mL ropivacaine 0.75%. Ampoules were labelled with respect to which volume to administrate to which side. Due to the volume difference, it was possible to visualize which side would be given the larger dose. The anesthesiologist (JKD) who administered the blocks could not be blinded and was therefore not further involved in the study. The preparation of the trial medicine was double-checked by a person not otherwise involved in the trial. To assure blinding of outcome assessors and participants, block performance took place behind a curtain and participants were blindfolded throughout the preparation and administration of the nerve blocks.

Nerve block procedure

Intravenous access, standard monitoring and baseline measurements were obtained before the block procedure. For the block procedure we used a Philips Sparq ultrasound system with a 4–12 MHz linear probe (Phillips, Netherlands) and a Pajunk SonoPlex 22G × 80 mm needle. With the patient in a supine position and the legs extended in neutral position, the transducer was placed parallel to the IL. With the femoral artery and vein as guidance the lateral part of the sartorius muscle and fascia latae was visualized. Approximately 3 cm inferior from this point, the branches of the lateral femoral cutaneous nerve was visualized in the hypoechoic fat-filled subfascial space between the sartorius muscle medially and the tensor fascia latae muscle laterally (Fig. 1). We used in plane approach and the needle was inserted at a shallow angle to reach the area of the nerve. The injection and spread of the local analgesics were visualized sonographically. The LFCN-block was performed on the right side first, immediately followed by the left side. Participants were monitored for 30 min after receiving the blocks. Failed blocks were predefined as preserved sensibility one hour after block performance when testing temperature discrimination in the examination area, described later.

Outcomes assessment

Participants were introduced to all assessment measurements and baseline values were recorded prior to block procedure.

Assessment of outcome measures was done one-hour post-block to ensure full onset of the block. The affected area (blocked area) was assessed using two tests – a temperature discrimination test and a mechanical discrimination test (pinprick). Temperature discrimination is the ability to sense coldness when applying an alcohol soaked gauze to the skin, and pinprick is the ability to recognize sharp sensation when stimulating with a Von Frey filament (Somedic Senselab, size 19, pressure 137.3 g/mm^2). To ensure a systematical exploration of the blocked areas, a line denoted "A" was drawn from the greater trochanter to the lateral epicondyle of the femur. This line was extended cranially. A line labelled "0A" was drawn perpendicular to line "A" at the point of the greater trochanter. Five cm above "0A" another line, also perpendicular to line "A", was drawn and denoted "-1A". Five cm beneath "0A" another line was drawn and denoted "1A". Lines up until "15A" where drawn (Fig. 2). Testing with temperature discrimination test and pinprick along the above described lines, ensured a standardized way of measuring the blocked area on each leg of each participant. The blocked areas were marked and mapped with both measurements before the incision lines were visualized. The length and coverage of the incision lines for both temperature discrimination test and pinprick were recorded.

Furthermore, maximum pain during tonic heat stimulation (THS) was assessed using the Visual Analogue Scale (VAS) score (0–100 mm) (No pain: VAS = 0, worst pain imaginable: VAS = 100) to mimic the postoperative pain from incisions. This was done using a computer-controlled thermode (Modular Sensory Analyzer Thermal Stimulator, 2.5 cm^2, Thermotest; Somedic A/B, Sweden) heated to 45^0 C for 30 s. Two distinct measurements were recorded for each incision, one for the superior (cranial) part of the incision, and one for the inferior (caudal) part of the incision (baseline values were obtained by stimulating the skin superficial to the greater trochanter).

The maximal voluntary isometric contraction (MVIC) of the quadriceps muscle was measured with the participant sitting in an upright position, with their arms across the chest and a dynamometer in fixed position slightly above the ankle anteriorly. MVIC of the quadriceps femoris muscle were calculated in kilograms of force for each leg by the mean of three consecutive measurements. We predefined a decrease in MVIC to < 80% of baseline as clinically relevant.

Outcome measures

All outcomes compared the sides given 8 mL ropivacaine with the sides given 16 mL ropivacaine. The primary outcome was: Difference in the percentage coverage of the posterior incision assessed by temperature discrimination test.

Secondary outcome measures were: Difference in percentage coverage of posterior incision assessed by pinprick (1 outcome); difference in the percentage coverage of the lateral incision assessed by both temperature discrimination test and pinprick (2 outcomes); difference in total blocked area assessed by temperature discrimination

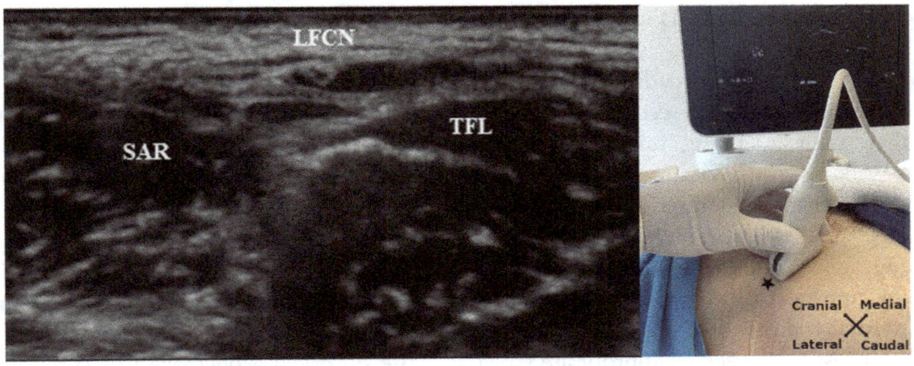

Fig. 1 Ultrasound image of the target nerve. The image is not from an actual trial participant. SAR = sartorius muscle. LFCN = lateral femoral cutaneous nerve. TFL = tensor facia latae muscle. * marks the anterior superior iliac spine

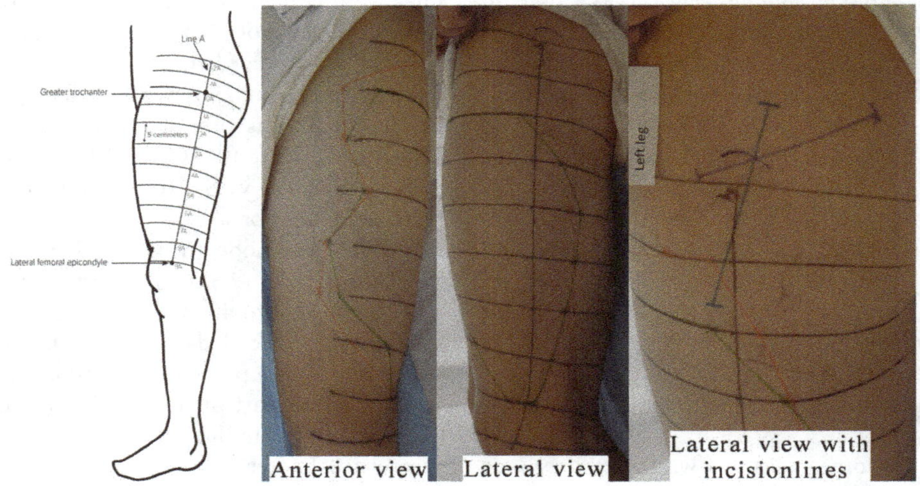

Fig. 2 Mapping of blocked areas. Sketch showing how to draw guiding lines for the mapping of the blocked area, 0A marks the point of the greater trochanter. Red lines border the blocked area which was mapped using temperature discrimination test. Green lines border the blocked area which was mapped using pinprick. The purple line corresponds to the posterior incision line. The blue line corresponds to the lateral incision line. The drawn sketch has previously been published in "Sensory distribution of the lateral femoral cutaneous nerve block – a randomised, blinded trial." Nersesjan M, Acta Anaesthesiologica Scandinavica volume 62 issue 6, Copyright© 2018, The Acta Anaesthesiologica Scandinavica Foundation. Published by John Wiley & Sons Ltd.

test and pinprick (2 outcomes); difference in number of patients feeling no pain (defined as VAS = 0 mm) assessed by maximum pain during THS test on the superior and inferior part of either incision lines (4 outcomes); and the difference in MVIC of the knee joint compared to baseline MVIC values (1 outcome).

Statistical analysis

In a study from 2014 the mean percentage coverages of the incision lines were reported to be between 10.1–21.3% with a standard deviation (SD) of 15.7–24.5% [11]. We aimed to show an increase in coverage of the incision line from 20 to 40% by doubling the volume of ropivacaine injected from 8 mL to 16 mL. In a paired design with a type 1 error rate of 5%, a type 2 error rate of 10%, and an estimated SD of 25%, 18 participants were needed to show an increase in coverage from 20 to 40%. Taking the unknown true SD into account, we chose to enroll 20 participants.

Data were entered into two spreadsheets by two authors (FV and MN) and thereafter cross-checked for typos before further analysis. Using histograms, QQ-plots, and Shapiro-Wilk test, the outcomes regarding the incision lines showed non-normal distribution, whereas all other outcome measures showed normal distribution. We used Wilcoxon-Signed rank test and Hodges-Lehmann estimator for non-normally distributed data and paired t-test for normally distributed data. Chi-squared test and Fisher's Exact test were used as appropriate (IBM SPSS statistics, release 24.0, IBM Corporation, Armonk, USA). The unblinding of the treatment allocation was done in two steps. First step unveiled the group allocation of participants. Calculations were completed, and conclusions drawn, before the final disclosure of the volumes administered in each group. A p-value of < 0.05 was considered statistically significant.

Results

Fifty individuals were screened for eligibility, 30 were excluded and 20 were enrolled (Fig. 3). Eleven participants were allocated to treatment A and nine to treatment B. All enrolled participants received the intervention and completed the trial. Demographics and baseline values are shown in Table 1. We observed one failed block (2.5%). The median coverage of the posterior incision assessed by temperature discrimination test was 0.0% (IQR 0.0 to 0.0) in the 8 mL group and 0.0% (IQR 0.0 to 2.5) in the 16 mL group with a difference of 0.0% (95% CI: 0 to 3.5; $p = 0.345$). The other outcomes regarding the incision lines are shown in Table 2.

The blocked sensory area was significantly larger in the 16 mL group compared with the 8 mL group when assessed by both temperature discrimination test and pinprick. The mean difference of the area assessed by temperature discrimination was 146.3 cm^2 (95% CI: 35.7–256.9; $p = 0.012$), while the mean difference of the area assessed by pinprick was 92.2 cm^2 (95% CI: 7.8–176.6; $p = 0.034$) (Table 2).

We observed a decrease in MVIC to less than 80% of baseline values in 2 of 20 legs receiving 8 mL ropivacaine and 2 of 20 legs receiving 16 mL ropivacaine (Table 2).

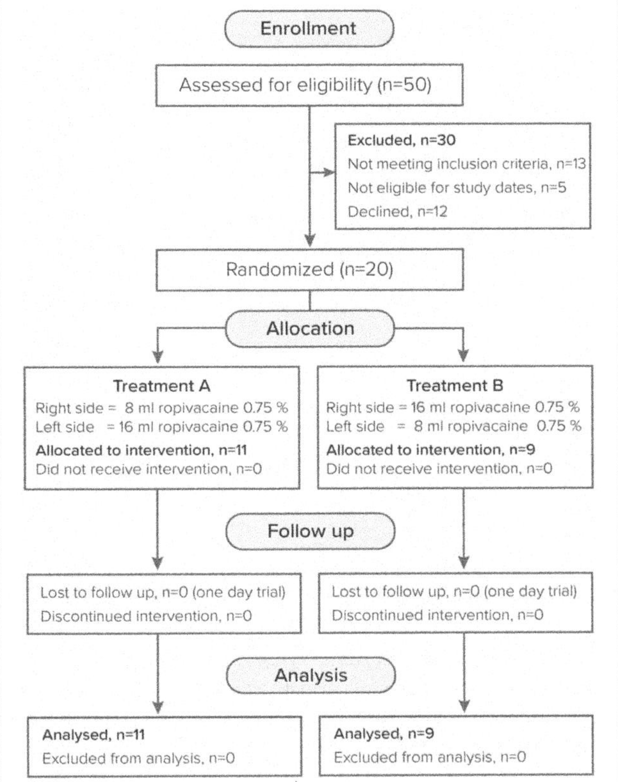

Fig. 3 Consort flowchart

None of the participants experienced bilateral decrease in MVIC to less than 80% of baseline.

No adverse events, both related or unrelated to the trial medication, were observed during the trial. Likewise, no participants reported any discomfort or paresthesia after the trial has ended.

Discussion

This trial showed that using 16 mL 0.75% ropivacaine instead of 8 mL 0.75% ropivacaine for LFCN-block did not result in a larger coverage of the posterior or lateral incision lines typically used for THA [19, 20]. However, we observed a larger sensorial blocked area on the side

Table 1 Demographics and baseline values

Variable	Mean (Range)		
Age, [years]	25		(19–49)
Sex, male/female	13/7		
Height, [cm]	176		(164–186)
Weight, [kg]	70		(55–85)
Quadriceps femoris, MVIC, [kg]	Right leg	41	(26–58)
	Left leg	44	(26–63)
Heat stimulation, VAS, [mm]	Right leg	41	(9–96)
	Left leg	44	(11–94)

MVIC = Maximum Voluntary Isometric Contraction, VAS=Visual Analogue Score

receiving 16 mL compared with 8 mL ropivacaine. There was no difference in the number of participants with a decrease of 20% or more in MVIC of the quadriceps femoris muscle compared with baseline values.

The analgesic effect of nerve blocks after THA surgery is well established [5], however, the role of the LFCN-block in this setting is uncertain. As stated, an 8 mL ropivacaine 0.75% LFCN-block may relieve movement related pain among THA patients with moderate to severe pain to a certain degree, but with a relatively high non-responder rate [8]. We found no increase in coverage of the incision lines using 16 mL compared with 8 mL in this clinical model of healthy volunteers. Based on these results, we find it unlikely that a larger volume would lower the non-responder rate in the setting of THA surgery using the investigated approaches. It is theoretically possible that minimally invasive THA procedures utilizing smaller incisions could benefit more, but this has yet to be investigated.

Injecting a larger volume of local anesthetics into the LFCN canal, however, did result in a larger blocked area, which may indicate the involvement of additional nerve branches. When dot plotting the blocked areas (Fig. 4) we saw that the blocks affected a generally larger area without spreading in any particular direction of the thigh. As hypothesized by Nielsen and colleagues [10] a larger volume injected in the LFCN-canal could spread to the proximal branch of LFCN. Our trial, however, did not confirm this hypothesis.

The increase in blocked area was approximately 30% and with no association between decrease in MVIC and a larger blocked area. The increase in area did not result in a better coverage of any of the tested incision lines for THA. Other types of surgery, as e.g., femoral fractures or plastic surgery procedures on the thigh may theoretically benefit from this larger blocked area.

This trial has the strengths of being blinded (participants, outcome assessors, and during statistical analyses) and designed with a bilateral setup, thereby limiting bias caused by anatomical variation between individuals. Furthermore, this trial (with respect to the 8 mL group) has the strength of reproducing the findings of Nersesjan and co-workers [12], which used the same methodology regarding block procedure and outcome assessment.

There are several limitations to this trial. First, the block technique used may not be ideal to block all branches of the LFCN, especially branches that cross posterior to the ASIS. A different technique (e.g. a more proximal approach to the LFCN) may yield a better coverage of the incision lines, or a larger area blocked.

Secondly, the incision lines drawn by the experienced orthopedic surgeon in this trial may not resemble the incision lines used by other surgeons. The surgeon was instructed to draw the incision lines as he would have if

Table 2 Outcomes

Variable	Group 8 mL		Group 16 mL		Difference and 95% CI		P
Coverage of posterior incision by temperature discrimination test, %	0.0	(0.0–0.0)	0.0	(0.0–0.0)	0.0	(0.0–3.5)	0.345
Coverage of lateral incision by temperature discrimination test, %	0.0	(0.0–19.3)	19.5	(0–45.3)	7.8	(−2.6–24.5)	0.221
Coverage of posterior incision by mechanical discrimination test, %	0.0	(0.0–0.0)	0.0	(0.0–0.0)	0.0	(0.0–0.0)	0.715
Coverage of lateral incision by mechanical discrimination test, %	0.0	(0.0–20.3)	0.0	(0.0–29.5)	3.9	(0.0–16.5)	0.110
Blocked area assessed by temperature discrimination test, cm^2	418	(225.0)	564	(182.7)	146.3	(35.7–256.9)	0.012
Blocked area assessed by mechanical discrimination test, cm^2	369	(211.4)	461	(156.0)	92.2	(7.8–176.6)	0.034
Post-block MVIC ≤80% of baseline, n	2		2				1.00
No pain during THS at superior portion of posterior incision, n	0		0				1.00
No pain during THS at superior portion of lateral incision, n	0		0				1.00
No pain during THS at inferior portion of posterior incision, n	0		1				1.00
No pain during THS at inferior portion of lateral incision, n	2		2				1.00

Coverage outcomes are reported as medians (IQR). Blocked areas are reported as means (SD). Maximal voluntary isometric contraction (MVIC) are reported as number of participants. Pain during tonic heat stimulation (THS) are reported as number of participants feeling no pain

he were to perform THA surgery. Incision lines may vary between surgeons due to different patient characteristics and experience, or preferences, of the surgeon. Furthermore, they may not exactly match examples in textbooks.

Thirdly, the spread of the local anesthetic and the occurrence of failed blocks may vary between patients who have undergone THA surgery and healthy volunteers. This could be due to demographical differences, e.g. Body Mass Index, the surgical trauma, and, perhaps, the indication for THA in the first place (femoral neck fracture, osteoarthritis, osteonecrosis, etc.). This trial had all nerve block administered by an anesthesiologist who specializes in peripheral nerve blocks, which could explain the low failed block rate (2.5%).

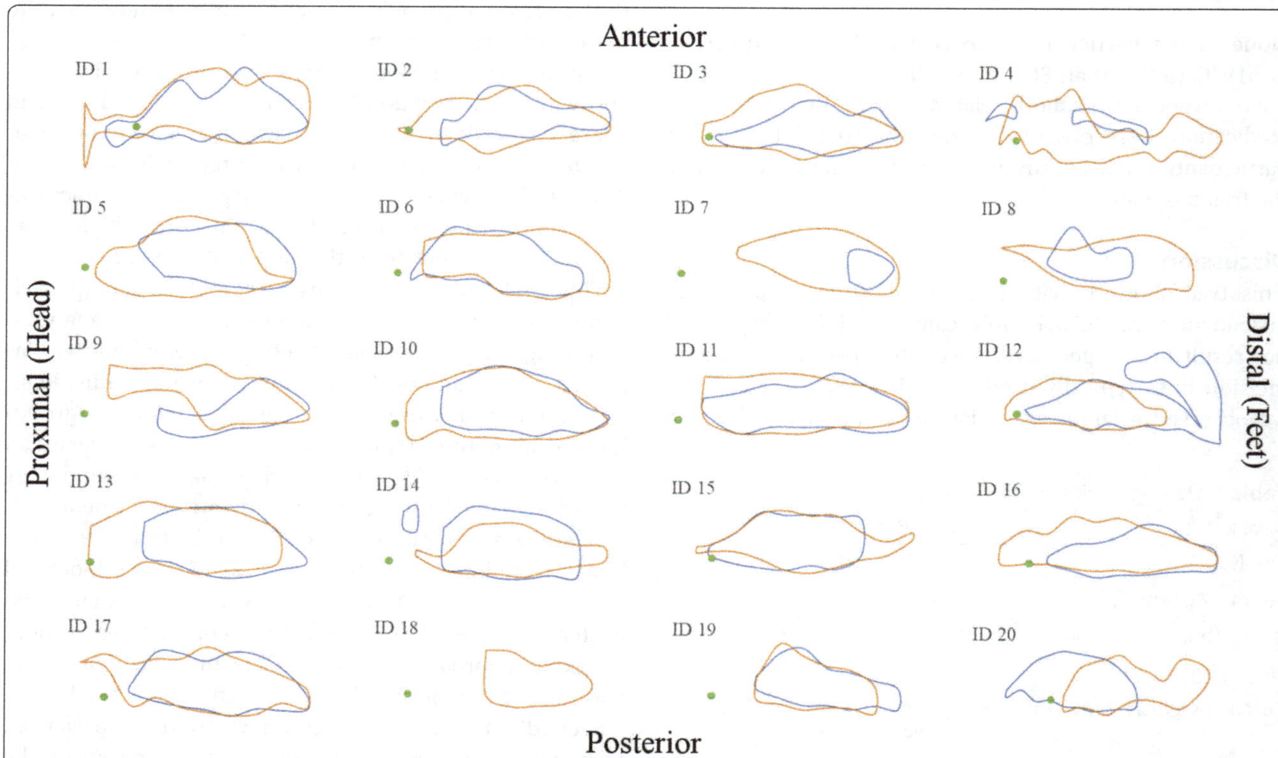

Fig. 4 Area dot-plots. Blocked areas assessed with temperature discrimination for each participant, identification number given. The green dot marks 0A (the point of the greater trochanter). Blue lines represent the side given 8 mL. Orange lines represent the side given 16 mL

Fourthly, the dose of ropivacaine was rather high in the 16 mL group (120 mg), especially if the LFCN-block were to be combined with other blocks. To resemble a clinical situation, a 16 mL diluted ropivacaine solution (i.e. 3.75 mg/mL) could have been used.

Lastly, this trial assumed that there were no intra-individual anatomical differences between the participants' right and left sides. This was not further investigated and therefore might have influenced the results.

Further research should focus on combining LFCN with other nerve block techniques (e.g. the transmuscular quadratus lumborum-block [21–23], posterior femoral cutaneous nerve block, or an iliohypogastric block) to obtain a better coverage of the posterior incision lines after THA, or clinical trials investigating the analgesic effects of LFCN-block in THA patients using the lateral approach.

Conclusions

In conclusion, a LFCN-block with 16 mL ropivacaine 0.75% did not result in a larger coverage of the posterior incision used for THA compared with a LFCN-block consisting of 8 mL ropivacaine 0.75%. It did, however, increase the blocked area. Based on results from this trial we cannot recommend increasing the volume of ropivacaine used in LFCN-blocks to achieve a larger coverage of incisions used in THA.

Abbreviations

ASA: American Society of Anesthesiologists physical status classification; ASIS: Anterior superior iliac spine; CI: Confidence interval; GCP: Good clinical practice; ID: Identification; IL: Inguinal ligament; IQR: Interquartile range; LFCN: Lateral femoral cutaneous nerve; mg: Milligrams; mL: Milliliters; MVIC: Maximal voluntary isometric contraction; SAR: Sartorius; SD: Standard deviation; TFL: Tensor fascia latae; THA: Total hip arthroplasty; THS: Tonic heat stimulation; UV: Ultraviolet; VAS: Visual analogue scale

Acknowledgements

Not applicable.

Author's contributions

Conceptualization: FV, MN, JHA, JKD, LB, DH, OM, KHT.. Data curation: FV, MN, JHA, JKD, LB, KHT. Formal analysis: FV, MN, KHT. Funding acquisition: DH, OM, KHT. Investigation: FV, MN, JHA, JKD, LB, KHT. Methodology: FV, MN, JHA, DH, OM, KHT. Project administration: FV, KHT. Resources: FV, MN, JHA, OM, KHT. Supervision: FV, OM, KHT.Visualization: FV, MN, KHT. Writing – original draft: FV, KHT. All authors have read and approved this manuscript.

Author details

[1]Department of Anesthesiology, Naestved Hospital, Naestved, Denmark. [2]CAR, Department of Anesthesiology, Centre of Anaesthesiological Research –ZealandUniversity Hospital, Koege, Denmark. [3]Department of Orthopedics, Zealand University Hospital, Koege, Denmark.

References

1. Gerbershagen HJ, Aduckathil S, van Wijck AJ, Peelen LM, Kalkman CJ, Meissner W. Pain intensity on the first day after surgery: a prospective cohort study comparing 179 surgical procedures. Anesthesiology. 2013;118(4):934–44.
2. Kehlet H, Dahl JB. Anaesthesia, surgery, and challenges in postoperative recovery. Lancet. 2003;362(9399):1921–8.
3. Hojer Karlsen AP, Geisler A, Petersen PL, Mathiesen O, Dahl JB. Postoperative pain treatment after total hip arthroplasty: a systematic review. Pain. 2015;156(1):8–30.
4. Fischer HB, Simanski CJ. A procedure-specific systematic review and consensus recommendations for analgesia after total hip replacement. Anaesthesia. 2005;60(12):1189–202.
5. Guay J, Johnson RL, Kopp S. Nerve blocks or no nerve blocks for pain control after elective hip replacement (arthroplasty) surgery in adults. The Cochrane database of systematic reviews. 2017;10:Cd011608.
6. Johnson RL, Kopp SL, Hebl JR, Erwin PJ, Mantilla CB. Falls and major orthopaedic surgery with peripheral nerve blockade: a systematic review and meta-analysis. Br J Anaesth. 2013;110(4):518–28.
7. Coad NR. Post-operative analgesia following femoral-neck surgery--a comparison between 3 in 1 femoral nerve block and lateral cutaneous nerve block. Eur J Anaesthesiol. 1991;8(4):287–90.
8. Thybo KH, Mathiesen O, Dahl JB, Schmidt H, Hagi-Pedersen D. Lateral femoral cutaneous nerve block after total hip arthroplasty: a randomised trial. Acta Anaesthesiol Scand. 2016;60(9):1297–305.
9. Jones SF, White A. Analgesia following femoral neck surgery. Lateral cutaneous nerve block as an alternative to narcotics in the elderly. Anaesthesia. 1985;40(7):682–5.
10. Nielsen TD, Moriggl B, Barckman J, Kolsen-Petersen JA, Soballe K, Borglum J, et al. The lateral femoral cutaneous nerve: description of the sensory territory and a novel ultrasound-guided nerve block technique. Reg Anesth Pain Med. 2018.
11. Davies A, Crossley A, Harper M, O'Loughlin E. Lateral cutaneous femoral nerve blockade-limited skin incision coverage in hip arthroplasty. Anaesth Intensive Care. 2014;42(5):625–30.
12. Nersesjan M, Hägi-Pedersen D, Andersen JH, Mathiesen O, Dahl JB, Broeng L, et al. Sensory distribution of the lateral femoral cutaneous nerve block – a randomised, blinded trial. Acta Anaesthesiol Scand. 2018.
13. Majkrzak A, Johnston J, Kacey D, Zeller J. Variability of the lateral femoral cutaneous nerve: an anatomic basis for planning safe surgical approaches. Clinical anatomy. 2010;23(3):304–11.
14. Tomaszewski KA, Popieluszko P, Henry BM, Roy J, Sanna B, Kijek MR, et al. The surgical anatomy of the lateral femoral cutaneous nerve in the inguinal region: a meta-analysis. Hernia. 2016;20(5):649–57.
15. Corujo A, Franco CD, Williams JM. The sensory territory of the lateral cutaneous nerve of the thigh as determined by anatomic dissections and ultrasound-guided blocks. Reg Anesth Pain Med. 2012;37(5):561–4.
16. Hanna A. The lateral femoral cutaneous nerve canal. J Neurosurg. 2017;126(3):972–8.
17. Hoppenfeld S, deBoer P, Buckley R. Surgical exposures in Orthopaedics : the anatomic approach. 4 ed. Philadelphia, PA: Wolters Kluwer Health; 2009. 767 p
18. Mulliken BD, Rorabeck CH, Bourne RB, Nayak N. A modified direct lateral approach in total hip arthroplasty: a comprehensive review. J Arthroplast. 1998;13(7):737–47.
19. Chechik O, Khashan M, Lador R, Salai M, Amar E. Surgical approach and prosthesis fixation in hip arthroplasty world wide. Arch Orthop Trauma Surg. 2013;133(11):1595–600.
20. Havelin LI, Fenstad AM, Salomonsson R, Mehnert F, Furnes O, Overgaard S, et al. The Nordic arthroplasty register association: a unique collaboration between 3 national hip arthroplasty registries with 280,201 THRs. Acta Orthop. 2009;80(4):393–401.
21. Hockett MM, Hembrador S, Lee A. Continuous Quadratus Lumborum block for postoperative pain in Total hip arthroplasty: a case report. A & A case reports. 2016;7(6):129–31.
22. Johnston DF, Sondekoppam RV. Continuous quadratus lumborum block analgesia for total hip arthroplasty revision. J Clin Anesth. 2016;35:235–7.
23. La Colla L, Ben-David B, Merman R. Quadratus Lumborum block as an alternative to lumbar plexus block for hip surgery: a report of 2 cases. A & A case reports. 2017;8(1):4–6.
24. World Medical Association. Declaration of Helsinki: ethical principles for medical research involving human subjects. Jama. 2013;310(20):2191–4.
25. ICH harmonized tripartite guideline. Guideline for good clinical practice. J Postgrad Med. 2001;47(1):45–50.

A randomized double-blind comparison of the double-space technique versus the single-space technique in combined spinal-epidural anesthesia for cesarean section

Eun Hee Chun[1], Sooyoung Cho[2], Jae Hee Woo[2] and Youn Jin Kim[2*]

Abstract

Background: Combined spinal-epidural anesthesia (CSEA) can be performed with either a single-space technique or a double-space technique for cesarean section. We performed a double-blind randomized controlled study to compare the effect of the double-space technique with that of the single-space technique on sensory block level and side effects.

Methods: Parturients undergoing elective cesarean section under regional anesthesia were randomized to receive CSEA with either the double-space technique (double group, $n = 20$) or the single-space technique (single group, n = 20). In the double group, an epidural catheter was inserted at the L1–2 interspace, and dural puncture was performed at the L3–4 interspace. In the single group, the procedure was performed at the L3–4 interspace using the needle-through-needle technique.

Results: There were no differences in time to readiness or intraoperative level of sensory block between the two groups. The postoperative sensory level was maintained at a higher level in the double group than in the single group (1 h postoperatively, $P = 0.029$; 6 h postoperatively, $P = 0.016$). There was no difference between the two groups in terms of side effects. The parturient satisfaction scores 48 h postoperatively were significantly different between groups (9.5 in the double group vs. 8 in the single group, $P = 0.004$).

Conclusions: We conclude that there were no differences in intraoperative variables between the double-space technique and the single-space technique for CSEA. However, double-space CSEA for cesarean section may be beneficial for controlling postoperative pain and improving parturient satisfaction.

Keywords: Cesarean section, Combined spinal-epidural technique, Obstetric anesthesia, Patient satisfaction, Regional anesthesia

* Correspondence: ankyj@ewha.ac.kr
[2]Department of Anesthesiology and Pain Medicine, College of Medicine, Ewha Womans University, 25 Magokdong-ro 2-gil, Gangseo-gu, Seoul, Republic of Korea 07084

Background

Combined spinal-epidural anesthesia (CSEA) has advantages that compensate for the shortcomings of spinal or epidural anesthesia alone for cesarean section. It combines the best features of spinal anesthesia (rapid onset, intense blockade, and a decreased drug requirement) and epidural anesthesia (titratable anesthesia levels, the ability to extend duration, postoperative analgesia supplementation), and it avoids the disadvantages of each, including different levels between individuals in spinal anesthesia and incomplete motor blocks and missed segments in epidural anesthesia.

CSEA can be performed using either the single- or double-space technique; the double-space technique was introduced first. Brownridge's first report of CSEA in obstetric anesthesia in 1981 described epidural catheter placement at L1–2 followed by a subarachnoid block at L3–4 [1]. The needle-through-needle technique was described independently by Coates and Mumtaz in 1982 [2]. At that time, the technique was performed with an ordinary epidural needle and a long spinal needle. Currently, a large number of commercial kits are available, designed specifically for needle-through-needle CSEA. The single-space technique, also called the needle-through-needle technique, is the most widely reported CSEA technique in the literature and is likely the most frequently used [3]. However, there is no recent comparison of the two methods, and the method used is chosen according to the anesthesiologist's preference in clinical settings. In previous studies, the double-space technique had a greater success rate than the single-space technique [4, 5] and a low complication rate [6], but there were also conflicting reports on the success rate [7]. Furthermore, we have found few reports about the comparisons between the two techniques that include block characteristics, side effects, and parturient satisfaction. It is time to think about the meaningful use of the two techniques rather than the kits.

We hypothesized that CSEA with either the single- or double-space technique would make a differences in the sensory block level, the incidence of side effects and the perioperative outcomes.

Methods

The study was approved in July 2014 by the local Institutional Review Board of Ewha Womans University Hospital, Seoul, Republic of Korea (EUMC 2014–05–032-007) and registered with the Clinical Trial Registry of Korea (https://cris.nih.go.kr) under the trial ID KCT0002514. Written informed consent was obtained from all patients. A prospective randomized, double-blind study was performed at term pregnancy scheduled for elective cesarean section. Parturients with pregnancy-induced hypertension, multiple pregnancies, placenta previa, cardiac diseases, or contraindications to regional anesthesia were excluded. A total of 40 parturients were randomized to receive CSEA with either the double-space technique (double group, $n = 20$) or single-space technique (single group, $n = 20$). The random allocation sequence was created by an anesthesiologist who did not participate in the study using a computer-generated randomization schedule (www.randomization.com). On arrival at the operating room, all parturients were rapidly infused with 10 ml kg^{-1} of lactated Ringer's solution. Oxygen was administered at a flow rate of 3 l min^{-1} through a nasal cannula. Electrocardiogram, non-invasive blood pressure and pulse oximetry monitoring were performed, and baseline values were recorded. After taking the right lateral position, preprocedural ultrasound scanning was performed in a nonsterile manner. Using a 2–5 MHz curved probe (M-TurboTM; SonoSite Canada Inc., Canada), the sacrum was identified first; then, the transducer was moved cephalad, and the intervertebral level was marked with a skin marker. All parturients received local anesthetic infiltration at the L1–2 and L3–4 interspaces using 1% lidocaine prior to CSEA.

In the double group, an 18-gauge Tuohy needle (Perifix®; B. Braun, Melsungen, Germany) was introduced, using a loss of resistance to air to confirm the epidural space. Dural puncture was performed at the L3–4 interspace with a 25-gauge Quincke tip spinal needle (Tae Chang Industrial Co., Ltd., Kongju, Korea). Next, 0.5% hyperbaric bupivacaine 6 mg mixed with fentanyl 25 μg was given intrathecally after the free flow of cerebrospinal fluid was observed. A 20-gauge epidural catheter was inserted through the epidural needle, 3–4 cm into the epidural space. After the Tuohy needle had been removed, the catheter was firmly fixed and covered with gauze so that the level of catheter entry could not be distinguished. For the epidural test dose, 3 ml of 0.375% levobupivacaine with epinephrine (1:200,000) was injected.

In the single group, the procedure was performed at the L3–4 interspace. An 18-gauge Tuohy needle (Espocan®; B. Braun, Melsungen, Germany) was introduced using a loss of resistance to air, and the dura was punctured with a 27-gauge Sprotte needle using the needle-through-needle technique. When free flow of cerebrospinal fluid was observed, 0.5% hyperbaric bupivacaine 6 mg and fentanyl 25 μg were administered. After withdrawal of the spinal needle, a 20-gauge epidural catheter was inserted through the epidural needle, 3–4 cm into the epidural space. The Tuohy needle was removed, and epidural catheter fixation and an epidural test dose injection were performed in the same manner as in the double group.

CSEA was performed by one investigator (YJK). The parturients and the investigator (EHC) were unaware of which group they had been assigned to, and the investigator (EHC) performed all assessments.

The primary outcome measures for this study were time spent on the procedure, time to readiness, and sensory block level. The secondary outcomes included the failure of the block, the incidence of side effects (e.g., hypotension, bradycardia, nausea, dizziness), neonatal outcomes, parturient satisfaction scores (0–10, 0 = unsatisfied, 10 = satisfied; at the end of the procedure, upon arrival at the postanesthesia care unit (PACU), and 48 h postoperatively) and variables associated with postoperative recovery (e.g., pain scores, motor blockade, and sensory level). The total procedure time was defined as the time interval between local infiltration to the skin and the intrathecal injection. Time to readiness was defined as the time from intrathecal injection to the T4 sensory block. The point of intrathecal injection was taken as time 0 min in both groups. Maternal blood pressure was recorded every minute for 10 min and at 5-min intervals for the remaining time. Hypotension was defined as a 20% or greater decrease below the preinduction level or a systolic pressure below 95 mmHg, which was treated immediately with ephedrine 5 mg, i.v., and repeated whenever necessary. Bradycardia (heart rate < 50 bpm) was treated with 0.5 mg of atropine.

At the end of surgery, parturients received an epidural bolus injection: 10 ml of a solution of ropivacaine 0.2% with morphine sulfate 1 mg. Postoperative analgesia was provided with an epidural infusion at 5 ml h^{-1} of a solution containing ropivacaine 2 mg ml^{-1} and fentanyl 4 μg ml^{-1}.

The sensory block was tested every minute for 10 min and 1, 6, 12, 24, and 48 h after the operation. The motor block was checked 1 and 6 h after the operation. Sensory levels were checked by cold sensation using an alcohol sponge, and the motor block was assessed using a modified Bromage scale (0 = no block; 1 = weak or absent hip flexion, able to move knees and ankles; 2 = unable to move hips or knees, able to move ankles; and 3 = unable to move any joint). Postoperative pain scores using numeric rating scales (NRS) (0–10; 0 = no pain, 10 = the most severe pain imaginable) were recorded postoperatively at 1, 6, 12, 24, and 48 h.

It was recorded when the patients started urination after foley catheter removal and when the patients observed the first flatus. The time to start walking was also recorded independently.

Statistical analysis

Statistical comparisons of the continuous variables between the two groups were analyzed with Student's *t*-test, and sensory and motor block variables were compared using the Mann-Whitney U test. Differences between the two groups in the incidences of side effects such as hypotension, pain, nausea and vomiting and dizziness were analyzed with chi-square tests and Fisher's exact test when appropriate. A repeated measures analysis of variance was used to test the difference between the two groups in blood pressure. $P < 0.05$ was considered to be statistically significant. SPSS (ver. 18.0, Chicago, IL, USA) was used for the statistical analysis. The data are expressed as numbers, percentages, and medians [range] or means ± standard deviation. From our experience and a previous study [8], using a two-sided design at a significance level of 5% with a power of 80%, an estimated 16 parturients per group were needed to detect a sufficient effect size. Assuming a 20% drop-out rate, we designed the study with 20 parturients in each group.

Results

Forty parturients scheduled for cesarean sections were enrolled in and analyzed for this study. Figure 1 presents the allocation of parturients into the study groups. No intergroup differences were identified with regard to individual characteristics, duration of surgery, anesthesia time, or total fluid intake and output (Table 1).

Table 2 shows variables associated with the procedures, including procedural time and anesthesia level. There were no differences between the two groups in procedural time. The time from intrathecal injection to T4 sensory block (time to readiness) was 7.5 ± 2.7 min in the single group and 6.6 ± 2.6 min in the double group. The level of sensory block from 1 to 10 min after induction was not different between the two groups. Failure of the block did not occur in either group.

There were no differences in systolic blood pressure between the two groups during the first 10 min after induction ($P = 0.248$, Fig. 2). There were no differences in Apgar scores between the two groups (Apgar score 1 min: 9.6 ± 0.6 in the double group vs. 9.4 ± 0.8 in the single group; Apgar score 5 min: 9.9 ± 0.3 in the double group vs. 10.0 ± 0.2 in the single group).

During the intraoperative period, the two groups were similar with regard to the occurrence of complications. Hypotension and bradycardia occurred only during the operation (Table 3).

The NRS scores for postoperative pain, which were measured at 1, 6, 12, 24, and 48 h, were not different between the groups. The pain scores 12 and 48 h postoperatively showed that pain was well controlled; the NRS scores were 1 in both groups. There were no differences in motor block recovery; however, the sensory block levels of the single group were lower than those of the double group 1 and 6 h postoperatively. The median values were T8 in the double group and T10 in the single group 1 h postoperatively ($P = 0.029$) and T12 in the double group and L1 in the single group 6 h postoperatively (Table 4).

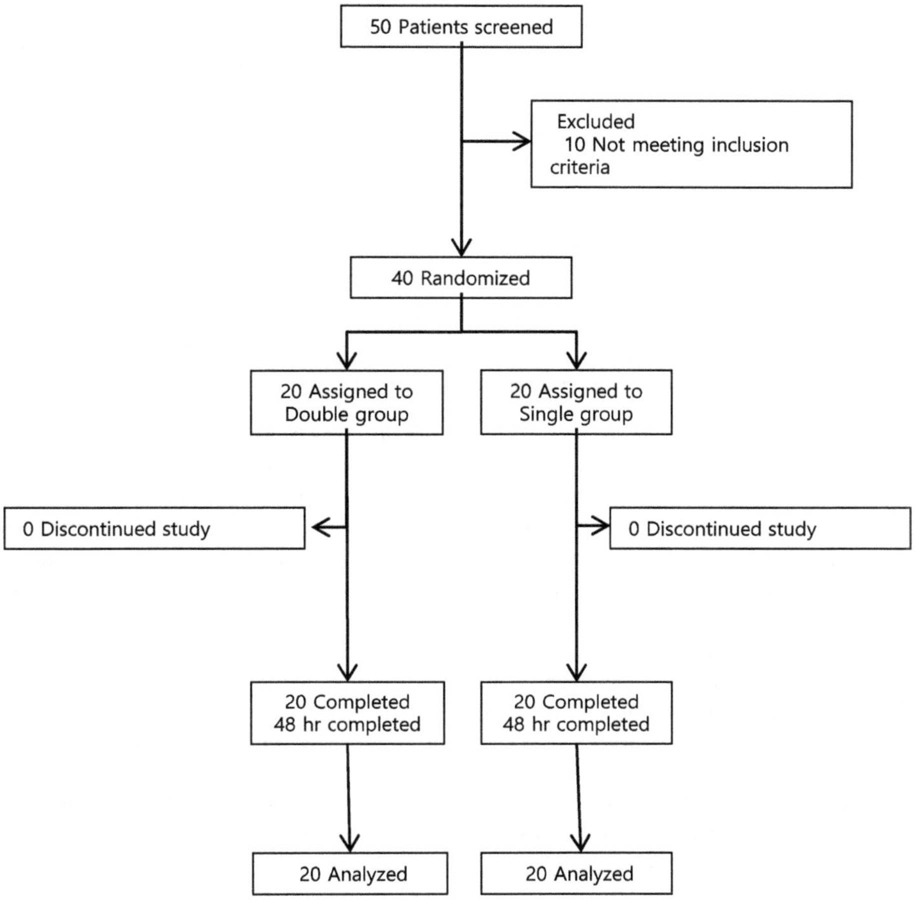

Fig. 1 CONSORT chart

Table 1 Patient characteristics and clinical features

	Double Group (n = 20)	Single Group (n = 20)
Age (years)	33.4 ± 2.9	34.0 ± 3.6
Sex (M/F)	0/20	0/20
Height (cm)	159.4 ± 4.6	160.9 ± 4.2
Weight (kg)	67.7 ± 8.6	66.7 ± 7.4
Gestational age (days)	270.8 ± 5.7	265.9 ± 22.7
Operation time (min)	62.5 ± 12.5	55.8 ± 8.5
Anesthesia time (min)	95.0 ± 17.0	87.3 ± 11.9
Fluid intake (ml)	2166 ± 709.3	1990.0 ± 456.7
Output (ml)	1310.0 ± 381.7	1115.0 ± 233.8

Data are presented as the number or mean ± SD. There were no differences between the two groups. Double group = patients who received combined spinal-epidural anesthesia with the double-space technique, Single group = patients who received combined spinal-epidural anesthesia with the single-space technique

*: $P < 0.05$, compared with the single group

The incidence of unilateral leg numbness during epidural patient-controlled analgesia (PCA) infusion was 2 (18%) in the double group and 6 (54%) in the single group, but there was no significant difference ($P = 0.235$).

The time required to start walking independently was 21.8 ± 4.2 h in the double group and 24.1 ± 7.5 h in the single group ($P = 0.241$). The time required to start urination after foley catheter removal was 25.1 ± 4.1 h in the double group and 27.4 ± 7.8 h in the single group ($P = 0.250$). The time required to observe the first flatus was 29.8 ± 10.8 h in the double group and 32.6 ± 11.3 h in the single group ($P = 0.427$). Two parturients in the single group observed the first flatus 2 days after the operation. Mild ileus was observed in their abdominal X-rays, and they recovered without any complications.

The parturient satisfaction scores after procedure completion (satisfaction score OR) and parturient satisfaction scores upon arrival at the PACU (satisfaction score RR) were not different. However, the parturient satisfaction score 48 h postoperatively (satisfaction score 48 h) was higher in the double group than in the single group (9.5 vs. 8, $P = 0.009$, Table 5).

Table 2 Variables associated with the procedures

	Double Group ($n = 20$)	Single Group ($n = 20$)	P value
Total procedure time (min)	5.0 ± 1.2	5.9 ± 2.4	0.135
Time to readiness (min)	6.6 ± 2.6	7.5 ± 2.7	0.241
Level of sensory block at 1 min	T6 [T3-T11]	T7 [T4-T10]	0.209
Level of sensory block at 3 min	T4 [T2-T9]	T4 [T2-T8]	0.769
Level of sensory block at 5 min	T4 [T1-T7]	T4 [T2-T5]	0.965
Level of sensory block at 10 min	T4 [T1-T5]	T4 [T2-T4]	0.976
Ephedrine dose (mg)	5 [0–30]	10 [0–30]	0.477

Data are presented as the mean ± SD or median values [range]. There were no differences between the two groups: double group = patients who received combined spinal-epidural anesthesia with the double-space technique; single group = patients who received combined spinal-epidural anesthesia with the single-space technique; total procedure time: time interval between local infiltration to skin and the intrathecal injection; time to readiness: time from intrathecal injection to T4 sensory block; the point of intrathecal injection was taken as time 0 min in both groups

Discussion

The present study was a randomized controlled trial comparing two CSEA methods: the single- and double-space techniques after the use of a developed commercial kit for the needle-through-needle technique. The main findings of the present study are that there were no differences in the intraoperative level of sensory block and the incidence of side effects between the two groups. However, the parturient satisfaction score 48 h postoperatively was higher in the double group than in the single group.

Lyons and colleagues reported that separate-needle CSEA had a lower spinal failure rate (4 vs. 16%) and was associated with less hypotension than needle-through-needle CSEA and that the separate-needle group had higher blocks than the needle-through-needle group [9]. However, the anesthesia level during the first 10 min after induction was not different between the two groups, and there were no cases of unsuccessful dural puncture or additional epidural injection during the operation. There were no differences in time from intrathecal injection to T4 sensory block (time to readiness) or systolic blood pressure between the two groups. The main factor determining the intraoperative anesthetic level was the intrathecal injection; furthermore, the site of the indwelling epidural catheter did not make differences in the anesthetic level in this study. In the report of Lyons and colleagues [9], the intrathecal injection

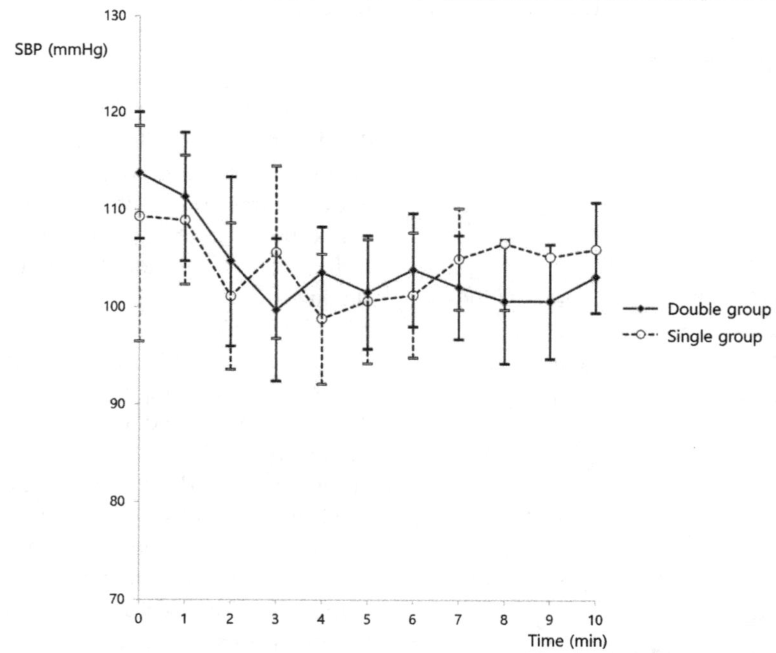

Fig. 2 Systolic blood pressure changes after induction. There were no differences between the two groups ($P = 0.248$); SBP = systolic blood pressure; double group = patients who received combined spinal-epidural anesthesia with the double-space technique; single group = patients who received combined spinal-epidural anesthesia with the single-space technique. The point of intrathecal injection was taken as time 0 min for both groups

Table 3 Incidence of side effects

	Double Group ($n = 20$)	Single Group ($n = 20$)	P value
Hypotension	7 (35%)	10 (50%)	0.337
Intraoperative	7	10	
Postoperative	0	0	
Bradycardia	1 (5%)	0 (0%)	1.000
Intraoperative	1	0	
Postoperative	0	0	
Nausea	1 (5%)	3 (15%)	0.605
Intraoperative	0	1	
Postoperative	1	2	
Dizziness	3 (15%)	3 (15%)	1.000
Intraoperative	0	0	
Postoperative	3	3	

Values are numbers (%). There were no differences between the two groups: double group = patients who received combined spinal-epidural anesthesia with the double-space technique; single group = patients who received combined spinal-epidural anesthesia with the single-space technique

drug and parturient position were not described. This point seems to be the cause of the difference in anesthetic level between the present study and Lyons' study.

A modification of the CSEA technique, for example, epidural volume extension, affects the block height [10]. In the present study, the double-space technique used the L1–2 lumbar interspace, and the single-space technique used the L3–4 interspace for insertion of the epidural catheter. We hypothesized that CSEA with either the single- or double-space technique would affect the sensory block level and side effects; however, there were no significant differences in intraoperative sensory block level and side effects. The mechanism of a higher sensory block with epidural volume extension has been explained as the intrathecal drug being pushed cephalad by the epidural injection [11]. The reasons why augmentation of the sensory block level was not observed in this study were as follows: first, the epidural injection doses were smaller than the epidural volume extension doses. Second, the intrathecal doses were small, so the cephalad spread of the drug was limited.

There were no differences in procedural time between the two groups, and this aspect seems to have little impact on the clinical choice of CSEA technique for anesthesiologists. Casati and colleagues reported that the needle-through-needle technique requires less time, has no greater failure rate, and results in greater parturient satisfaction than the double-space technique [7]. At that time, the development of a spinal needle with a locking mechanism may have contributed to the result. Currently, several commercial kits are commonly used, and the procedural skill in using them has been highly developed. The procedural time depends on the physician's proficiency rather than on the method.

There was no difference between the groups in the incidences of hypotension, bradycardia, nausea, or dizziness. Although some of these factors are known to affect patient satisfaction [12], there was no difference between the two groups in this study. Therefore, these side effects are not considered to have caused the difference in satisfaction scores between the groups.

We attempted to find aspects to improve maternal satisfaction 48 h postoperatively by reviewing the subjective and objective outcomes. We did not use questionnaires because there is no widely accepted questionnaire for parturients undergoing cesarean section. Some

Table 4 Variables associated with postoperative recovery

	Double Group ($n = 20$)	Single Group ($n = 20$)	P value
Bromage scale 1 h (0–3)	1 [0–2]	1 [0–3]	0.774
Bromage scale 6 h (0–3)	0 [0–1]	0 [0–2]	0.762
Sensory level 1 h	T8 [T4-T11]	T10 [T4-T11]	0.029*
Sensory level 6 h	T12 [T6-L1]	L1 [T8-L5]	0.016*
Pain 1 h NRS (0–10)	0 [0–2]	0 [0–4]	0.281
Pain 6 h NRS (0–10)	1 [0–3]	0.5 [0–3]	0.300
Pain 12 h NRS (0–10)	1 [0–7]	1 [0–8]	0.801
Pain 24 h NRS (0–10)	1.5 [0–4]	1 [0–7]	0.694
Pain 48 h NRS (0–10)	1 [0–3]	1 [0–7]	0.672
Time required to start ambulation (h)	21.8 ± 4.2	24.1 ± 7.5	0.241
Time required to start urination after foley catheter removal (h)	25.1 ± 4.1	27.4 ± 7.8	0.250
Time required to observe the first flatus (h)	29.8 ± 10.8	32.6 ± 11.3	0.427

Data are presented as median values [range] or means ± SD. NRS; Numeric rating scale, Bromage scale (0 = no block, 1 = weak or absent hip flexion, able to move knees and ankles, 2 = unable to move hips or knees, able to move ankles, 3 = unable to move any joint)

There were no differences between the two groups in postoperative pain score or motor block. The sensory level was significantly higher in the double group than in the single group. *: $P < 0.05$, compared with the single group

Table 5 Parturient satisfaction scores

	Double Group (n = 20)	Single Group (n = 20)	P value
Satisfaction score OR (0–10)	10 [8–10]	10 [8–10]	0.298
Satisfaction score RR (0–10)	10 [7–10]	10 [8–10]	0.089
Satisfaction score 48 h (0–10)	9.5 [8–10]	8 [6–10]	0.009*

Data are presented as median values [range]. Satisfaction score OR: the parturient satisfaction score at the end of the procedure; satisfaction score RR: the parturient satisfaction score after arrival at the postanesthesia care unit (PACU); satisfaction score 48 h: the parturient satisfaction score 48 h postoperatively. *: $P < 0.05$, compared with the single group

questionnaires are based on subjective discomfort; these were not suitable for this study, which compared the features of two anesthetic techniques [12, 13]. Among the factors affecting maternal satisfaction in previous studies [12, 13], several were investigated in the present study, including procedural time, nausea, dizziness, postoperative pain, motor blockade, time required to start waking independently, time required to start urination after foley catheter removal, time required to observe the first flatus, and unilateral leg numbness. In a retrospective study of labor epidural analgesia, the clinical determinants associated with parturient dissatisfaction were headache, backache, urinary retention, and neural deficit [14]. There were statistically insignificant differences between the two groups for these factors. Furthermore, satisfaction is multidimensional and could be influenced by many factors, such as family support, environmental changes, and mood changes [15]. Although analgesic effectiveness contributes to satisfaction, it is not the only contributor [16]. Among the investigated factors, only unilateral leg numbness developed during postoperative epidural PCA infusion. Therefore, it is presumed to be the cause of the difference in satisfaction scores 48 h postoperatively.

It has been shown that the double-space technique is more advantageous for postoperative pain control. The double group did not show a more profound motor block than the single group; nevertheless, the postoperative analgesic level was higher in this group. CSEA offers advantages, including the ability to eliminate a motor blockade and to achieve a highly selective sensory blockade and optimize analgesia [17]. Our comparison of postoperative pain scores (NRS) did not show a significant difference because the epidural bolus, 10 ml of a solution containing 0.2% ropivacaine and morphine sulfate 1 mg injected in the recovery room, was so effective. Postcesarean pain has at least two components: somatic pain and visceral pain. These are transmitted via T10-L1 spinal nerves [18]. In this respect, the double-space technique is more useful for achieving appropriate postoperative analgesia levels than the single-space technique.

The enhanced recovery after surgery (ERAS) concept has been widely adopted, and there has been great interest in early recovery after a cesarean section [19]. The important aspects of patient recovery were investigated, including the time required to start walking independently, the time required to start urination after foley catheter removal, and the time required to observe the first flatus. These times were shorter in the double group than in the single group; however, the difference was not significant. The factors that affect the time required to start independent ambulation varied. The presence of unilateral leg numbness may affect ambulation. The incidence of unilateral leg numbness during the first 48 h postoperatively was lower in the double group than in the single group, but the difference was not significant. However, the difference between the two groups suggests that the double-space technique may be beneficial for ERAS. Anesthetic considerations for ERAS include postoperative analgesia, fluid management, respiratory function restoration, fasting, and rapid recovery from the motor block. It is believed that there is evidence to support the use of epidurals in ERAS colorectal surgery, but there is no established ERAS guideline for cesarean section. We suggest that these techniques for epidural catheter indwelling can lead to differences in parturient satisfaction and recovery time.

In the present study, the factors affecting parturient recovery were not controlled. Parturients may delay starting ambulation independently without any problems unless they are actively encouraged to walk. This limits the understanding of the anesthetic technique's effect on a parturient's recovery. Therefore, additional research is needed to understand the benefits of the double-space technique in ERAS.

Conclusions

We conclude that there were no differences in intraoperative variables between the double-space technique and single-space technique for CSEA. However, double-space CSEA for cesarean section may be beneficial for controlling postoperative pain and improving parturient satisfaction.

Abbreviations

CSEA: Combined spinal-epidural anesthesia; ERAS: Enhanced recovery after surgery; NRS: Numeric rating scales; PACU: Postanesthesia care unit; PCA: Patient-controlled analgesia

Acknowledgements

Not applicable.

Authors' contributions

EHC collected data and wrote the manuscript. SC generated the random allocation sequence and analyzed data. JHW helped conduct the study and data collection. YJK designed the study. All authors read and approved the final manuscript.

Author details

[1]Department of Anesthesiology and Pain Medicine, Kangnam Sacred Heart Hospital, Hallym University College of Medicine, Seoul, Republic of Korea. [2]Department of Anesthesiology and Pain Medicine, College of Medicine, Ewha Womans University, 25 Magokdong-ro 2-gil, Gangseo-gu, Seoul, Republic of Korea 07084.

References

1. Brownridge P. Epidural and subarachnoid analgesia for elective caesarean section. Anaesthesia. 1981;36:70.
2. Coates MB, Mumtaz MH, Daz M, Kuz M. Combined subarachnoid and epidural techniques. Anaesthesia. 1982;37:89.
3. Blanshard HJ, Cook TM, Blanshard HJ, Cook TM, Blanshard HJ, Cook TM. Use of combined spinal-epidural by obstetric anaesthetists. Anaesthesia. 2004;59:922.
4. Backe S, Sheikh Z, Wilson R, Lyons G. Combined epidural/spinal anaesthesia: needle-through-needle or separate spaces? Eur J Anaesthesiol. 2004;21:854–7.
5. Sadashivaiah J, Wilson R, McLure H, Lyons G. Double-space combined spinal-epidural technique for elective caesarean section: a review of 10 years' experience in a UK teaching maternity unit. Int J Obstet Anesth. 2010; 19:183–7.
6. Cook T. 201 combined spinal–epidurals for anaesthesia using a separate needle technique. Eur J Anaesthesiol. 2004;21:679–83.
7. Casati A, D'ambrosio A, De Negri P, Fanelli G. A clinical comparison between needle-through-needle and double-segment techniques for combined spinal and epidural anesthesia. Reg Anesth Pain Med. 1998;23: 390–4.
8. Ithnin F, Lim Y, Sia AT, Ocampo CE. Combined spinal epidural causes higher level of block than equivalent single-shot spinal anesthesia in elective cesarean patients. Anesth Analg. 2006;102:577–80.
9. Lyons G, Macdonald R, Mikl B. Combined epidural/spinal anaesthesia for caesarean section. Anaesthesia. 1992;47:199–201.
10. McNaught AF, Stocks GM. Epidural volume extension and low-dose sequential combined spinal-epidural blockade: two ways to reduce spinal dose requirement for caesarean section. Int J Obstet Anesth. 2007;16:346–53.
11. Tyagi A, Girota G, Kumar A, Kumar S, Sethi AK, Mohta K. Single-shot spinal anaesthesia, combined spinal-epidural and epidural volume extension for elective caesarean section: a randomized comparison. Int J Obstet Anesth. 2009;18:231–6.
12. Morgan P, Lo J, Halpern S. The development of a maternal satisfaction scale for caesarean section. Int J Obstet Anesth. 1999;8:165–70.
13. Sindhvananda W, Leelanukrom R, Rodanant O, Sriprajittichai P. Maternal satisfaction to epidural and spinal anesthesia for cesarean section. J Med Assoc Thail. 2004;87:628–35.
14. Tan DJA, Sultana R, Han NLR, Sia ATH, Sng BL. Investigating determinants for patient satisfaction in women receiving epidural analgesia for labour pain: a retrospective cohort study. BMC Anesthesiol. 2018;18:50.
15. Robinson PN, Salmon P, Yentis SM. Maternal satisfaction. Int J Obstet Anesth. 1998;7:32–7.
16. Richardson MG, Lopez BM, Baysinger CL, Shotwell MS, Chestnut DH. Nitrous oxide during labor: maternal satisfaction does not depend exclusively on analgesic effectiveness. Anesth Analg. 2017;124:548–53.
17. Rawal N, Van Zundert A, Holmström B, Crowhurst JA. Combined spinal-epidural technique. Reg Anesth Pain Med. 1997;22:406–23.
18. McDonnell NJ, Keating ML, Muchatuta NA, Pavy TJ, Paech MJ. Analgesia after caesarean delivery. Anaesth Intensive Care. 2009;37:539–51.
19. Wrench IJ, Allison A, Galimberti A, Radley S, Wilson MJ. Introduction of enhanced recovery for elective caesarean section enabling next day discharge: a tertiary Centre experience. Int J Obstet Anesth. 2015;24:124–30.

14

Risk of postoperative nausea and vomiting in hip and knee arthroplasty

Antonio Moraitis[1*], Magnus Hultin[2] and Jakob Walldén[1]

Abstract

Background: The overall risk of postoperative nausea and vomiting after general anaesthesia is approximately 30% even with prophylactic medications. Studies exploring the risk after regional anaesthesia including intrathecal morphine are limited but indicate that intrathecal morphine is highly emetogenic and is additive to the PONV risk associated with other forms of anaesthesia. The aim of this observational study was to investigate the risk of PONV after spinal blockade combined with intrathecal morphine and to explore associations with patient and perioperative factors, including given PONV-prophylaxis. We hypothesized that a large number of patients in a clinical setting receive less prophylaxis than the recommendations in guidelines *(suboptimal prophylaxis)*, leading to a higher risk for PONV compared to those receiving adequate PONV prophylaxis.

Methods: The study was conducted as a prospective observational cohort study regarding PONV in patients undergoing hip/knee replacement under spinal anaesthesia including intrathecal morphine. Patients were included at a county hospital in Sweden during April–November 2013 ($n = 59$) and September 2014–June 2015 ($n = 40$). One hundred eight patients entered the study with 99 patients analysed in the final cohort. Patients were followed the first three postoperative days with a questionnaire regarding PONV and peri- and postoperative data was collected. PONV risk is presented as the proportion of patients (%) with PONV and was related to the level of perioperative PONV-prophylaxis (suboptimal/optimal). Univariate analysis was used to analyse factors associated with PONV.

Results: Forty-six patients (46%) experienced PONV during the 3-day study period whereof 36 patients (36%) until noon the first day after the procedure. 19/27 patients (70%) that received suboptimal PONV-prophylaxis experienced PONV compared to 27/72 (38%) that received optimal PONV-prophylaxis ($p = 0.015$). Further, female gender and/or a history of motion sickness were associated with an increased PONV-risk.

Conclusions: There was a high risk for PONV after spinal anaesthesia including morphine. PONV risk was associated with the level of prophylaxis and with known risk factors for PONV. Our findings suggest that a more liberal use of PONV prophylaxis might be motivated.

Keywords: Postoperative nausea and vomiting, Injections, Spinal, Prevention & Control, Arthroplasty, Morphine

* Correspondence: antonio.moraitis@umu.se
[1]Department of Surgical and Perioperative Sciences, Anaesthesiology and Intensive Care Medicine (Sundsvall), Umeå University, Sundsvall, Sweden

Background

The overall risk of postoperative nausea and vomiting (PONV) after general anaesthesia is reported to be approximately 30% even with prophylactic medications, but studies exploring the risk after regional anaesthesia including intrathecal morphine are limited [1, 2]. Hip and knee arthroplasty can be performed under regional anaesthesia using a spinal blockade, and postoperative pain can be reduced by adding intrathecal morphine [3, 4]. However, this method might be associated with a high risk of PONV [5, 6].

In Apfel's model for assessing PONV risk, developed for general anaesthesia, significant risk factors are being female, non-smoker, having prior history of PONV and/or motion sickness, need of opioids for postoperative analgesia. If all factors are present, the risk of PONV can be as high as 80% [7].

Apfel's risk score is often used for procedures under regional anaesthesia and prophylaxis given according to guidelines. Commonly used prophylactic drugs acting via different pharmacological targets are corticosteroids (anti-inflammatory), ondansetron (5-hydroxytriptamine 3 (5-HT_3) receptor antagonist) and droperidol (dopamine D_2 receptor antagonist), which are equally effective and each independently reduce PONV with approximately 25% [8]. Despite increased awareness and the introduction of new antiemetics, PONV is still a problem in the perioperative period. Risk stratification and a multimodal approach are key elements but are only effective if implemented and complied with, especially in high-risk patients [9–12]. Screening for PONV and a multimodal prophylaxis and treatment have a moderate evidence level and a strong recommendation grade [13].

The aim of this observational study was to investigate the risk of PONV in spinal blockade combined with intrathecal morphine and to explore factors associated with PONV with a focus on if the level of given PONV prophylaxis adhered to the guidelines. We hypothesized that a large proportion of patients receive less prophylaxis than recommended in a clinical setting, leading to a higher risk for PONV compared to those receiving adequate PONV prophylaxis.

Methods

Study design

The study cohort was part of a prospective observational cohort study regarding PONV. After obtaining written informed consent from the patients, data were collected from patient medical charts and through a standardized form with questions regarding PONV. The study was approved by the Regional Ethics Committee in Umeå, University Campus, Umeå, Sweden, on May 8, 2012 (Chairperson A. Iacobaeus, Dnr 2012/146-31 M).

Study cohort

Our study cohort consisted of patients at Sundsvall Hospital, Sweden, undergoing hip/knee replacement under spinal anaesthesia including intrathecal morphine. Inclusion criteria were, besides the criteria for the cohort, age ≥ 18 years and being able to participate. Due to research resources, the inclusion was performed during two periods, April–November 2013 ($n = 59$) and September 2014–June 2015 ($n = 40$).

Anaesthesia and PONV prophylaxis

The choice of anaesthesia, PONV prophylaxis and pain management was based on clinical routines and at the discretion of the attending anaesthesiologist. At the time of the study, the clinical routine for hip and knee arthroplasty was spinal anaesthesia with bupivacaine 15–20 mg, morphine 0.12 mg and clonidine 30 µg. PONV prophylaxis during anaesthesia were given according to local guidelines which stipulates that patients should be given a number of PONV prophylaxes equal to one less than the value of each patients Apfel-score. Drugs used for PONV prophylaxis were betamethasone 4 mg, ondansetron 4 mg, and droperidol 0.5–1 mg intravenously with a priority in that same order. Further, paracetamol (1 g × 4) and an oral depot opioid (oxycodone 10–20 mg/day) was given as base analgesics. Some patients also received a cox-2 inhibitor (etoricoxib 90–120 mg) in the premedication and some patients received gabapentin (600–900 mg/day) postoperatively for up to 7 days. As rescue analgesic, either intravenous morphine or peroral oxycodone were used. For all patients, an enhanced recovery pathway was used including early nutrition and mobilisation.

Patient classification according to PONV risk and given prophylaxis

The simplified PONV risk score, developed by Apfel et al., was used to calculate the predicted the PONV risk [7]. Factors included in the model were female gender, non-smoking status, history of previous PONV and/or motion sickness, and use of postoperative opioids yielding a risk score of maximum 4. According to published guidelines, the optimal number of PONV prophylaxis to be given is related to the risk score [8]. To classify if patients had received PONV-prophylaxis according to our local guidelines, we (ourselves) defined *optimal prophylaxis* as the number of PONV prophylaxes needed being one less than the value of the risk score. When the number of prophylactic drugs given were less than *optimal prophylaxis*, patients were classified as having received *suboptimal prophylaxis*. Thus, *suboptimal prophylaxis* indicates that patients receives less PONV-prophylaxis than recommended. Our model is a simplification of the consensus guidelines published in 2014 [8], with the main difference that with four risk factors, where the guidelines states two or more interventions, we considered three interventions as optimal.

Data collection

Preoperatively, patients were asked questions regarding risk factors for PONV. Postoperatively, patients answered a questionnaire with standardized questions regarding PONV at 2, 4, and 6 h after arrival at the recovery unit and at noon on postoperative days 1–3. The PONV questions were based on a validated scale for assessing PONV [14]. With the patient form, data regarding vomiting, retching, and nausea were obtained for each evaluation period, as well as the frequency of nausea [sometimes /often /most of the time /all the time] and if any rescue medications were given. Patients were also instructed to estimate any pain and to specify if any extra pain-relieving medicine had been taken. Further study data were obtained from the patients' medical records and the perioperative charts.

Primary outcome variables

PONV was defined as the presence of nausea and/or vomiting.

- Cumulative number of patients (%) with PONV over the observation intervals.
- Number of patients (%) with PONV during the postoperative intervals 0–2 h (hours), 2–4 h, 4–6 h, 6 h - Day 1, Day 1 - Day 2 and Day 2-Day 3.
- Number of patients with *suboptimal* or *optimal* PONV-prophylaxis.
- Number of patients (%) with PONV in relation level of prophylaxis (suboptimal/optimal).

Secondary outcome variables

Patient and perioperative factors associated with PONV risk.

Statistical methods

PONV risk is presented as the proportion of patients (%) with PONV, and a corresponding 95% confidence interval was calculated for PONV risk using the method recommended by Newcombe and Altman [15].

To explore factors associated with PONV risk, we performed univariate analysis on dichotomized data with Pearson's chi-squared test and calculated odds ratios (ORs) with the corresponding 95% confidence intervals.

Data were entered in spreadsheets (Excel, Microsoft, Redmond, Washington, USA), and statistical analysis was performed with SPSS (IBM Corp. Released 2016, IBM SPSS statistics for Mac, Version 24, Armonk, New York, USA). Bar charts were created with MATLAB (Release 2018b, The MathWorks, Inc., Natick, Massachusetts, USA).

We did not perform any power calculation, although we considered the final study cohort of 99 patients to be an appropriate size for an observational study of a standardized procedure.

Results

Patient characteristics

Preoperatively, 109 patients were screened and asked for participation in the study, with 108 patients included. Seven patients did not receive spinal morphine and two patients had not answered any of the questions in the questionnaire, thus a final cohort of 99 patients were analysed.

The patients had a median age of 67 years (range 38–87 years), and 57% were female. Seventy-eight patients (79%) underwent hip arthroplasty and 21 (21%) underwent knee arthroplasty. The median dose of intrathecal morphine was 0.12 mg (range 0.08–0.20), and all patients received 30 μg intrathecal clonidine. Fifty-five patients (55%) had a high predicted risk for PONV (Apfel-score 3 or 4). For further patient characteristics see Table 1.

PONV prophylaxis

Ninety-four patients (94%) received betamethasone, 53 (54%) received ondansetron, and 20 (20%) received droperidol as PONV prophylaxes. Of those given only one prophylactic drug, 42 patients received betamethasone and 3 received ondansetron. The 31 patients given two prophylaxes all received betamethasone and ondansetron.

Twenty-seven patients (27%) received suboptimal prophylaxis in relation to their PONV risk score, and there was a significant difference between women and men in given suboptimal prophylaxis (45% [19 of 42 women] vs. 14% [8 of 57 men], $p < 0.001$; Table 2).

The risk of PONV in relation to the number of PONV-risk factors and the amount of PONV-prophylaxis given are presented in Table 3.

Cumulative PONV risk

During the first 2 h, 9% (CI: 5–16%) experienced PONV with an increase to 26% (CI: 19–36%) in the first 6 h. At Day 1, 36% (CI: 28–46%) had experienced PONV, and at Day 3 46% (CI: 37–56%). Further details of PONV risk over time including each observation period are presented in Fig. 1 and Table 4.

Factors associated with PONV-risk

A higher incidence of PONV was observed during the first day among those who received suboptimal prophylaxis. On the third postoperative day, 70% of patients with suboptimal prophylaxis had experienced any PONV compared to 38% with optimal prophylaxis ($p < 0.01$; Table 4).

Being female (OR 2.33 (1.01–5.38)), having previous history of PONV (OR 5.37 (1.82–15.8)), and suboptimal

Table 1 Patient characteristics ($n = 99$)

	Value
Gender, *female sex*	42 (42%)
Age, *years*	67 (37–87)
BMI, m^2kg^{-1}	28 (19–43)
ASA-class	
1	26 (26%)
2	60 (61%)
3	13 (13%)
Smokers	1 (1%)
History of motion sickness	19 (19%)
Previous PONV	19 (19%)
Preoperative treatment with opioids	12 (12%)
COX-2 inhibitor in premedication	9 (9%)
Apfel-score	
0–1	0 (0%)
2	44 (44%)
3	35 (35%)
4	20 (20%)
Hip prosthesis surgery, *numbers*	78 (79%)
Knee prosthesis surgery, *numbers*	21 (21%)
Spinal anaesthesia combined with intrathecal morphine and clonidine	99 (100%)
Duration of anaesthesia, *minutes*	170 (105–336)
Duration of surgery, *minutes*	95 (57–256)
PONV prophylaxis	
Betamethasone	93 (94%)
Ondansetron	54 (55%)
Droperidol	20 (20%)
Number of prophylaxes given	
0	3 (3%)
1	45 (45%)
2	31 (31%)
3	20 (20%)
Rescue antiemetics until noon Day 1	27 (27%)
Gabapentin included in postoperative medication	36 (36%)

Values are presented as numeric values (% of total) or median (SD). *ASA* American Society of Anaesthesiologists Classification, *PONV* postoperative nausea and vomiting, *BMI* body mass index. PONV, number of prophylaxis given: Of those receiving only 1 prophylactic drug, 42 patients received betamethasone and 3 received ondansetron. For those given two prophylaxis, all received betamethasone and ondansetron. No missing data except BMI of one patient

Table 2 Proportion of males vs. females receiving suboptimal prophylaxis

	Men ($n = 57$)	*Female* ($n = 42$)	*p-value*
Suboptimal prophylaxis *(n = 27)*	8 (14%)	19 (45%)	
Optimal prophylaxis *(n = 72)*	49 (86%)	23 (55%)	$p < 0.001$

p-value for comparisons between gender and suboptimal or optimal prophylaxis with Pearson's chi-squared test

PONV prophylaxis (OR 3.04 (1.22–7.57)) had higher odds for PONV until noon Day 1 (Table 5).

Discussion

The main finding in our observational study in patients receiving intrathecal morphine was a high risk of PONV. The cumulative risk during the first three postoperative days showed that nearly half of the patients experienced

Table 3 Risk of PONV (%) at 0–24 h in relation to PONV risk factors and number of PONV-prophylaxis given

Number of risk factors	Number of PONV-prophylaxis 0	1	2	3
2	100% (1/1)	23% (6/26)	27% (3/11)	33% (2/6)
3	100% (2/2)	31% (4/13)	27% (4/15)	20% (1/5)
4	- (0/0)	83% (5/6)	60% (3/5)	56% (5/9)

Values are risk of PONV (number of patients with PONV in subgroup / total number of patients in subgroup). Grayshaded subgroups are considered given optimal prophylaxis in accordance to the definitions in the study

PONV. Every fourth patient were given less PONV-prophylaxis than the recommendations in general guidelines, and these patients had an almost doubled risk for PONV. Further, females were given less prophylaxis to a greater extent and also had a higher risk of PONV.

The PONV risk found in our cohort are in accordance with previous studies. A meta-analysis evaluating intrathecal morphine (0.05–0.25 mg) in caesarean section found an overall PONV-risk of number needed to harm (NNH) of 6.3 for nausea and 10.1 for vomiting [5]. Another study investigating side effects in a randomized, double-blind, dose-response study concluded that nausea was present at even low doses of intrathecal morphine (0.015 mg) with an risk of 56% compared to a control group with a risk of 4% [6]. The absolute risks vary between studies and might be dependent on study settings and PONV prophylaxis, but many studies with intrathecal morphine report high risk for PONV [16–19].

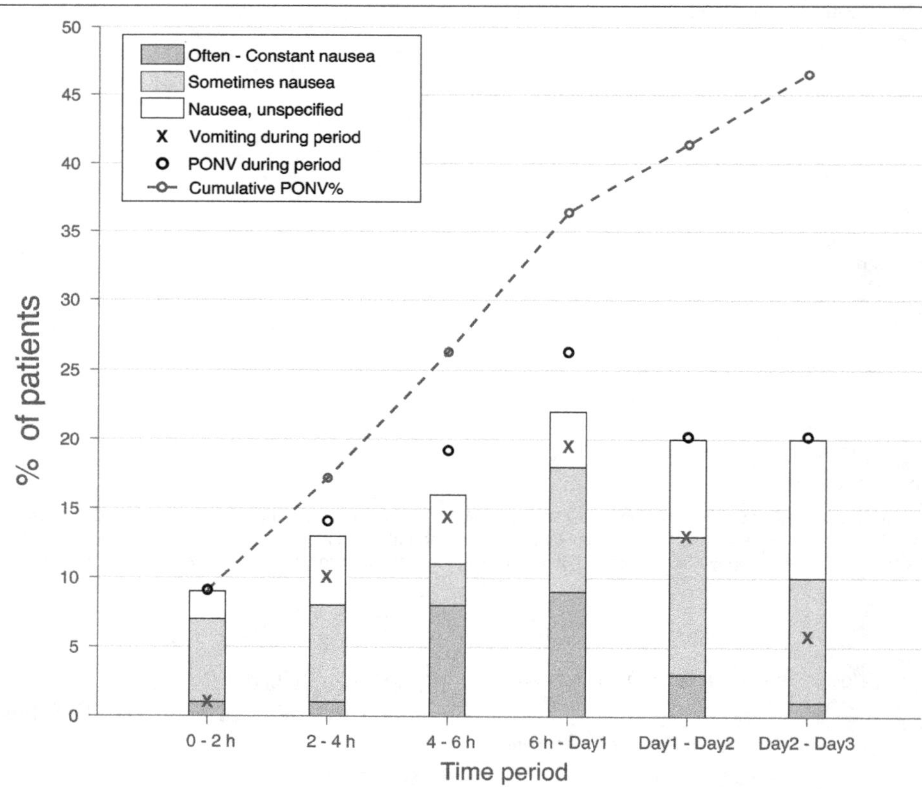

Fig. 1 Cumulative risk of PONV and risk of nausea (including frequency), vomiting, and PONV during the different observation periods. Bars represent risk for nausea, and grey parts of the bars represent nausea that affected the patient's activity (getting out of bed, moving in bed, walking normally, and eating or drinking) and was graded as sometimes (light grey) and often/constant (dark grey). The dashed line shows the cumulative incidence of PONV and accounts for the total number of patients with any event of nausea or vomiting

Table 4 PONV risk in relation to the level of prophylaxis

Number of patients (%) with PONV	All patients (*n* = 99)	*Suboptimal PONV prophylaxis (n = 27)*	*Optimal PONV prophylaxis (n = 72)*	*p-value*
0 h–6 h	26 (26%)	9 (33%)	17 (24%)	$p = 0.44$
6 h–Day 1	26 (26%)	12 (44%)	14 (19%)	$p < 0.05$
Day 1–Day 2	20 (20%)	12 (44%)	8 (11%)	$p < 0.01$
Day 2–Day 3	20 (20%)	8 (30%)	12 (17%)	$p = 0.17$
0 h–Day 1	36 (36%)	15 (56%)	21 (29%)	$p < 0.05$
0 h–Day 3	46 (46%)	19 (70%)	27 (38%)	$p < 0.01$

PONV postoperative nausea and vomiting; comparison between suboptimal and optimal prophylaxis with Pearson's chi-squared test. Data collected with a standardized questionnaire answered at 2, 4 and 6 h after arrival at the recovery unit and at noon on postoperative days 1–3. Risk of PONV during different postoperative periods after hip or knee arthroplasty under spinal anaesthesia including intrathecal morphine. Day 1 = first day after surgery

Almost 80% of our patients *with PONV* during the three-day study period presented with their first episode of PONV during the first 24 h, indicating that there should be an awareness regarding symptoms of PONV and readiness for rescue treatments during the first postoperative day.

The third consensus guidelines from 2014 recommended that PONV-prophylaxis should be given according to individual PONV-risk and is based on the presence of PONV risk factors. With a higher risk score, the number of prophylactic interventions is increased [8]. The guideline states, that with 0, 1, 2, 3 or 4 risk factors, the minimum number of prophylactic agents to be 0, 0, 1, 2, 2, respectively. We simplified the model to a linear relationship and defined optimal prophylaxis as at least 0, 0, 1, 2, 3 agents with 0, 1, 2, 3, or 4 risk factors, respectively. The small differences between the models are that high-risk patients with four risk factors should be given three prophylaxis with our model, whereas the consensus guidelines recommend a minimum of two prophylaxis. As the highest risk for PONV were found in patients with four risk factors (Table 3), the results indicates that we used an acceptable model as there were differences between patients with three and four risk factors. Patients with four risk factors might be considered more prophylaxis than patients with three risk factors.

We found that almost one third of our patients were given *suboptimal* PONV-prophylaxis, even though there were local guidelines stating the optimal level of prophylaxis. Further, patients with suboptimal prophylaxis had an almost doubled risk for PONV. We cannot conclude if it was the suboptimal prophylaxis per se, the factors the classification was based on (i.e. female gender, previous PONV) or other unknown factors that actually caused the increased risk. Our findings agree with others that, even if guidelines are implemented in a clinical setting, there are major difficulties for clinicians to adhere to the guidelines [20]. A recent study showed that simplification of the risk assessment with a guidance to prophylaxis increased the number of patients receiving adequate PONV-prophylaxis and reduced the risk for PONV [21, 22].

We found that female gender and previous PONV were associated with a higher risk of PONV. Known risk factors for PONV are female gender, non-smoker, history of PONV or motion-sickness, and postoperative use of opioids [7]. With only one patient being a smoker and intrathecal opioids being given to all patients, it was not possible to evaluate the latter factors. Based on our findings, we suggest that factors associated with increased PONV risk after general anaesthesia might be relevant for predicting PONV risk after regional anaesthesia when intrathecal opioids are used as an adjuvant.

The use of opioids is one of the main factors that contribute to PONV [23]. All of our patients received intrathecal morphine, most of the patient's postoperative oral opioids and some rescue opioids. With our observational study design, it was not possible to evaluate the effect of each type of opioid administration. However, patients with severe pain had a tendency to a higher PONV-risk and we might speculate that this is due to an increased number of opioids given to these patients.

As our study was an observational study, we did not interfere with the treatments given to the patients. Even if there were local guidelines, patients received different postoperative analgesic and we found differences in the doses of intrathecal opioids, some patients were given Cox-2 inhibitors before the procedure and one third of the patients received oral gabapentin postoperatively. We did not find any major association to an altered risk for PONV with these factors.

Our primary outcome variable (PONV) were based on reported events of nausea and vomiting. Except reporting the frequency of PONV, we did not put the PONV

Table 5 Factors associated with risk for PONV until noon the first postoperative day

	Number of patients	Number of patients with PONV (%)	Unadjusted OR (CI)	*p*-value
Gender				
Female	42	20 (48%)	2.33 (1.01–5.38)	0.046
Male	57	16 (28%)		
BMI				
< 35 kg/m^2	88	30 (34%)	1.93 (0.52–7.20)	0.32
≥ 35 kg/m^2	10	5 (50%)		
History of PONV				
Yes	19	13 (68%)	5.37 (1.82–15.8)	0.003
No	80	23 (29%)		
History of motion sickness				
Yes	19	8 (42%)	1.35 (0.49–3.75)	0.56
No	80	28 (35%)		
Non-smoker				
Yes	98	36 (36%)	NA	0.184
No	1	1 (100%)		
Preoperative treatment with opioids				
Yes	12	4 (33%)	0.90 (0.24–3.08)	0.81
No	87	32 (37%)		
COX-2 inhibitor in premedication				
Yes	9	3 (33%)	0.86 (0.21–3.68)	0.84
No	90	33 (37%)		
Suboptimal PONV prophylaxis				
Yes	27	15 (56%)	3.04 (1.22–7.57)	0.015
No	72	21 (29%)		
Type of prosthesis surgery				
Hip	78	27 (35%)	0.71 (0.26–1.88)	0.49
Knee	21	9 (43%)		
Intrathecal morphine, dose				
80–100 µg	11	5 (45%)	1.51 (0.42–5.42)	0.79
120 µg	76	27 (35%)	reference	
140–200 µg	12	4 (33%)	0.91 (0.25–3.29)	
Gabapentin given postoperatively				
Yes	36	13 (39%)	1.22 (0.52–2.88)	0.66
No	63	23 (35%)		
Given oral or parenteral opioids until noon Day 1				
Yes	97	35 (36%)	0.56 (0.03–9.3)	0.68
No	2	1 (50%)		
Maximal NRS ≥5 for pain until noon Day 1.				
Yes	39	17 (44%)	1.67 (0.72–3.84)	0.23
No	60	19 (32%)		

Number of patients is the total number in the subgroup. PONV risk is presented as the number of patients in the subgroup with PONV (%). Unadjusted OR, unadjusted odds ratio; *CI* 95% confidence interval, *NRS* Numeric Rating Scale, *Day 1* first day after surgery, *NA* not available for calculation

in the overall context of postoperative recovery. Today there are several validated tools to follow the postoperative quality of recovery, for example QoR-15 [24, 25], that includes several domains of recovery. Further, there are other factors, like fluid management and ambulation [26], that were not included in our study protocol and that may have impact on PONV. In future studies regarding PONV we believe it is of value to include these factors and an extensive quality of recovery tool.

A weakness in our study could be missing data, even though it was a prospective design. We might have missed PONV events that had not been identified or documented on the questionnaires, and thus the "true" result might be a higher risk for PONV. Further, there might be missed documentation of given PONV prophylaxis resulting in classification as suboptimal instead of optimal prophylaxis. This might have had an impact on the number of patients with suboptimal prophylaxis, but this would not have affected the observed high risk of PONV observed in our study.

The high risk of PONV in our study might suggest that patients undergoing hip and knee arthroplasty, including intrathecal morphine in the analgesic regime, might need more PONV prophylaxis. A main argument against a more liberal approach to PONV prophylaxis is an increased risk for side effects from the prophylactic drugs [2, 8]. However, antiemetics are generally well tolerated [27], and the benefits from adequate prophylaxis are desirable for patients, including increased well-being and a smoother postoperative recovery. Currently there is not enough evidence to make any firm conclusions, and more clinical studies are needed to evaluate the effects of liberal PONV prophylaxis.

Recently, the fourth consensus guidelines for the management of PONV were published [12]. The major change is a more liberal approach to PONV-prophylaxis with a recommendation to give two agents to patients with 1–2 risk factors and three or four agents when more than two risk factors are present. If generalised, the new guidelines propose that patients with any risk factors for PONV should be given 1–2 additional prophylactic intervention compared to our model used in this study. Our conclusion that more prophylaxis might be needed, are in line with these new recommendations.

Conclusion

The risk for PONV after spinal morphine was high even with prophylaxis, and the increased risk was associated with known risk factors for PONV (female, previous PONV) and when a lower amount of PONV prophylaxis was given in relation to the risk. Our findings suggest that a more liberal use of PONV prophylaxis might be motivated.

Abbreviations

ASA-class: American Society of Anesthesiologists classification; BMI: Body mass index; CI: Confidence interval; h: Hours; kg: Kilogram; mg: Milligram; µg: Microgram; NA: Not available; NNH: Number needed to harm; NRS: Numeric rating scale; OR: Odds ratio; PONV: Postoperative nausea and vomiting; QoR-15: Quality of recovery-15; SD: Standard deviation

Acknowledgements

Not applicable.

Authors' contributions

MH and JW are the main contributors to the conception and design of this study. AM is the main author working with the compilation, analysis and interpretation of the raw data and presenting it in the form of this article. AM have drafted this article with substantial revisions and feedback from MH and JW. JW are the main contributor to the design of the figure/tables presented in this article. All authors, (AM, MH, JW), have approved the submitted version and have agreed both to be personally accountable for the author's own contributions and to ensure that questions related to the accuracy or integrity of any part of the work, even ones in which the author was not personally involved, are appropriately investigated, resolved, and the resolution documented in the literature.

Author details

[1]Department of Surgical and Perioperative Sciences, Anaesthesiology and Intensive Care Medicine (Sundsvall), Umeå University, Sundsvall, Sweden. [2]Department of Surgical and Perioperative Sciences, Anaesthesiology and Intensive Care Medicine (Umeå), Umeå University, Umeå, Sweden.

References

1. Franck M, Radtke FM, Apfel CC, Kuhly R, Baumeyer A, Brandt C, et al. Documentation of post-operative nausea and vomiting in routine clinical practice. J Int Med Res. 2010;38(3):1034–41.
2. Watcha MF, White PF. Postoperative nausea and vomiting. Its etiology, treatment, and prevention. Anesthesiology. 1992;77(1):162–84.
3. Rathmell JP, Pino CA, Taylor R, Patrin T, Viani BA. Intrathecal morphine for postoperative analgesia: a randomized, controlled, dose-ranging study after hip and knee arthroplasty. Anesth Analg. 2003;97(5):1452–7.
4. Bowrey S, Hamer J, Bowler I, Symonds C, Hall JE. A comparison of 0.2 and 0. 5 mg intrathecal morphine for postoperative analgesia after total knee replacement. Anaesthesia. 2005;60(5):449–52.
5. Dahl JB, Jeppesen IS, Jørgensen H, Wetterslev J, Møiniche S. Intraoperative and postoperative analgesic efficacy and adverse effects of intrathecal opioids in patients undergoing cesarean section with spinal anesthesia: a qualitative and quantitative systematic review of randomized controlled trials. Anesthesiology. 1999;91(6):1919–27.
6. Raffaeli W, Marconi G, Fanelli G, Taddei S, Borghi GB, Casati A. Opioid-related side-effects after intrathecal morphine: a prospective, randomized, double-blind dose-response study. Eur J Anaesthesiol. 2006;23(7):605–10.
7. Apfel CC, Läärä E, Koivuranta M, Greim CA, Roewer N. A simplified risk score for predicting postoperative nausea and vomiting: conclusions from cross-validations between two centers. Anesthesiology. 1999;91(3):693–700.
8. Gan TJ, Diemunsch P, Habib AS, Kovac A, Kranke P, Meyer TA, et al. Consensus guidelines for the management of postoperative nausea and vomiting. Anesth Analg. 2014;118(1):85–113.
9. Kaye AD, Cornett EM, Chalabi J, Naim NZ, Novitch MB, Creel JB, et al. Pharmacology of Antiemetics: update and current considerations in anesthesia practice. Anesthesiol Clin. 2017;35(2):e41–54.
10. Kovac AL. Updates in the Management of Postoperative Nausea and Vomiting. Adv Anesth. 2018;36(1):81–97.
11. Walldén J, Flodin J, Hultin M. Validation of a prediction model for post-discharge nausea and vomiting after general anaesthesia in a cohort of Swedish ambulatory surgery patients. Eur J Anaesthesiol. 2016;33(10):743–9.
12. Gan TJ, Belani KG, Bergese S, Chung F, Diemunsch P, Habib AS, et al. Fourth consensus guidelines for the Management of Postoperative Nausea and Vomiting. Anesth Analg. 2020;131(2):411–48.
13. Wainwright TW, Gill M, McDonald DA, Middleton RG, Reed M, Sahota O, et al. Consensus statement for perioperative care in total hip replacement and total knee replacement surgery: enhanced recovery after surgery (ERAS((R))) society recommendations. Acta Orthop. 2020;91(1):3–19.
14. Myles PS, Wengritzky R. Simplified postoperative nausea and vomiting impact scale for audit and post-discharge review. Br J Anaesth. 2012;108(3):423–9.
15. Altman DG, Gardner MJSwc. Statistics with confidence: confidence intervals

and statistical guidelines. In: Altman DG, et al., editors. [Great Britain]: BMJ Books. 2nd edn. London: British Medical Journal; 2000.

16. Karlsen AP, Wetterslev M, Hansen SE, Hansen MS, Mathiesen O, Dahl JB. Postoperative pain treatment after total knee arthroplasty: a systematic review. PLoS One. 2017;12(3):e0173107.
17. Hess SR, Lahaye LA, Waligora AC, Sima AP, Jiranek WA, Golladay GJ. Safety and side-effect profile of intrathecal morphine in a diverse patient population undergoing total knee and hip arthroplasty. Eur J Orthop Surg Traumatol. 2019;29(1):125–9.
18. Pinsornsak P, Teeyaphudit M, Ruetiwarangkoon C, Chaiwuttisak A. Comparison of Ramosetron with Ondansetron for prevention of Intrathecal morphine-induced nausea and vomiting after primary Total knee Arthroplasty: a randomized control trial. J Arthroplast. 2017;32(3):1040–3.
19. Cheah JW, Sing DC, Hansen EN, Aleshi P, Vail TP. Does Intrathecal morphine in spinal anesthesia have a role in modern multimodal analgesia for primary Total joint Arthroplasty? J Arthroplast. 2018;33(6):1693–8.
20. Kranke P, Eberhart LH. Possibilities and limitations in the pharmacological management of postoperative nausea and vomiting. Eur J Anaesthesiol. 2011;28(11):758–65.
21. Dewinter G, Staelens W, Veef E, Teunkens A, Van de Velde M, Rex S. Simplified algorithm for the prevention of postoperative nausea and vomiting: a before-and-after study. Br J Anaesth. 2018;120(1):156–63.
22. Kappen TH. Risk-tailored prophylaxis for postoperative nausea and vomiting: has the big little problem gotten any smaller? Br J Anaesth. 2018;120(1):9–13.
23. Horn CC, Wallisch WJ, Homanics GE, Williams JP. Pathophysiological and neurochemical mechanisms of postoperative nausea and vomiting. Eur J Pharmacol. 2014;722:55–66.
24. Lyckner S, Boregard IL, Zetterlund EL, Chew MS. Validation of the Swedish version of quality of recovery score −15: a multicentre, cohort study. Acta Anaesthesiol Scand. 2018;62(7):893–902.
25. Stark PA, Myles PS, Burke JA. Development and psychometric evaluation of a postoperative quality of recovery score: the QoR-15. Anesthesiology. 2013;118(6):1332–40.
26. Jewer JK, Wong MJ, Bird SJ, Habib AS, Parker R, George RB. Supplemental perioperative intravenous crystalloids for postoperative nausea and vomiting. Cochrane Database Syst Rev. 2019;3:CD012212.
27. De Hert S, Staender S, Fritsch G, Hinkelbein J, Afshari A, Bettelli G, et al. Pre-operative evaluation of adults undergoing elective noncardiac surgery: updated guideline from the European Society of Anaesthesiology. Eur J Anaesthesiol. 2018;35(6):407–65.

Effects of bupivacaine or levobupivacaine on cerebral oxygenation during spinal anesthesia in elderly patients undergoing orthopedic surgery for hip fracture

Roser Vives[1*], Diana Fernandez-Galinski[2], Francisca Gordo[2], Alberto Izquierdo[2], Joan C. Oliva[3], Carmen Colilles[2] and Caridad Pontes[1]

Abstract

Background: Bupivacaine and levobupivacaine have similar pharmacokinetic and pharmacodynamic characteristics, and are used regularly in spinal anesthesia. Whether potential differences in their hemodynamic and anesthetic profiles could determine a differential risk of complications in elderly subjects, is controversial. The main objective was to compare the effects of intrathecally administered levobupivacaine (LB) versus bupivacaine (B), on regional cerebral O_2 saturation during spinal anesthesia, cognitive status and neurological complications in elderly patients undergoing surgery for hip fracture.

Methods: This was a randomized, controlled, single blind study. 58 patients aged 70 or older undergoing surgery for hip fracture with spinal anesthesia were allocated with a 1:1 ratio to receive LB or B, combined with fentanyl 15 µg, by intrathecal route. The primary outcome was the proportion of intraoperative time with regional cerebral desaturation (≥20% reduction in regional cerebral oxygen saturation from baseline), monitored by near –infrared spectroscopy. Secondary endpoints included hemodynamic parameters, level of sensory and motor block, changes in Short Portable Mental Status Questionnaire (SPMSQ), and neurological complications.

Results: The mean percentage of intraoperative time with desaturation in the B group was 6.1% (SD: 17.5) and 4.7% (SD: 11.9) in the left and right hemisphere respectively; in the LB group the mean was 4.8% (SD: 11.4) in the left hemisphere and 2.4% (SD: 8.3) in the right one. No statistically significant differences were found between treatment groups. The level of sensory block at the start of surgery was lower for LB than for B (Th10 vs Th8, p:0.047) and motor block at 15 min was lower for LB (2.5 vs 3, p:0.009). No differences in postoperative SPMSQ were observed. Neurological complications such as confusional state, agitation or disorientation were reported in 50% of patients in the B group and 21.4% of patients in the LB group, $p = 0.05$.

(Continued on next page)

* Correspondence: Roser.vives@uab.cat
[1]Departament de Farmacologia, de Terapèutica i de Toxicologia, UAB, Clinical Pharmacology Unit, Parc Taulí Hospital Universitari, Institut d'Investigació i Innovació Parc Taulí I3PT, Universitat Autònoma de Barcelona, Parc Taulí 1, 08028 Sabadell (Barcelona), Spain

(Continued from previous page)

Conclusions: No statistically significant differences in regional cerebral oxygen saturation or hemodynamic parameters were observed between both treatment groups. Bupivacaine and levobupivacaine differed in sensory and motor block achieved. While no differences were observed in cognitive impairment measured by the SPMSQ between treatment groups neurological complications reported by the physician were more frequent with bupivacaine.

Keywords: Spinal anesthesia, Regional cerebral oxygen saturation, Bupivacaine, Levobupivacaine

Background

Decline in cognitive function in elderly patients during hospitalization has been, in part, attributed to sudden changes in the usual environment of the patient, but also, to the acute morbidity or exacerbation of pre-existing conditions. Geriatric patients suffering a hip fracture who undergo surgery are an especially frail population, because of concomitant morbidity, polypharmacy and bleeding. A multi-factorial intervention aimed to preserve cognitive function in this population during the acute hospital stay has shown good results [1]. Spinal anesthesia would be part of this multi-factorial interventions [1], although the evidence on the differential effects of spinal and general anesthesia on cognition is controversial. Shorter length of hospitalization, which could result in fewer complications, has been described for regional anesthesia, but it does not reduce mortality [2].

Intraoperative hypotension is an undesirable and frequent effect of spinal anesthesia, which may complicate a pre-existing coronary heart disease, worsen previous mental impairment or precipitate a cerebral stroke. Different strategies to maintain the hemodynamic stability of the patient include the choice of anesthetic drugs with the most favorable hemodynamic profile, and use of reduced doses of local anesthetic [3]. Racemic bupivacaine (B) and levobupivacaine (LB) are closely related local anesthetic agents; controversial reports suggest that they have different anesthetic profiles, with B inducing higher blockade, more hypotension, and consequently, potentially more cerebral desaturation [4, 5].

Clinical monitoring of CNS is rarely performed during spinal anesthesia. Instead, indirect parameters such as arterial pressure, heart rate and arterial O_2 saturation are registered [6]. Regional cerebral oxygen saturation ($rCSO_2$) through near –infrared spectroscopy, a non invasive monitoring that reflects a balance between supply and consumption of O_2 to the brain, has been proposed as a tool that may provide relevant information on CNS ischemic stress, and may be potentially useful to guide the clinical management of the patient during spinal anesthesia [7]. Thus, $rCSO_2$ might also be useful to assess the CNS consequences of the differences in the hemodynamic and anesthetic profile between two different anesthetic agents used in spinal anesthesia.

Currently, both B and LB are used interchangeably for spinal anesthesia in our hospital. Our working hypothesis was that cerebral desaturation would be higher in patients treated with B than in those receiving LB, and that this could be related to worse neurological outcomes. In order to test the hypothesis, we designed the present pragmatic randomized clinical trial to compare the effect of B and LB on regional cerebral oxygen saturation, during spinal anesthesia in elderly patients undergoing surgery for hip fracture repair, both administered by spinal route and according to routine clinical practice. We also compared the effects of both anesthetics on postoperative cognitive status and incidence of nervous system related adverse events.

Methods

Design

This was a randomized, controlled, single-center, single blind trial conducted at Hospital de Sabadell. The protocol was approved by the Ethics Committee of the Centre on March 2013 (*CEIC Corporació Sanitaria Parc Taulí, Sabadell,* reference number 2013/015). The study was registered at the European Union Clinical Trials Registry (EudraCT 2013–000846 -20) on April 9th, 2013 and at ClinicalTrials.gov (NCT01960543) on September 23rd, 2013. All patients received comprehensive information by the investigator on the study objectives, procedures and risks and signed the informed consent form before inclusion. Informed consent in front of a witness was allowed for patients unable to write or read due to physical impairment but with preserved cognitive function.

Patients

Patients aged 70 years and older requiring surgery for hip fracture repair that were suitable to receive spinal block,were included. Prior to inclusion, patients underwent cognitive examination by means of the Short Portable Mental Status Questionnaire (SPMSQ) [8, 9] and those with low scores (≥ 8 failures if elementary school, ≥ 7 failures if higher education), were excluded. Patients were excluded if they had any contraindication to B or LB (hypersensitivity to amide local anesthetics, severe aortic stenosis, heart failure or coagulopathies) or if they refused the regional anesthetic technique.

Methodology

A random list was generated by the clinical pharmacology unit using Winpepi V2.67 [10]. Sequentially numbered sealed opaque envelopes were produced containing the treatment identity for each patient. The list and a copy of the codes were kept in a file not accessible to the study team. Inclusion was confirmed by the anesthetist, who opened the first available sequentially numbered sealed code to randomize the patient. The study was blind for patients and for the anesthesiologists who evaluated the postoperative SPMSQ questionnaire.

Patients were not pre-medicated. Antihypertensive drugs were discontinued on the day of surgery and restarted at 48 h after surgery. Patients were randomly allocated (ratio 1:1) to receive treatment with racemic bupivacaine (Bupivacaine Braun 0.5%®, B. Braun Medical, S. A, Spain) or levobupivacaine (Chirocane®, Abbvie Spain S.L.U, Spain), both combined with fentanyl 15 µg, by intrathecal route. Both B and LB were isobaric. Spinal anesthesia was administered through a 25 gauge spinal needle using the midline or paramedial approach. The B and LB dose administered was 7 mg if height was < 160 cm and 9 mg if height was ≥160 cm, or when the surgical procedure was a hip prosthesis. Low doses were used with the objective to maintain the hemo dynamic stability and minimize intra-operative hypotension. Supplemental oxygen administration was started after spinal injection. As per the protocol, if the anesthesia was not sufficient to initiate surgery, midazolam 1 mg and propofol 30 mg could be administered, and if not effective, general anesthesia was induced and the patient was withdrawn from the study. In the operating room patients received 300 ml of Lactated Ringer's over 20 min. Electrocardiography, cuff for non-invasive blood pressure measurement, and pulse oximetry (Philips Intellivue MP70 Anesthesia) were used for routine monitoring. Hypotension (systolic blood pressure (SBP) < 100 mmHg) was treated with iv phenylephrine 50–75 µg, and ephedrine 5 mg in case the hypotension did not revert after two doses of phenylephrine. Bradycardia (heart rate (HR) < 50 beats/min) was treated with atropine 0.5–1 mg.

Outcomes and measurements

Patient characteristics such as ASA physical status, patient's pathologies and treatments, type of fracture and surgery, SPMSQ and preoperative hemoglobin were recorded. In the operating room, and after spinal anesthesia, the level of sensory block (SB) was evaluated by pinprick, and motor block (MB) by the modified Bromage scale 15 min after the spinal injection, before and at the end of the surgery. The modified Bromage scale is used to measure the intensity of motor block based on the ability of the patients to move their lower extremities (0 = no paralysis, 1 = able to move knees, unable to raise extended legs, 2 = able to flex ankles unable to flex knees, 3 = unable to flex ankles, knees or hips). After surgery, SB was evaluated every 30 min until regression to L5 level.

Regional cerebral oximetry was measured by near–infrared spectroscopy using INVOS 5100 C, 7.00.0014 version (Somanetics Inc., Troy, MI, 48084 - USA). A first measure of $rSCO_2$ was performed at entry in the operating room. A second measurement taken 2 min later was considered as the reference baseline value for each hemisphere, and values were recorded throughout the study. Regional cerebral desaturation was defined as a 20% or larger reduction in $rCSO_2$ with respect to the ipsilateral baseline value. Routine monitoring of SBP, mean arterial pressure (MAP), HR and O_2 saturation (O_2 Sat) monitoring, volume of crystalloid infused, intraoperative use of vasoconstrictor drugs, postoperative hemoglobin and the need for blood transfusions, were also recorded.

The primary outcome measure was the mean proportion of intra-operative time with regional cerebral oxygen desaturation, defined as an $rSCO_2$ relative reduction of 20% from baseline value. The area under the curve (AUC) for the intraoperative time below the desaturation threshold was also calculated (AUC $rCSO_2$ reduced by ≥20% from baseline). Similar calculations were done using an absolute value of 50% as a cutoff point (AUC $rCSO_2$ < 50%). Minimum values (trough $rCSO_2$) and time to first saturation drop under the different cut off points were also recorded.

Postoperative cognitive impairment was evaluated after 5 to 7 days, by changes in the SPMSQ scores from baseline. Any adverse events related to nervous system disorders, reported by the responsible physician within 30 days after surgery were also recorded.

Statistical methods

A sample size of 28 patients per group was calculated assuming an expected clinically relevant difference between treatments of 0.15 or higher on the mean proportion of intraoperative time with desaturation, with a standard deviation (SD) of 0.2, an alpha of 0.05 and 80% power.

Qualitative variables were described by the number of valid values and the frequency and percentage of each category, and compared between groups using Fisher exact tests. Quantitative variables were described by measures of central tendency and dispersion, and compared between groups using a Student T test or Mann-Whitney's test, as appropriate. A post-hoc bivariate analysis using the above mentioned statistical tests was performed to explore the relationship of selected variables with intraoperative desaturation, postoperative cognitive impairment and neurological complications. Variables showing statistical significance in the bivariate analysis were included in logistic regression multivariate analyses to explore predictors of regional cerebral desaturation, cognitive impairment or neurological complications.

Results

From September 2013 to December 2014, 58 patients meeting all the eligibility criteria were randomized. In two patients, the spinal anesthesia was not feasible and they were converted to general anesthesia; they were excluded from the analysis. At the start of surgery, three patients in the LB group needed midazolam + propofol and one patient in each group received midazolam alone. Figure 1 displays the disposition of patients, and Table 1 shows the baseline characteristics of patients.

Most patients (57.1%) had at least 3 comorbidities at hospital admission. Table 1 shows the most frequent concomitant diseases per treatment group. 78.3% of patients were taking 3 or more different medications on a regular basis, and 53.6% more than 4. Table 1 shows the treatments most frequently used by patients per treatment group. The majority of patients were operated on within 2 days after admission, and the time from admission to surgery was evenly distributed in both treatment groups.

No significant differences were observed between treatment groups in the proportion of intraoperative time with desaturation, nor in any of the secondary variables based on the measurement of $rCSO_2$ (Table 2). Overall, 46% of patients (13 B; 13 LB) presented a relative reduction in $rCSO_2 > 20\%$ from baseline in either one or both hemispheres; considering absolute values of $rCSO_2$ below 50, 64.3% (B) and 53.6% (LB) showed desaturation at some time point. Hemodynamic parameters (SBP, MAP and HR) were comparable between the two groups, as well as the need for vasoconstrictor drugs, although a trend to a lower SBP for patients was observed in B group (Table 3). The anesthetic profile for each treatment group is shown in Table 3. Intraoperative red blood cell transfusion was required in 3 patients in the B group and in 4 patients in the LB group. The mean (SD) volume of crystalloid infused were 605.4 (321.6) in the B group and 589.3 (240.5) mL in the LB group ($p = 0.83$).

Postoperative SPMSQ scores were overall better than those observed at baseline (Table 4), and no statistically significant differences were detected between treatment groups. Worsening in the SPMSQ score after surgery was observed in 23.1% of patients in the B group, and in

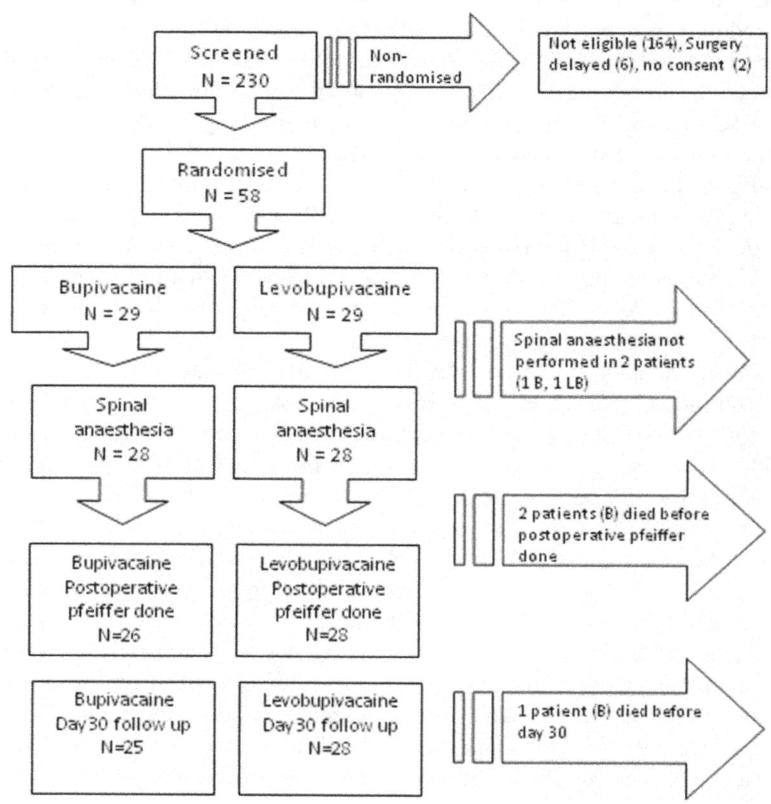

Fig. 1 Disposition of patients

Table 1 Baseline characteristics

Description of patients	*Bupivacaine (n = 28)*		*Levobupivacaine (n = 28)*	
	N	%	N	%
Gender				
Female	19	67.9	24	85.7
ASA physical status				
1	0	0	1	3.6
2	2	7.1	9	32.1
3	26	92.9	18	64.3
Education				
Elementary school	26	92.9	27	96.4
High school/University degree	2	7.1	1	3.6
Concomitant diseases				
Hypertension	18	64.3	18	64.3
Diabetes Mellitus	13	46.4	6	21.4
Dyslipidemia	7	25.0	8	28.6
Arrhythmia	7	25.0	5	17.9
Renal Failure	7	25.0	3	10.7
Cerebrovascular disease	1	4.2	4	16.7
Depression	1	3.6	6	21.4
Concomitant treatments				
Diuretic	14	50.0	11	39.3
ACE inhibitors	10	35.7	7	25.0
AR Blockers	6	21.4	8	28.6
Calcium antagonists	7	25.0	4	14.3
Beta-blockers	5	17.9	6	21.4
CNS drugs	19	67.9	25	89.3
Benzodiazepines	11	39.3	11	39.3
Antidepressants	8	28.6	12	42.9
Fracture type				
Pertrochanteric	17	60.7	11	39.3
Subtrochanteric	1	3.6	5	17.9
Femoral neck	8	28.6	7	25
Periprosthetic	1	3.6	2	7.1
Supracondylar	1	3.6	1	3.6
Distal diaphyseal	0	0	2	7.1
Surgery type				
Intramedullary internal fixation	16	57.1	14	50.0
Extramedullary internal fixation	5	17.9	8	28.6
Total hip arthroplasty	3	10.7	1	3.6
Cemented arthroplasty	4	14.3	3	10.7
Cementless hemiarthroplasty	0	0	2	7.1
Local anesthetic doses				
7 mg	8	28.6	7	25.0
9 mg	20	71.4	21	75.0
Right rCSO2 lower than Left rCSO2	14	50.0	11	39.3

Table 1 Baseline characteristics *(Continued)*

Description of patients	*Bupivacaine (n = 28)*		*Levobupivacaine (n = 28)*	
	N	%	N	%
	Mean (SD)	n	Mean (SD)	N
Age (years)	83.1 (5.5)	28	83.7 (6)	28
Weight (Kg)	66 (10.3)	28	67.6 (11.7)	28
Height (cm)	161 (7)	28	159.1 (6.3)	28
Baseline hemoglobin (g/L)	112.6 (19)	28	116.2 (18.1)	28
Duration on surgical intervention (min)	60.6 (24.7)	28	78.9 (35.5)	28
Baseline SBP (mmHg)	150.8 (24.7)	28	148.7 (21.8)	28
Baseline MAP (mmHg)	87.1 (14.2)	27	87.8 (14.4)	27
Baseline HR (bpm)	78.7 (11.7)	28	81.5 (11.5)	28
Baseline oxygen saturation (%)	92.4 (6.6)	28	93.9 (2.7)	28
Baseline rCSO2 (%) Left	59.8 (7.8)	28	59.7 (10.4)	28
Baseline rCSO2 (%) Right	58.8 (9.1)	28	60.1 (11.2)	28

ASA American Society of anesthesiologists, *bpm* beats per minute, *HR* heart rate, *MBP* mean blood pressure, *SBP* systolic blood pressure, *SD* standard deviation, *rCSO₂* regional cerebral oxygen saturation

28.6% of patients in the LB group. No differences in changes from baseline in SPMSQ scores were observed between treatment groups, even after adjusting by baseline SPMSQ scores.

Three patients from the B group died, and none in the LB group ($p = 0.24$). Reasons were aspiration pneumonia followed by heart failure, worsening of a pre-existing chronic renal failure, and sepsis following a respiratory infection, respectively. None of the deaths were considered related to the study treatment by the investigators.

Neurological complications were reported more often in patients in the B group (14, 50%) compared to the LB group (6, 21.4%), $p = 0.0496$. Confusional state was reported in 10 patients (7 B, 3 LB), agitation in 3 patients (2 B, 1 LB), cognitive impairment in 2 patients (1 B, 1 LB) and disorientation in 2 patients (1 B, 1 LB); three patients experienced agitation and disorientation (1 B), bradypsychia-dysartria (1 B) and encephalopathy related to hypercalcemia (1 B).

Baseline mean hemoglobin values were similar in both treatment groups (112.6 g/L and 116.2 g/L for B and LB respectively), and the drop in hemoglobin post-surgery was comparable in both groups (106.2 g/L for B and 110.4 g/L for LB). Anemia was reported as an adverse event in 80.4% of patients, and was similar for B and LB groups, with 9 and 6 patients in B and LB groups respectively, requiring postoperative transfusion ($p = 0.546$). Urinary infections were reported in 4 and 5 patients, renal failure in 8 and 5 patients, and respiratory infections and/or respiratory failure in 3 and 3 patients in B and LB groups, respectively.

The multivariate exploratory analysis showed that intraoperative desaturation was associated with low $rCSO_2$ in the right hemisphere at baseline, so that the risk of desaturation, increased by 61 fold in patients with baseline $rCSO_2$ in the lowest quartile, and by 38 fold in those in the second quartile, as referred to the highest $rCSO_2$ quartile (Table 5 and Fig. 2). Similarly, subjects in the lower quartile for trough intraoperative MAP had a 29 fold increased risk of desaturation, as compared to the highest quartile (Table 5 and Fig. 2). No variable was found to be significantly predictive of postoperative cognitive impairment, defined as a worsening in the SPMSQ score. In the multivariate analyses, only low SPMSQ scores at baseline predicted neurological complications (OR = 1.58 for each additional incorrect answer in the baseline SPMSQ score, 95%CI: 1.14–2.21).

Discussion

Our study found no significant differences between B and LB in any of the endpoints based on regional cerebral oxygen saturation. Cognitive impairment assessment by SPMSQ did not show mental decline for most subjects, but patients receiving B had significantly more reported neurological complications. The population included in our study was a very aged population (mean age of 83.5 years, with 8 (14%) patients aged 90 or older). Patients receiving LB had lower sensory and motor blockades, as expected, and those receiving B had a trend towards lower SBP. This is consistent with the results reported by Erdil et al. comparing B and LB (7.5 mg) in urologic procedures [5] and can be explained by a higher density of LB compared with bupivacaine [11].

$rCSO_2$ is determined by a balance between cerebral oxygen supply and demand, and cerebral oxygen supply is related to hemoglobin concentration, arterial O_2 saturation and blood volume; all of them are factors that can be adversely affected during spinal anesthesia. Some

Table 2 Intraoperative regional cerebral oxygen saturation with bupivacaine and levobupivacaine

	All patients			Patients with any desaturation		
	B	LB		B	LB	
Desaturation > 20% below baseline						
Left hemisphere	($n = 28$)	($n = 28$)		($n = 9$)	($n = 12$)	
AUC (min %)	14.93 (42.60)	12.43 (30.86)	ns	69.67 (72.28)	34.80 (44.63)	ns
Time below 20% from baseline (min)	5.57 (14.47)	5.21 (13.14)	ns	17.36 (21.84)	12.14 (18.21)	ns
% of time with desaturation	6.07 (17.47)	4.82 (11.40)	ns	18.9 (27.52)	11.25 (15.49)	ns
Time to first deep (min)	–	–	ns	23.67 (22.31)	32.66 (30.27)	ns
Right hemisphere	($n = 28$)	($n = 28$)	ns	($n = 9$)	($n = 10$)	ns
AUC (min %)	14.32 (35.34)	4.32 (14.98)	ns	57.29 (52.43)	15.3 (26.05)	ns
Time below 20% from baseline (min)	4.74 (11.87)	2.44 (8.30)	ns	14.75 (17.58)	6.84 (13.15)	ns
% of time with desaturation	4.01 (9.33)	2.16 (7.08)	ns	14.02 (13.24)	6.04 (11.15)	ns
Time to first deep (min)	–	–	–	29.28 (25.65)	45.97 (22.56)	ns
Desaturation < 50% (absolute values)						
Left hemisphere	($n = 28$)	($n = 28$)		($n = 15$)	($n = 13$)	
AUC (min %)	53.07 (108.82)	158.29 (440.69)	ns	114.31 (138.06)	340.92 (607.88)	ns
Time below 20% from baseline (min)	12.82 (24.37)	16.59 (36.85)	ns	23.93 (29.32)	35.75 (48.11)	ns
% of time with desaturation	11.62 (19.38)	13.65 (30.69)	ns	21.68 (22.24)	29.41 (40.20)	ns
Time to first deep (min)	–	–	ns	20.71 (30.77)	30.57 (35.09)	ns
Right hemisphere	($n = 28$)	($n = 28$)	ns	($n = 17$)	($n = 13$)	ns
AUC (min %)	77.54 (152.84)	134.14 (422.71)	ns	127.71 (180.6)	288.9 (594.63)	ns
Time below 20% from baseline (min)	15.84 (30.14)	13.32 (31.68)	ns	26.09 (35.34)	28.68 (42.20)	ns
% of time with desaturation	13.08 (23.03)	11.12 (26.55)	ns	21.54 (26,49)	23.94 (35.40)	ns
Time to first deep (min)	–	–	–	28.80 (34.42)	19.12 (27.98)	ns
Lowest values rCSO2 (%)						
	($n = 28$)	($n = 28$)				
Left hemisphere	49.46 (8.59)	48.32 (11.71)	ns			
Right hemisphere	48.18 (10.60)	49.86 (11.87)	ns			

B Bupivacaine, *LB* Levobupivacaine, *AUC* area under the curve, *rCSO2* regional cerebral oxygen saturation, *ns* not significant *p* value. Values expressed as mean (Standard Deviation) for all patients of the treatment group and for patients who presented desaturation of the measured hemisphere

studies comparing spinal versus general anesthesia have shown varying incidences of cerebral desaturation related to the anesthetic technique [12, 13]. During spinal anesthesia in urologic surgery, Nishikawa observed a 10% reduction in $rCSO_2$ in patients with higher levels of sensory block (>Th4.7) [14]. Also, in a randomized study in elderly patients undergoing abdominal surgery under general anesthesia, the use of $rCSO_2$ monitoring avoided cerebral desaturation and was associated with a reduced incidence of postoperative cognitive decline [6].

We have predefined two cutoff points for assessment of desaturation: a relative change ≥20% from baseline, and an absolute saturation below 50%. We compared the percentage of time that patients spent below these thresholds, and also the lowest values achieved. These variables have not previously been reported for very elderly patients with spinal anesthesia, and in our study, we did not observe any difference between the treatment groups, although differences in the anesthetic profile and rate of complications between B and LB were observed, suggesting that both anesthetic agents are not equivalent in efficacy.

During surgery, we provided tailored prehydration and supplementary oxygen, transfused red blood cells and used vasoconstrictor drugs (mainly phenylephrine) to manage hypotension in every patient presenting SPB measures lower than 100mmHg [15]. Despite intensive management, 46% of patients had at least one drop of $rCSO_2$ of 20% below the baseline value, in at least one cerebral hemisphere. Reference values of $rCSO_2$ range from 60 to 80% [16]. At baseline our patients had mean $rCSO_2$ values around 60%, so that drops below 50% were easily and quickly reached, while reductions of $rCSO_2 \geq 20\%$ from baseline were less frequent. These findings are consistent with the baseline $rCSO_2$ of $63 \pm 8\%$ described by Casati et al. for relatively healthy patients aged around 70 [5],

Table 3 Anesthetic and intraoperative hemodynamic profile of bupivacaine and levobupivacaine

Anesthetic profile	*N*	*Bupivacaine*	*N*	*Levobupivacaine*	
Sensory Block (*median – range*)					
15 min after SI	25	Th9 (Th4-Th12)	20	Th11 (Th5-TL2)	p: 0.14
Start of surgery	23	Th8 (Th4-T12)	22	Th10 (Th5 – L2)	p: 0.047*
End of surgery	24	Th11 (Th5-L5)	21	Th11 (Th7- L5)	p: 0.61
Duration of SB (min) (mean ± SD)	24	178.25 ± 44.89	22	175.18 ± 42.53	p: 0.81
Motor Block (*median – range*)					
15 min after SI	25	3 (2–3)	20	2.5 (1–3)	p: 0.009*
Start of surgery	24	3 (2–3)	22	3 (1–3)	p: 0.057
End of surgery	25	3 (0–3)	21	1 (0–3)	p: 0.21
Duration of MB (min) (mean ± SD)	25	157.04 ± 41.71	23	141.65 ± 56.02	p: 0.29
Time (min) (Mean ± SD)					
SI to Start of surgery	25	21.32 ± 6.80	23	19.78 ± 7.45	p: 0.46
SI to End of surgery	25	80.75 ± 27.88	23	97.67 ± 35.97	p: 0.055
Surgery	28	60 ± 24.6	28	78.6 ± 35.4	p: 0.03*
Hemodynamic profile					
Patients with hypotension (n/%)	28	19 / 67.8%	28	20 / 71.4%	p: 0.99
Minimum values (Mean ± SD)					
Lowest SBP (mmHg)	28	84.0 ± 26.43	28	96.03 ± 21.31	p: 0.06
Lowest MAP (mmHg)	28	53.03 ± 14.11	28	56.96 ± 14.20	p: 0.31
Lowest HR (beats/min)	28	65.57 ± 10.66	28	65.57 ± 12.68	p: 0.52
Use of Vasoconstrictor drugs					
Phenylephrine n° patients / mean dose (ug) ± SD	28	17 / 258.82 ± 181.12	28	16 / 239.06 ± 153.83	p: 0.73
Ephedrine n° patients / mean dose (mg) ± SD	28	6 / 11.83 ± 5.19	28	7 / 15.57 ± 13.62	p: 0.52
Atropine 0.5 mg (n/%)	28	0/0.0%	28	3/10.7%	p:0.24

SB sensory block, *MB* motor block, *SI* spinal injection, *SBP* systolic blood pressure, *MAP* mean arterial pressure, *HR* heart rate. *SD* standard deviation. Motor Block (0 = no paralysis, 1 = able to move knees, unable to raise extended legs, 2 = able to flex ankles unable to flex knees, 3 = unable to flex ankles, knees or hips)

and Carlson et al. described that, awake elderly, with marginal $rCSO_2$ levels (50–60%), had the greatest changes in $rCSO_2$ during sleep that may affect subject's cognition [17]. Moreover, we observed a wide inter-patient variability in the number and duration of drops below our proposed thresholds of $rCSO_2$, especially in subjects already showing some degree of baseline desaturation. Such variability may have compromised the power of the study for the main hypothesis, and may be indicative of either the lack of suitability of $rCSO_2$ as a surrogate of cerebral oxygen saturation during spinal anesthesia, or of a choice of thresholds unable to discriminate clinically relevant desaturation. Future studies should consider including a more homogeneous population in terms of $rCSO_2$ and the definition of more stringent thresholds for the main variables.

Table 4 SPMSQ scores at baseline and after 5–7 days

	Baseline			Post-op		
	B	LB		B	LB	
	(*n* = 28)	(*n* = 28)		(*n* = 26)	(*n* = 28)	
SPMSQ			ns			ns
0–2 errors	9 (32.1%)	13 (46.4%)		14 (53.8%)	16 (57.1%)	
3–4 errors	12 (42.9%	9 (32.1%)		8 (30.8%)	8 (28.6%)	
5–7 errors	7 (25.0%)	6 (21.4%)		4 (15.4%)	3 (10.1%)	
8 or more errors	0	0		0	1 (3.7%)	
SPMSQ change, mean (SD)				0.50 (1.96)	0.32 (1.63)	ns

B Bupivacaine, *LB* Levobupivacaine, *SPMSQ* Short Portable Mental Status Questionnaire, *SD* standard deviation, ns not significant p value

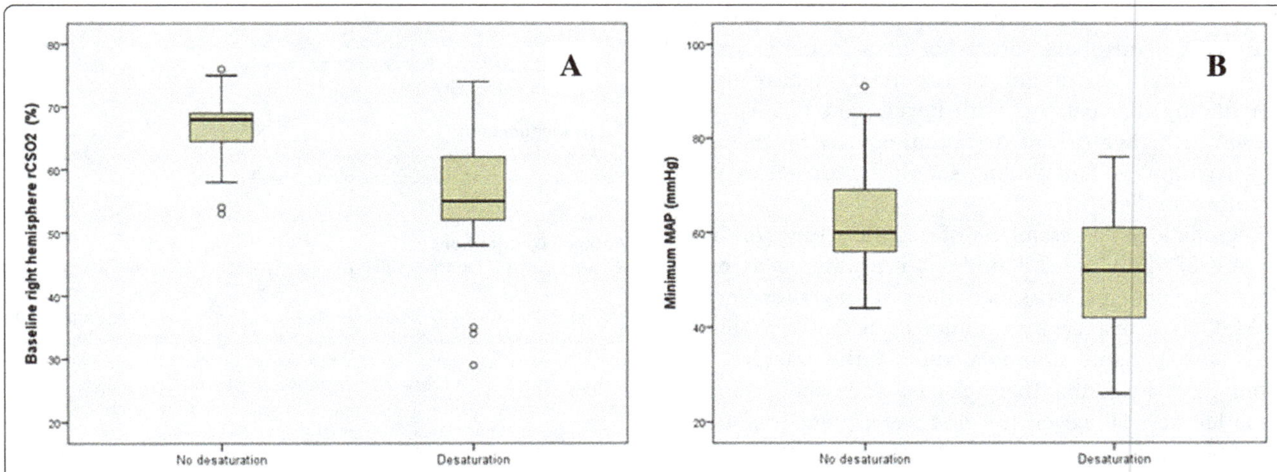

Fig. 2 Mean values and dispersion for (A) baseline right hemisphere $rCSO_2$ and (B) minimum intra-operative MAP in patients with and without intraoperative desaturation. Footer: $rCSO_2$: regional cerebral saturation of oxygen. MAP: Mean arterial pressure

While in some studies intraoperative cerebral desaturation has been found to be significantly associated with an increased risk of cognitive decline [6, 18], a recent review did not show evidence of a relationship between a low $rCSO_2$ and neurological complication [19]. Besides, intrasubject differences in $rCSO_2$ between L and R during anesthesia has been also been suggested as a risk factor for neurological impairment [20]. In our study, the desaturation variables studied did not prove to be useful as predictors of cognitive decline; however, we found that neurological complications were more frequent with B. Such observation could be due to chance, but could also be due to the trends towards lower values of SBP and MAP in B group than in LB group [21], since a higher sympathetic block may exaggerate hypotension after spinal anesthesia. In our study, no standardized method to assess and report neurological complications was considered, and this variable was only based on the clinical observation of the physicians. This is a limitation of the study and may be the reason for this finding.

Our post-hoc multivariate analyses also found significant associations between preoperative SPMSQ scores and NC, and the risk of intraoperative desaturation was substantial and increasingly higher for patients in the lower quartiles of baseline $rCSO_2$ in the right hemisphere. Preoperative SPMSQ has been widely reported in the literature as a risk factor of cognitive decline [1], but low baseline $rCSO_2$ in the right hemisphere as a risk factor for desaturation could be further explored as a potential marker of subjects in whom more preemptive hemodynamic management could be indicated. Salazar et al. found that, in patients undergoing total knee replacement, right $rCSO_2$ values lower than left $rCSO_2$ was a factor associated with the presence of memory

Table 5 Multivariate model for intraoperative desaturation risk

	N	Mean	SD	OR (CI 95%)	*p* value
rCSO2 –Right[a] (overall)	*56*	*59.41*	*10.128*		0.020
1st quartile	15	47.53	7.954	61.1 (3.3 to 1127.9)	0.006
2nd quartile	14	55.79	1.626	37.6 (2.2 to 635.2)	0.012
3rd quartile	12	64.00	2.000	2.1 (0.4 to 12.1)	0.429
4th quartile	15	71.00	2.803	(Ref)	
MAPmin[b] (overall)	*54*	*55.00*	*14.17*		0.145
1st quartile	13	36.23	7.33	28.7 (1.4 to 604.8)	0.031
2nd quartile	15	51.80	2.98	9.9 (0.8 to 122.3)	0.074
3rd quartile	13	59.92	1.89	4.3(0.4 to 51.3)	0.244
4th quartile	13	72.54	8.07	(Ref)	
Exp				0.085	0.045

OR Odds Ratio, *CI* Confidence interval, *MAP* Mean Arterial Pressure, *SD* Standard Deviation
[a]Baseline regional Cerebral Saturation of Oxygen in Right Hemisphere; [b]Minimum value for Mean Arterial Blood pressure, intraoperative

decline. We did not explore the asymmetry between left and right hemisphere saturation as a factor associated with cerebral desaturation or cognitive impairment, but our finding that patients with lower right $rCSO_2$ values present a higher risk of desaturation may be related to this asymmetry. This finding should be further explored in future studies.

Regarding the assessments of cognitive function based on the SPMSQ, we did not observe differences either, since few patients worsened their scores after surgery. SPMSQ is a test easy to administrate and suitable for very aged patients immobile due to the fracture, who often have forgotten their glasses and who often had poor literacy. However, the first assessment was after a hip fracture and hospital admission, when the patients were in a estrange environment, in pain and anxious and were being treated with analgesic and sedating drugs. Thus, this assessment may not represent the true cognitive status of the patients before hospital admission; in turn, the second assessment was done after fracture stabilization, control of pain and beginning of rehabilitation. Resolution of the previous painful conditions may explain why most patients presented better scores in comparison to baseline. A population undergoing elective surgery would be a more appropriate setting to check the relationship between $rCSO_2$ and cognitive decline.

Finally, 3 (10.3%) subjects died in the B group and none in LB group. The reported rate of death in this particular population is 5.3% [2], and the observation is consistent with these figures, considering the small sample size of our study that does not have power enough as to detect statistically significant differences in mortality.

Conclusions

This prospective, randomized, clinical trial in very elderly patients could not show differences in cerebral oxygenation between B and LB during spinal anesthesia, but lower sensory and motor blockade was seen with LB than with B, and a trend to lower MAP and SPB was observed for B. While no differences were observed in cognitive impairment measured by the SPMSQ between treatment groups, postoperative neurological complications as reported by the physician were more frequent in B. An increased risk for intraoperative cerebral oxygen desaturation was observed for patients with lower trough intraoperative MAP and lower baseline $rCSO_2$ values in the right hemisphere, and neurological complications were associated to lower cognitive status at the preoperative assessment. Finally, $rCSO_2$ was not found as a predictive factor for cognitive impairment or late neurological complications.

Abbreviations

ASA: American Society of Anesthesiologists; AUC: Area under the curve; B: Bupivacaine; HR: Heart rate; LB: Levobupivacaine; MAP: Mean arterial pressure; MB: Motor block; NC: Neurological complication; O2 Sat: O2 saturation; rCSO2: Regional cerebral oxygen saturation; SB: Sensory block; SD: Standard deviation; SPB: Systolic blood pressure; SPMSQ: Short Portable Mental Status Questionnaire

Acknowledgements

Novella Caló, Carolina García-Bartolo, Cristian Hernández-Delgado, Anna Valle-Beltran, Susana Fernández-Galinski, Marc Fradera.

Authors' contributions

RV participated in protocol writing, statistical analysis, interpretation of results and manuscript writing. DFG conceived the study, participated in protocol writing, recruited and assessed patients and participated in the interpretation of results and manuscript writing. FG recruited and assessed patients and participated in the interpretation of results and reviewed the manuscript. AI recruited and assessed patients and participated in the interpretation of results and reviewed the manuscript. JCO did the statistical analysis and reviewed the manuscript. CC recruited and assessed patients and participated in the interpretation of results and reviewed the manuscript. CP participated in protocol writing, statistical analysis, interpretation of results and manuscript writing. All authors read and approved the final manuscript.

Author details

[1]Departament de Farmacologia, de Terapèutica i de Toxicologia, UAB, Clinical Pharmacology Unit, Parc Taulí Hospital Universitari, Institut d'Investigació i Innovació Parc Taulí I3PT, Universitat Autònoma de Barcelona, Parc Taulí 1, 08028 Sabadell (Barcelona), Spain. [2]Anesthesiology Department, Parc Taulí Hospital Universitari, Institut d'Investigació i Innovació Parc Taulí I3PT, Universitat Autònoma de Barcelona, Parc Taulí 1, 08028 Sabadell (Barcelona), Spain. [3]Statistics Unit, Parc Taulí Hospital Universitari, Institut d'Investigació i Innovació Parc Taulí I3PT, Universitat Autònoma de Barcelona, Parc Taulí 1, 08028 Sabadell (Barcelona), Spain.

References

1. Björkelund KB, Hommel A, Thorngren KG, Gustafson L, Larsson S, Lundberg D. Reducing delirium in elderly patients with hip fracture a multi-factorial intervention study. Acta Anaesthesiol Scand. 2010;54:678–88.
2. Neuman MD, Roenbaum PR, Ludwig JM, Zubizarreta JA, Silber JH. Anesthesia technique, mortality and length of stay after hip fracture surgery. JAMA. 2014;311:2508–17.
3. Ben David B, Frankel R, Arzumonov T, Marchevsky Y, Volpin G. Minidose bupivacaine-fentanyl spinal anesthesia for surgical repair of hip fracture in the aged. Anesthesiology. 2000;92:6–10.
4. Gautier P, De Kock M, Huberty L, Demir T, Izydorczic M, Vanderick B. Comparison of the effects of intrathecal ropivacaine, levobupivacaine, and bupivacaine for caesarean section. Br J Anaesth. 2003;91:684–9.
5. Erdil F, Bulut S, Demirbilek S, Gedik E, Gulhas N, Ersoy MO. The effects of intrathecal levobupivacaine and bupivacaine in the elderly. Anesthesia. 2009;64:942–6.
6. Casati A, Fanelli G, Pietropaoli P, Proietti R, Tufano R, Danelli G, et al. Continuous monitoring of cerebral oxygen saturation in elderly patients undergoing abdominal surgery minimizes brain exposure to potential hypoxia. Anesth Analg. 2005;101:740–7.
7. Murkin JM, Arango M. Near infrared spectroscopy as an index of brain and tissue oxygenation. Br J Anaesth 2009;103 Suppl I: i3-i13.
8. Pfeiffer E. A short portable mental status questionnaire for the assessment of organic brain deficit in elderly patients. J Am Geriatr Soc. 1975;23:433–41.
9. Martinez de la Iglesia J, Dueñas Herrero R, Onis Vilches MC, Aguado Tabemé C, Albert Colomer C, Luque Luque R. Cross cultural adaptation and validation of Pfeiffer's test (short portable mental status questionnaire [SPMSQ]) to screen cognitive impairment in general population aged 65 or older. Med Clin (Barc). 2001;117:129–34.
10. WinpepiV2.67. At: http://www.brixtonhealth.com/pepi4windows.html, last accessed on August 14th, 2015.
11. McLeod GA. Density of spinal anesthetic solutions of bupivacaine, levobupivacaine, and ropivacaine with and without dextrose. Br J Anaesth. 2004;92:547–51.
12. Hoppenstein D, Zohar E, Ramaty E, Shabat S, Fredman B. The effects of general vs spinal anesthesia on frontal cerebral oxygen saturation in geriatric patients undergoing emergency surgical fixation of the neck of femur. J Clin Anesth. 2005;17:431–8.

13. Papadopoulus G, Karanikolas M, Liarmakopoulou A, Papathanakos G, Korre M, Beris A. Cerebral oximetry and cognitive dysfunction surgery for hip fractures: a prospective observational study. Open Orthop J. 2012;6:400–5.
14. Nishikawa K, Hagiwara R, Nakamura K, Ishizeki J, Kubo K, Saito S, et al. The effects of the extent of spinal block on the BIS score and regional cerebral oxygen saturation in elderly patients: a prospective, randomized and double-blinded study. J Clin Monit Comput. 2007;21:109–14.
15. Nakasuji M, HakSuh S, Nomura M, Nakamura M, Imanaka N, Tanaka M, et al. Hypotension from spinal anesthesia in patients aged greater than 80 years is due to a decrease in systemic vascular resistance. J Clin Anesth. 2012;24:201–6.
16. Tosh W, Patteril M. Cerebral Oxymetry. BJA Educ. 2016;16:417–21.
17. Carlson BW, Neelon VJ, Carlson JR, Hartman M, Bliwise DL. Cerebral oxygenation in wake and during sleep and its relationship to cognitive function in community- dwelling older adults without sleep disordered breathing. J Gerontol A Biol Sci Med Sci. 2011;66:150–6.
18. Slater JP, Guarino T, Stack J, Vinod K, Bustami RT, Brown JM 3rd, et al. Cerebral oxygen desaturation predicts cognitive decline and longer hospital stay after cardiac surgery. Ann Thorac Surg. 2009;87:36–45.
19. Zheng F, Sheinberg R, Yee MS, Ono M, Zheng Y, Hogue CW. Cerebral near infrared spectroscopy monitoring and neurologic outcomes in adult cardiac surgery patients: a systematic review. Anesth Analg. 2013;116:663–76.
20. Salazar F, Doñate M, Boget T, Bogdanovich A, Basora M, Torres F, et al. Relationship between intraoperative regional oxygen saturation trends and cognitive decline after total knee replacement: a post hoc analysis. BMC Anesthesiol. 2014;14:58.
21. The American Geriatrics Society Expert Panel on Postoperative Delirium in Older Adults. Postoperative Delirium in Older Adults: Best Practice Statement from the American Geriatrics Society. At: https://doi.org/10.1016/j.jamcollsurg.2014.10.019, last accessed August 14th, 2015.

16

The application of a neural network to predict hypotension and vasopressor requirements non-invasively in obstetric patients having spinal anesthesia for elective cesarean section (C/S)

Irwin Gratz[1*], Martin Baruch[2], Magdy Takla[1], Julia Seaman[3], Isabel Allen[4], Brian McEniry[1] and Edward Deal[1]

Abstract

Background: Neural networks are increasingly used to assess physiological processes or pathologies, as well as to predict the increased likelihood of an impending medical crisis, such as hypotension.

Method: We compared the capabilities of a single hidden layer neural network of 12 nodes to those of a discrete-feature discrimination approach with the goal being to predict the likelihood of a given patient developing significant hypotension under spinal anesthesia when undergoing a Cesarean section (C/S). Physiological input information was derived from a non-invasive blood pressure device (Caretaker [CT]) that utilizes a finger cuff to measure blood pressure and other hemodynamic parameters via pulse contour analysis. Receiver-operator-curve/area-under-curve analyses were used to compare performance.

Results: The results presented here suggest that a neural network approach (Area Under Curve [AUC] = 0.89 [$p < 0.001$]), at least at the implementation level of a clinically relevant prediction algorithm, may be superior to a discrete feature quantification approach (AUC = 0.87 [$p < 0.001$]), providing implicit access to a plurality of features and combinations thereof. In addition, the expansion of the approach to include the submission of other physiological data signals, such as heart rate variability, to the network can be readily envisioned.

Conclusion: This pilot study has demonstrated that increased coherence in Arterial Stiffness (AS) variability obtained from the pulse wave analysis of a continuous non-invasive blood pressure device appears to be an effective predictor of hypotension after spinal anesthesia in the obstetrics population undergoing C/S.
This allowed us to predict specific dosing thresholds of phenylephrine required to maintain systolic blood pressure above 90 mmHg.

Keywords: Arterial stiffness, Cesarean section, Finger cuff, Hypotension, Neural network, Non-invasive, Predictive algorithm

* Correspondence: gratz-irwin@cooperhealth.edu
[1]Cooper University Hospital, 1 Cooper Plaza, Camden, NJ 08103, USA

Background

Intraoperative hypotension has been reported to occur in between 5 to 99% of cases depending on the specific surgical population and it is associated with complications that can harm patients [1]. A particularly vulnerable population are obstetric patients undergoing spinal anesthesia for Cesarean sections (C/S).

Spinal anesthesia in this population is associated with hypotension incidence as high as 70% and hypotension remains a common and clinically-important problem that is associated with morbidity for both mother and child. Even brief episodes of hypotension can result in lower fetal Apgar scores and acidosis [2–4].

Detection and management of maternal hemodynamic instability during C/S remains a primary clinical and research focus as early recognition can enhance clinical decision making [5]. The latest developments in monitoring of arterial waveforms invasively allow for the prediction of hypotension to possibly improve patient outcomes [6, 7]. However, prediction of hypotension based on a noninvasive technique would expand our monitoring and diagnostic capabilities. For the purpose of the study, hypotension in this population was defined as a systolic blood pressure < 90 mmHg, this blood pressure was chosen because it is our institution's current standard for the C/S population. Furthermore, it aligns with other investigators, the consideration being that spinal sympathectomy primarily affects systolic blood pressure [8]. Additionally, systolic and diastolic blood pressures are the two most often reported parameters used in both clinical practice and clinical research studies as they are proven markers of cardiovascular disease [9].

We evaluated the CareTaker® (CT) continuous noninvasive blood pressure device (Caretaker Medical LLC, Charlottesville, Virginia) which has been described in detail elsewhere [10, 11]. Briefly, the CT is a physiological sensing system that communicates physiological data wirelessly via Bluetooth. The device uses a low pressure (35–45 mmHg), pump-inflated, cuff surrounding the middle phalange of the middle finger that pneumatically couples arterial pulsations via a pressure line to a custom-designed piezo-electric pressure sensor for detection and analysis.

The use of pulse analysis of the arterial pressure pulse offers a potential tool to investigate physiological markers for the prediction of hypotension, without impacting clinical workflow. A plausible physiological candidate for predicting the likelihood of hypotension in C/S patients undergoing spinal anesthesia is arterial stiffness (AS), which has been investigated in the separate contexts of hypotension and pregnancy, and can be assessed using pulse contour analysis [12]. Recent work on the prediction of imminent hypotension has focused on identifying changes in the variability of physiological signals, among them AS [13, 14]. Variability changes are due to compensatory mechanisms in the cardiovascular system as it attempts to maintain stability [10, 15]. In the context of pregnancy, significant longitudinal changes in AS have been documented [13]. It is therefore reasonable to investigate whether underlying compromised physiological compensatory reserve can be predicted prior to spinal anesthesia induction.

The CT is FDA-cleared for the measurement of heart rate, continuous noninvasive blood pressure, and respiration. Blood pressure monitoring is accomplished via a pulse contour analysis algorithm called Pulse Decomposition Analysis (PDA), which analyzes the component pulses, specifically the left ventricular ejection pulse (P1) and its reflections, the renal reflection pulse (P2) and the iliac reflection pulse (P3), that constitute the arterial pressure pulse [16]. Part of the PDA framework is the AS parameter which quantifies the spectral content of the arterial pressure pulse that is due to the component pulses [10]. The spectral content in turn is related to arterial stiffness as it is the mechanical filtering of the arterial wall that determines to what extent the structure of the component pulses is resolved. As determined in other studies, this filtering limits the upper observable frequency components in the peripheral arterial pressure pulse to approximately 20 Hz [17]. Preliminary validation tests indicate that the AS parameter tracks expected trends after the introduction of vaso-active agents as well as age-related population trends [10].

The aim of the present study was to develop a preoperative model that could predict the development of severe post spinal hypotension noninvasively using AS as a hemodynamic marker.

Methods

This study was approved by the Institutional Review Board of Cooper University Hospital (IRB #17–119) and all patients provided written informed consent. The study population was a subset of a larger study which compared the agreement of blood pressures obtained from the CT non-invasive blood pressure measurement device to those from intermittent oscillometric cuff inflations during abdominal and obstetric surgeries.

Forty nine patients (> 34 weeks gestation) with an American Society of Anesthesiologists status II who were undergoing elective C/S under spinal anesthesia were enrolled in this study. All patients had an intravenous catheter started in the preoperative preparation room. Lactated Ringer's solution was slowly infused to keep the vein open.

Measurements were started in the preoperative preparation room approximately 90 min prior to initiation of spinal anesthesia and continued throughout the entire procedure. The CT device provides physiological data, including systole, diastole, mean arterial pressure (MAP), heart rate and the AS parameter, on a beat-by beat basis. The data is transmitted wirelessly from the central, wrist-worn, processing unit to a nearby Android-based tablet (Samsung Galaxy Tab. A, Samsung Group, Seoul, South Korea) that is part of the FDA-cleared CT system.

Anesthesia procedure

For the purposes of this study hypotension is defined as systolic blood pressure < 90 mmHg. In this prediction study, a 30-min data window after the start of data collection was used for analysis, starting approximately 90 min prior to induction. All patients underwent spinal anesthesia with a 24-gauge spinal needle in sitting position based on the classic midline method with the administration of 10.5 mg bupivacaine solution 0.5%. We quickly (within 3 min) placed patients in the supine position after the injection and this practice should have limited the development of hypotension immediately after the spinal injection. Intra-operatively, systolic blood pressure was maintained above 90 mmHg with boluses of phenylephrine (100 mcg). Boluses were repeated at 5 min intervals until a systolic blood pressure of > 90 mmHg was achieved as per our standard protocol. The blood pressure and heart rate were measured, separate from the beat-by-beat CT-based measurements, using an upper arm cuff (Critikon Soft-Cuf, model SFT-A2-2A, GE Healthcare, Chicago, Illinois, USA) initially every 2 min for 10 min, and every 5 min thereafter. All patients were pre-hydrated with 1000 ml of lactated Ringers just prior to the spinal injection. The anesthesia level was determined in all patients and was between thoracic levels 4 to 6 as measured by a pin prick. All patients were placed in the left lateral position to ensure avoidance of compression of the vena cava by the gravid uterus.

Arterial stiffness assessment

The AS parameter that is part of the pulse analysis PDA framework has been described in detail elsewhere [10]. Briefly, the parameter quantifies the spectral content of the arterial pressure pulse envelope and is driven primarily by the resolution of the section of overlap of the renal pulse (P2), and the iliac pulse (P3). This section incorporates the pulse region that was examined by others and was found to correlate with expected age- and drug-related changes in arterial stiffness [18].

Visual examination of AS data of patients scheduled to undergo spinal anesthesia as part of a C/S procedure suggested that subjects who later required higher phenylephrine dosages to stabilize their persistent hypotension exhibited larger variability in the 30-min time-window 90 min prior to induction. Specifically, these patients would exhibit AS modulations, sometimes distinctly oscillatory, with time scales on the order of 3 min. From these observations arose the hypothesis that the likelihood of post-induction severe hypotension, defined by the need for the administration of significant dosages of phenylephrine, albeit at an as yet underdetermined threshold, could be predicted by a measure of the amplitude or duration of the observed modulations in the AS data. The benefit of choosing this indication of hypotension, as opposed to for example the time duration for which systole < 90 mmHg, is that, even on cursory examination, it provided less ambiguity than the interpretation of blood pressure readings near a threshold, which clinicians based on their extensive experience do routinely, would have introduced.

Signal pre-processing

As was stated above, the AS data is provided by the CT system on a beat-by-beat basis, i.e. at a non-uniform heart rate. For most signal-processing approaches, non-uniformly spaced data presents a significant challenge. This includes correlation schemes which involve the digital mapping of data sections onto other data sections, with highly unpredictable results if data time intervals are not equal. The data were therefore linearized at a frequency to preserve the spectral content of the inter-beat variations, which in this cohort, at heart rates between 70 and 103 bpm, resides in the 1–2 Hz frequency band. To assure oversampling at a factor of 5, as opposed to the Nyquist limit of 2, times the highest frequency embedded, a linearization frequency of 10 Hz was chosen and implemented using spline resampling. Figure 1b, which displays an example of the time evolution of the AS response of patient 07, also displays a highly enlarged, about 9 s, data section for comparison of the original and the resampled data trace, which without the enlargement would be indistinguishable.

Since inspection of the observed modulations revealed limited coherency and because of the very low frequency regime involved, spectral analysis approaches were not considered. Instead the data were analyzed using auto-correlation spectra that provide information on signal coherence. Cross- and auto-correlation-based analyses have been used for pattern recognition in the context of physiological signals such as, for example, blood pressure, heart rate variability, and respiration [19–21]. Specifically, for a signal that is self-coherent on some time scale, the autocorrelation will exhibit correlation coefficients of significant amplitude and the coefficients will change sign, i.e. exhibit zero-crossings, with different lag-times as the signal's time components constructively and destructively interfere with each other.

For each patient, the autocorrelation spectrum was calculated for a 2000 s window, or about 33 min of 10 Hz resampled AS data, corresponding to 20,000 data points. This yields a same-sized autocorrelation spectrum with

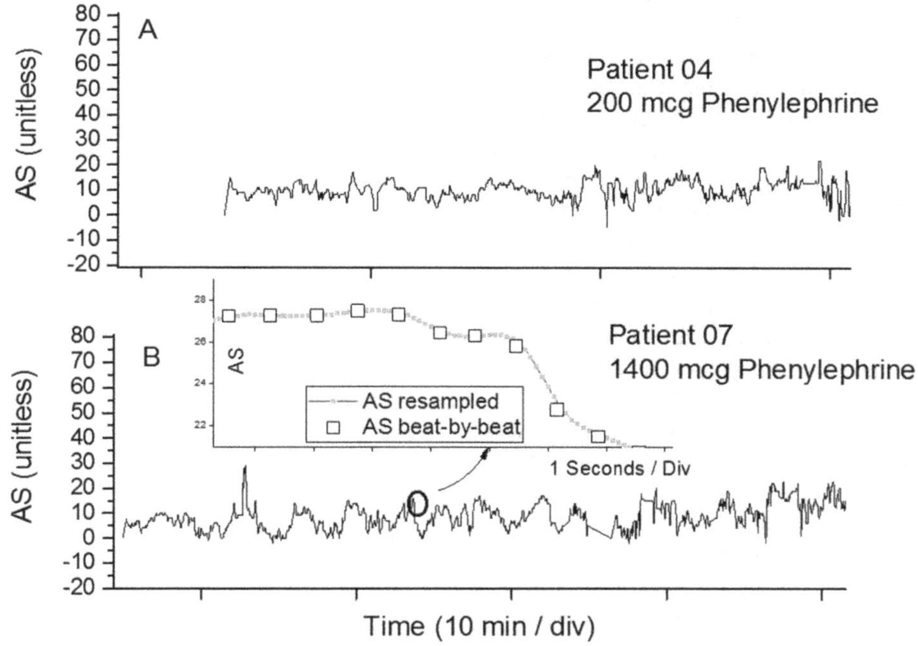

Fig. 1 a. Time evolution of the AS response of patient 04, 60 min prior to induction, who subsequently required minimal phenylephrine intervention, 200 ml. **b**. Time evolution of the AS response of patient 07, 60 min prior to induction, who subsequently required significant phenylephrine intervention, 1400 ml. The graph of patient 07 also shows an inset with an expansion and overlay of about 15 s of the original beat-by-beat AS data as well as the AS data re-sampled at 10 Hz

time lags from 0 to 2000 s at the resampled resolution. Visual inspection was used to select the specific analysis window for each patient so as to avoid data in the patient session that was clearly motion artifact-contaminated due to the patient settling in, which usually occurred in the first 5 min of recorded data.

Single-feature extraction and classification assessment

The observed modulations were quantified by integrating over the absolute-value of the lag times of the auto-correlation spectra from 100 s to the maximum time lag of 2000 s, the goal being to isolate the observed longer-time scale modulations from shorter-range lag times. Analyses were performed in Matlab 2017b (MathWorks, Natick, MA, USA).

Using the value obtained from the absolute AS auto-correlation area integration for each patient as a metric, ROC analyses were used to assess whether the metric could classify those patients that developed severe hypotension, characterized by requiring higher dosages of phenylephrine, from those who developed no or less severe hypotension, as indicated by lower dosages or the absence of any drug administration. The cumulative phenylephrine dosage administered to the respective patient was considered, irrespective of stepped administrations. Classification accuracy was assessed for different phenylephrine dosage thresholds.

Neural network classification assessment

In a separate analysis approach, a single hidden layer neural network (NN) of 12 nodes, using back-propagation and gradient descent, was tasked with the same classification for the different phenylephrine thresholds. The basic configuration of the fully interconnected feed-forward NN used here and the basic equations describing its functionality are as follows:

Equation 1

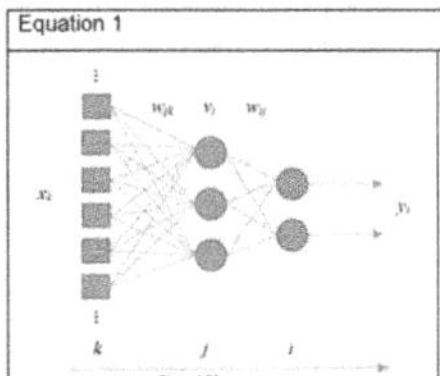

$$h(j) = \sum_k w_{jk} x_k$$

$$v_j = f_{sigmoid}(-h_j)$$

$$s_i = \sum_j w_{ij} v_j$$

$$y_i = f_{sigmoid}(-s_i)$$

The input data elements x_k are individually weighted, summed, and the summation is the input to a sigmoidal activation function before the output is submitted to hidden nodes v_j, whose outputs in turn are weighted, summed and presented to another activation function before submission to the output nodes y_i. Additional hidden layers, with the commensurate interconnections, weighting and summing activating of each layer's outputs etc., can be inserted to analyze performance as a function of input signal combinations.

The motivation here was to assess the classification capability of a "black box" approach that would have access, in contrast to the single-metric approach described above, to any number and combination of distinguishing features hidden in the data. If a significant number of such features were to exist, the classification performance of the NN would be expected to significantly exceed that of the single-metric approach. Classification performance was assessed using distributions and means of classification runs, the number of which was determined based on error and classification accuracy convergence. The choice of nodes, as well as the single-layer configuration, was arrived at by an analysis of the error as well as the classification accuracy of differently sized networks at different phenylephrine thresholds in order to address the potential of over-fitting.

The sample size required to estimate an area under the curve (AUC) of 0.85 ± 0.025 was calculated to be at least 33 patients, assuming a Type 1 error of 0.01, a power of 0.95, and the same number of mild and severe hypotension cases, i.e. an allocation ratio of 1 [22].

Prediction attempt based on comorbidities and pre-Op systole

The possibility of predicting severe hypotension based on baseline patient conditions, comorbidities or pre-op systolic blood pressure cuff measurements was investigated.

Results

Forty-nine patients were monitored as part of the study, with data from 45 patients included in the analysis. Table 1 lists patient population characteristics as well distributions of patient conditions and comorbidities. The following four patients were excluded from the original 49: One patient did not receive a spinal injection, the pre-injection data session from one patient was too short and two other data sessions were too compromised due to motion artifacts. For the 45 patients considered, which includes 4 patients who did not require the administration of phenylephrine, the mean dosage was 462 mcg, standard deviation (SD) 299 mcg, to treat hypotension post induction. No other vasopressor was used.

Table 1 Patient characteristics

Age (years)	
Mean (SD)	31.7 (4.72)
Range	21–44
Height (cm)	
Mean (SD)	160.9 (6.83)
Range	149.9–180.3
Weight (kg)	
Mean (SD)	98.7 (20.48)
Range	62.6–136.5
BMI (kg/m^2)	
Mean (SD)	37.8 (7.76)
Range	23.7–55.2
Pre-op systole (mmHg)	
Mean (SD)	128.9 (19.14)
Range	74–194
Systole at induction (mmHg)	
Mean (SD)	131.2 (18.18)
Range	96–202
Systole at + 10 min (mmHg)	
Mean (SD)	115.4 (21.18)
Range	66–215
Minimum systole (mmHg)	
Mean (SD)	98.13 (14.89)
Range	61–137
Minutes until minimum systole	
Mean (SD)	12.68 (8.48)
Range	2–39
Medical history	
Prior C/S (Y/N), n	9/36
Hypertension (Y/N), n	6/39
Diabetes mellitus (Y/N), n	6/39
Chronic obstructive pulmonary disease (Y/N), n	0/39
Atrial fibrillation (Y/N), n	0/39

Figure 1a displays an example of the time evolution of the AS response, linearized and resampled to a rate of 10 Hz, of Patient 04, 90 min prior to induction, who subsequently required minimal phenylephrine intervention, 200 mcg, while Fig. 1b displays comparable results for Patient 07 who required 1400 mcg to stabilize her hypotension.

Examination of the AS autocorrelation spectrum of Patient 04, Fig. 2 (trace A), suggests minimal coherence in the AS signal as the excursions of the coherence amplitude from zero are very small. The autocorrelation spectrum for Patient 07, Fig. 2 (trace B, offset from trace A for clarity), displays a more coherent response. Here the positive and negative correlation coefficients display oscillatory and significant amplitudes, suggesting that significant coherent signal components are present with distinct phase relationships.

In order to parameterize the observed coherence response, an integration over the absolute value of each patient's coherence spectrum, starting from a time lag of 100 s, was performed, as previously described. Figure 3 displays the result of performing the absolute autocorrelation value integration, for each patient, and graphing the results as a function of the total phenylephrine dosage administered to the respective patient.

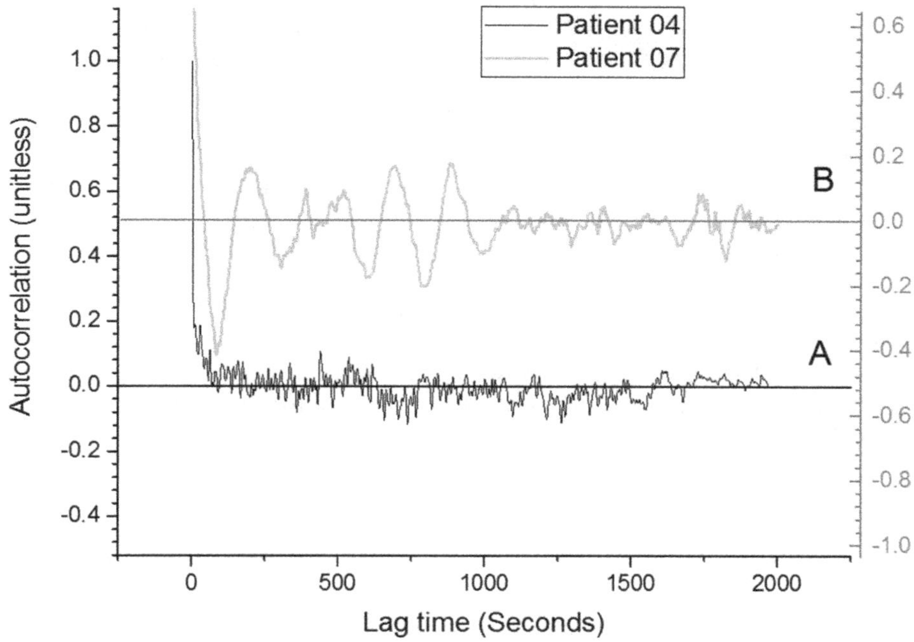

Fig. 2 Black trace (**a**): Normalized AS autocorrelation spectrum of patient 04 (Fig. 1a, 200 mcg) suggests minimal coherence in the AS signal due to highly unequal and low-amplitude positive and negative correlations. Gray trace (**b**): Normalized AS autocorrelation spectrum of patient 07 (Fig. 1b, 1400 mcg) suggests high coherence in the AS signal. Spectra are offset from each other for clarity

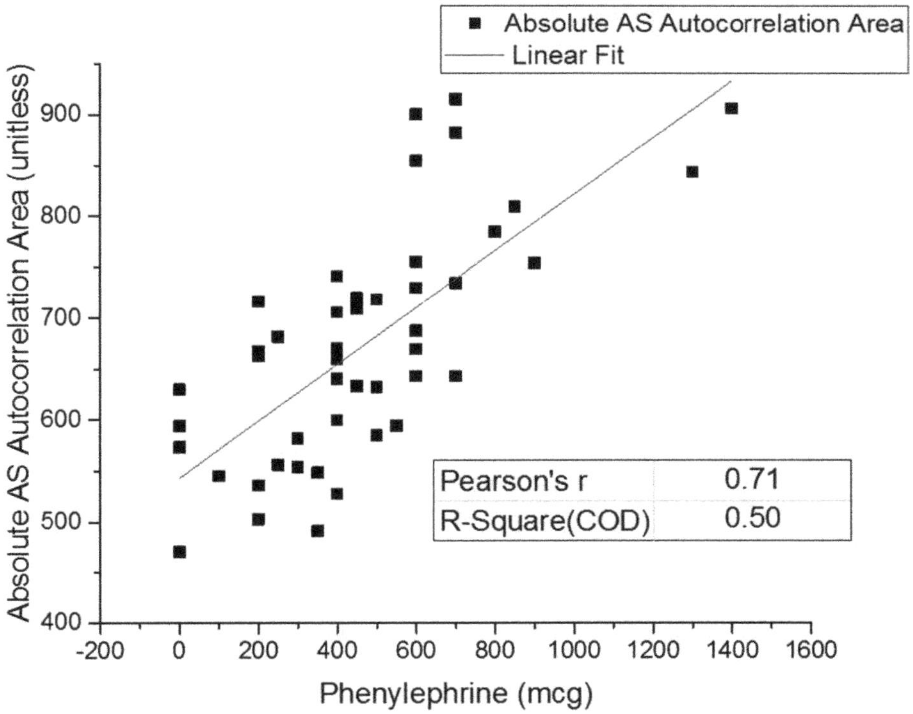

Fig. 3 Graph of the result of the absolute autocorrelation value integration, for each patient, as a function of the total phenylephrine dosage administered to the respective patient

A ROC analysis was performed to assess the ability of the absolute AS autocorrelation area metric, obtained 90 min pre-induction, to predict the likelihood of a given patient developing severe hypotension post-induction. In order to establish the optimal discrimination threshold, the Youden index, which is defined as sensitivity + specificity − 1 and provides a summary measure of a discriminatory test, was used. The AUC and resulting sensitivity/specificity were determined for different dosage thresholds of the data and are presented in Fig. 4, which presents the results for the Youden index (open circles) and AUC (solid squares) as a function of phenylephrine dosage threshold. The local maxima in the Youden index and AUC analysis suggest that 400 mcg is an optimal ROC threshold. The resulting ROC, with an AUC = 0.87 ($p < 0.001$), is presented in Fig. 5 (light gray curve). Specificity and sensitivity were calculated from the Youden index corresponding to that threshold and, respectively, are 0.68 and 0.93.

In order to validate these results and obtain a more comprehensive assessment of the classification potential of the feature set characterizing the AS autocorrelation spectra with regard to predicting severe hypotension, the spectra were submitted for classification to a 12-node single hidden layer NN. A detailed analysis, described below, was performed to assess the optimum number of nodes as well as the number of layers.

The following hyper parameters were used: the batch sized equaled the sample size, i.e. Fourty-five patient data sets; a learning rate of 0.01 was chosen since speed optimization was not a concern; a log-sigmoid transfer function was used for node activation. An analysis was performed to address the potential of over-fitting by assessing the classification accuracy and the classification error as a function of the number of network nodes and network layers.

Since training of a given NN amounted to gradient searches in very high dimensional spaces, some searches would terminate in local minima, with commensurately poor classification as reflected in low AUC values and significant classification errors. Other training runs would avoid local minima and yield good, in rare cases perfect, classification. Five hundred training runs were performed for each dosage threshold with randomized initialization of network weights. For each run, training data sets, validation data sets and test data sets were randomly chosen based on the ratios, respectively, of 0.7, 0.15, and 0.15. The optimum number of training runs was determined by extending their number until the standard deviation in the errors of a series of runs was

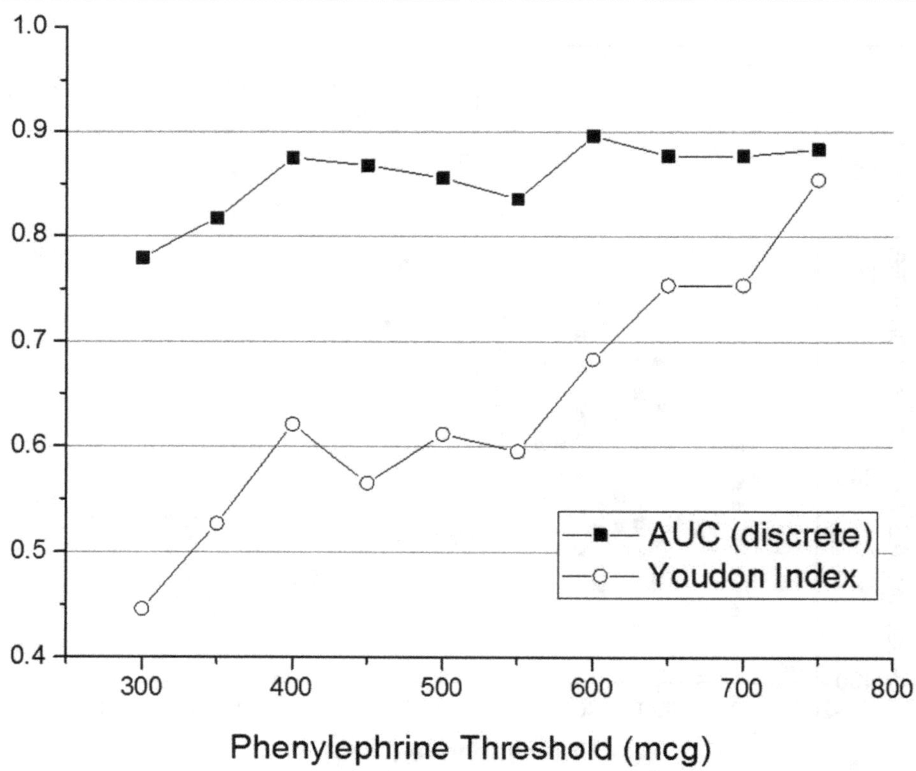

Fig. 4 Youden index (open circles) and AUC values (solid squares) as a function of phenylephrine dosage threshold for the single-feature analysis using the absolute autocorrelation value integration as a metric

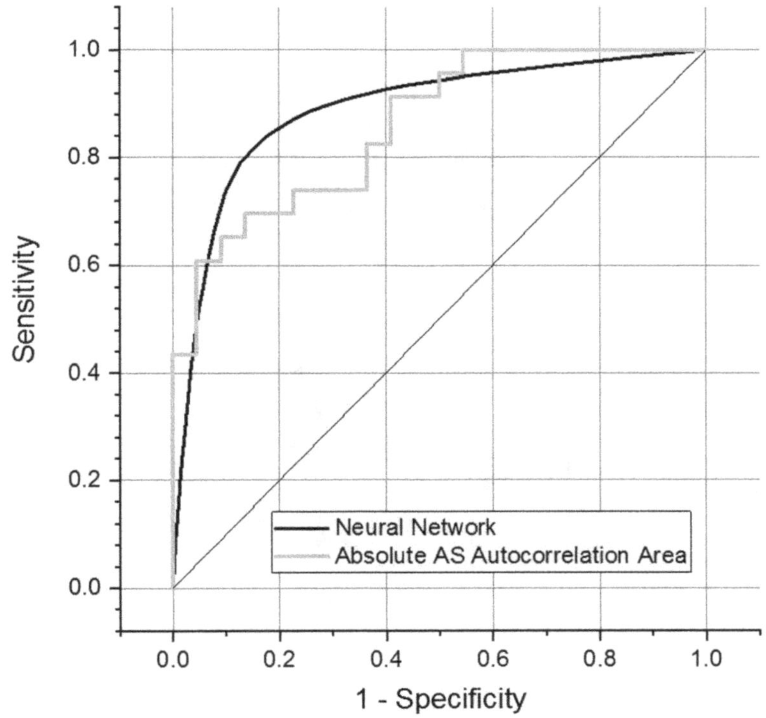

Fig. 5 Light gray trace: ROC analysis based on phenylephrine dosage <=400 mcg or > 400 mcg. AUC = 0.87 for autocorrelation area. Solid black line: ROC analysis based on average of 500 runs of 12 node NN based on phenylephrine dosage <=450 mcg or > 450 mcg, AUC = 0.89

approximately 1/10 the maximum range of errors observed at a fixed phenylephrine dosage. Each run was terminated once the validation score did not improve for 6 epochs. The error definition used here is the mean absolute classification error, where the classification error, with a continuous range from − 1 to 1, represents the difference between the NN output and the target designation, i.e. whether a given patient's total phenylephrine dosage is below (target = 0) or above (target = 1) the discrimination threshold. The absolute error range is continuous between 0 and 1, in contrast to the binary target designation, as the NN classification estimate is continuous.

In the context of assessing the categorization capability of the NN the optimum number of nodes and layers was determined, based on categorization error and mean AUC. Figure 6 presents three-dimensional graphs of the error (A) and AUC (B) evolution as a function of the number of nodes of a single hidden layer NN as well as the phenylephrine dosage. The network node axis is logarithmic to better reveal the dependence of the classification error and classification accuracy (AUC) for single-digit network nodes. The surface plots clarify that the classification error and the classification accuracy, after initially respectively decreasing/increasing with an increasing number of nodes, level off at approximately 12 nodes. This indicates that further increases in the number of nodes would only increase computational load but not enhance discrimination capability, providing the motivation for limiting the node number to 12.

The results of assessing the effect of including more NN layers on categorization performance are presented in Figs. 7 & 8, which present, respectively, the *difference* between the performance of a two-layer and a three-layer 12-node NN and that of the single-layer 12-node NN shown in Fig. 6. Specifically, Figs. 7 & 8 present the *subtraction* of the categorization error (A) and of the mean AUC (B) of the respective 2-layer/3-layer NN from that of the single-layer NN. Consequently, if the performance were identical, all 4 graphs would present a plane positioned at $z = 0$, which is approximately the case, for the performance of both the 2-layer and the 3-layer networks, in the range of nodes > 12. For the range < 12 nodes the performance of the higher layer number networks is poorer. This is indicated by the larger errors, i.e. for both Fig. 7A and Fig. 8A the difference in error in the range < 12 nodes is negative, meaning the subtracting higher-level network error is larger than the single-layer network's corresponding error, and by the positive AUC difference ranges displayed in Fig. 7B and Fig 8B, meaning the subtracting higher-level network AUC is smaller than that of the single-layer network, indicating the higher/better discrimination capability of the single-layer network.

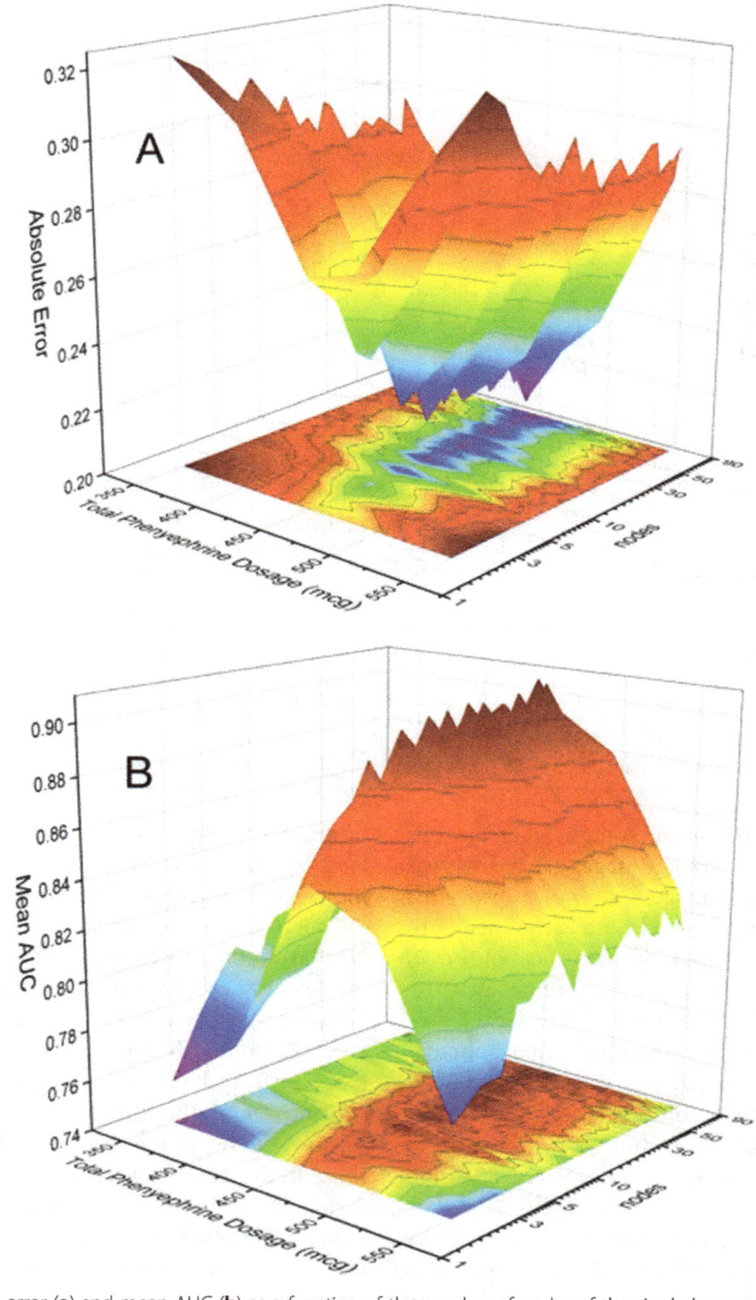

Fig. 6 Evolution of absolute error (**a**) and mean AUC (**b**) as a function of the number of nodes of the single-layer network as well as the phenylephrine dosage. The network node axis is logarithmic to better reveal the dependence of the classification error and classification accuracy (AUC) for single-digit network nodes

The general leveling-off response characteristic for the number of nodes > 12 is observed for all phenylephrine dosage levels, however, a distinct minimum/maximum in the classification error/classification accuracy (AUC) is observed for 450 mcg, where these quantities level off at, respectively, 0.28 and 0.89 for the single-layer network. For this threshold, AUC = 0.89 ($p < 0.001$) with specificity and sensitivity, respectively, equal to 0.91 and 0.84. The resulting ROC is presented in Fig. 5, solid black curve.

An attempt was made to predict hypotension based on patient baseline information and cuff-based pre-op systolic blood pressure. The results of correlating these parameters with phenylephrine dosage administered are presented in Table 2. None achieved statistical significance, precluding any effort to build a predictive model.

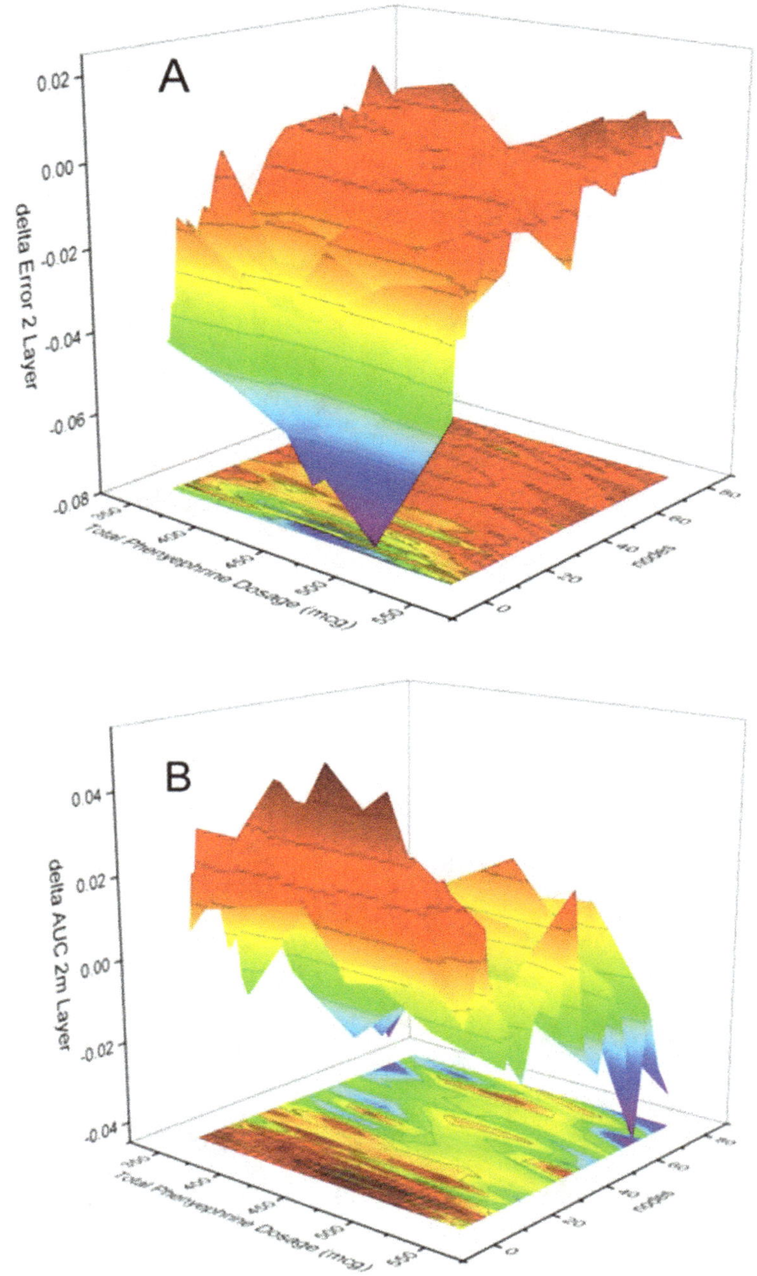

Fig. 7 Evolution of the difference of the absolute error (**a**) and mean AUC (**b**) between the single-layer network and the two-layer network as a function of the number of nodes of the network as well as the phenylephrine dosage. Note that the error difference (A) is negative for nodes< 12, indicating that the two-layer error is larger. For nodes< 12 the AUC is smaller for the two-layer network, as indicated by the positive AUC difference. For larger node numbers there is no difference in classification performance

Discussion

The significant findings of this study are: (1) it appears to be possible to assess the likelihood of significant post-spinal hypotension through the evaluation of coherencies in AS autocorrelation spectra and (2) this significant hemodynamic information can be obtained from non-invasive and readily obtained arterial pressure pulse information.

The results presented here add to the previous research in that multiple studies have identified changes in AS in comparisons of pregnant versus normal women as well as over the course of pregnancy. A prior study by Osman determined that arterial stiffness changes sinusoidally during pregnancy with an overall mean pulse wave velocity (PWV), the Gold Standard surrogate

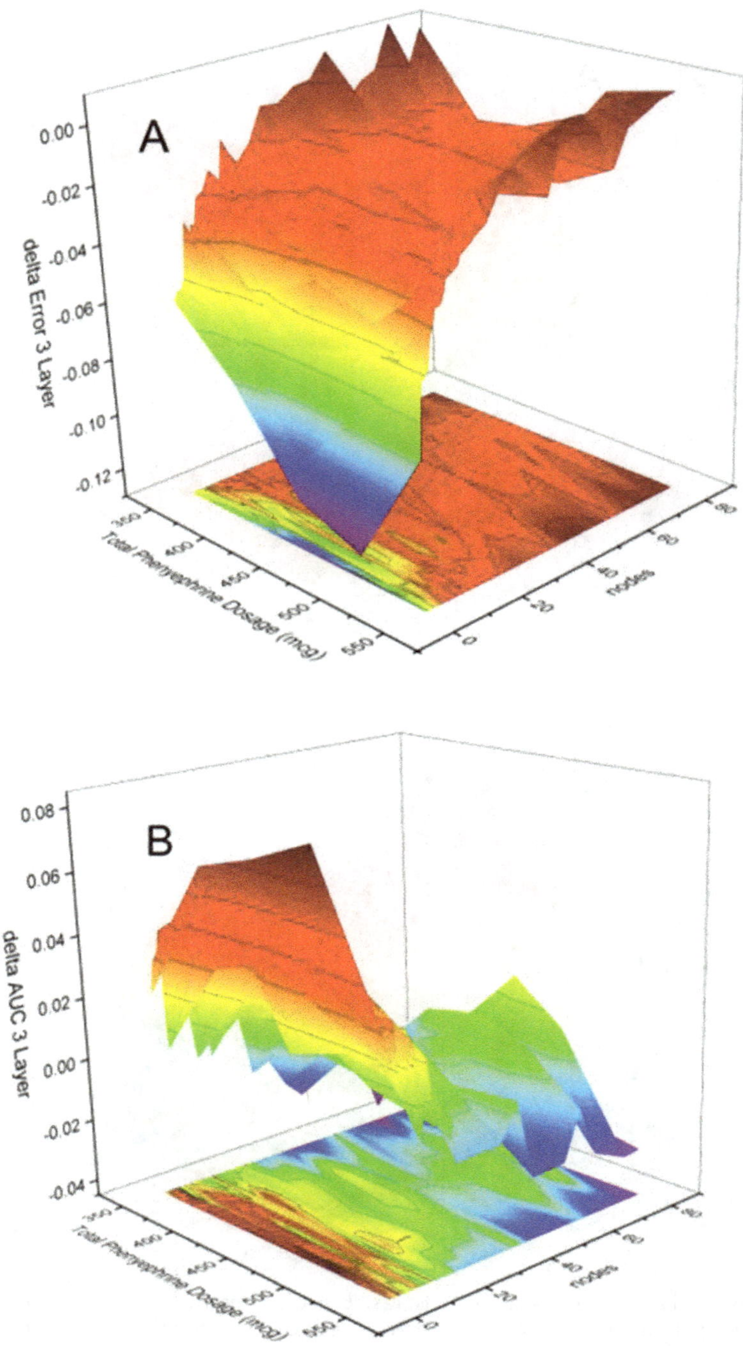

Fig. 8 Evolution of the difference of the absolute error (**a**) and mean AUC (**b**) between the single-layer network and the three-layer network as a function of the number of nodes of the network as well as the phenylephrine dosage. Note that the error difference (A) is negative for nodes< 12, indicating that the three-layer error is larger. For nodes< 12 the AUC is smaller for the three-layer network, as indicated by the positive AUC difference. For larger node numbers there is no difference in classification performance

parameter, of 7.81 m/s significantly lower than the measured 10.0 m/s in non-pregnant women [13]. Different mechanisms have been proposed to explain the changes in PWV throughout pregnancy. While the initial drop may be due to changes of vaso-active substances such as nitric oxide (NO) [23, 24], progesterone, relaxin, the changes may also be related to volume expansion [25], while the inhibition of NO, an increase in cardiac output

Table 2 Correlations of patient baseline information with phenylephrine dosage

Parameter	*Correlation (p-value)*
Pre-op Systole	−0.17 (0.26)
Prior C/S	−0.17 (0.27)
Hypertension	−0.13 (0.39)
Diabetes Mellitus	0.05 (0.75)
Chronic obstructive pulmonary disease	No positive patients
Atrial Fibrillation	No positive patients

or increased circulatory volume [26] could be responsible for the increase that is observed from mid-trimester to term [27].

A question in the context of these findings, which were obtained during normal gestational evolution, is whether these changes in AS, and probably other hemodynamic parameters, indicate that certain pregnant women are more prone to developing hemodynamic instabilities in response to a significant stressor, such as spinal anesthesia? Our results suggest that increased coherence in AS may be such a marker. If increased coherence is interpreted as decreased spontaneous variability, the concept of a predictive model of this specific case of hypotension becomes more plausible. Variabilities in different physiological parameters, heart rate variability for example, have been shown to decrease prior to hemodynamic crises, such as a hypotensive event, as compensatory mechanisms in the cardiovascular system try to maintain stability [28].

Comparing the classification performance of a discrete parameterization of a physiological data set such as the autocorrelation spectra used here with that of a generalized pattern recognition approach such as NNs is useful because the generalized approach can provide an assessment of the totality of available features that would aid successful classification. This is likely why the NN approach was more successful at classification than the discrete approach, although the small degree of improvement is also indicative, as is discussed below. The NN utilized a set of distinguishing features in its optimization of classification, as opposed to a single measure. As an example, we investigated utilizing the first crossing of the autocorrelation spectrum as a basis of classification. However, as a single-variable classification attempt the approach yielded only an AUC = 0.6. Other features to add to the discrete model could include, for example, distinct frequency components in autocorrelation spectrum. The NN likely identified a combination of these multiple features and others.

However, given that the discrete feature classification approach yielded comparable performance results with those of the NN suggests that the feature that the absolute value integration was designed to quantify, primarily the amplitude of the AS modulations, represents a significant portion of the classification potential available in the AS autocorrelation spectra. In fact, and this point was examined as part of the validation analysis for the number of nodes and layers used in the NN, the lack of significant improvement in the classification performance of the NN over that of the discrete feature suggests a dearth of additional available features overall. Specifically, increasing the number of nodes past the threshold value of 12 did not improve performance, i.e. both classification error and accuracy remained flat and significantly different from what would indicate perfect classification, addressing over-fitting concerns.

The same consideration applies to the results of expanding the NN to include multiple layers, which potentially provides access to more refined categorization opportunities in the combinations of inputs. The fact that these network expansions yielded no improvement in categorization capability again suggests that hidden features that could be used to improve performance are not present in the input AS autocorrelation spectra.

These considerations in turn suggest that the addition of complementary data sources, such as for example heart rate variability spectra, will be required to significantly enhance the classification capability of either the NN or the discrete approach.

The results presented here suggest that the NN approach, at least at the implementation level of a clinically relevant prediction algorithm, is somewhat superior to the discrete feature approach, providing implicit access to a plurality of features and, presumably, combinations thereof. In addition, the expansion of the approach to include the submission of other physiological data signals to the network can be readily envisioned and has been implemented in the context of general hypotension prediction by others [7]. In the context of gaining understanding of the underlying physiological mechanisms, however, discrete feature identification will continue to be relevant for reasons we present below.

The results presented here fit into the larger picture of the evolving and increasingly successful attempt to predict impending hypotension in critical clinical settings from arterial waveforms [6, 7]. However, these recent studies have focused on using the discrimination capability of NNs primarily because traditionally hemodynamic parameters such as heart rate variability [29, 30], stroke volume variability [31], arterial stiffness [32] or pulsatility indices [33] have been usually obtained as static single measurements that do not lend themselves to continuous, discrete monitoring. Nonetheless, it is very plausible that the NNs utilize the listed hemodynamic parameters in their categorization assessment through their effect on the arterial pulse, but the dependence is hidden. Problems arise when the NN approach fails in the absence of a more concrete underlying physiological model, because troubleshooting a NN is not an option, only to include more data and hope that a re-learned NN will perform better. Our work suggests that there may be a useful intersection between discrete assessments, particularly as the extraction of traditional hemodynamic parameters as beat-by-beat pulse features matures, and the general and considerable capabilities of the NN.

From the clinical point of view the incremental value of the proposed approach, be it based on discrete feature- or NN-based discrimination, is promising. Knowledge of pre-op blood pressures, specific patient conditions and/or comorbidities, which in general may or may not be completely available, in the cohort studied had no predictive value regarding post-induction hypotension, the blood pressure results specifically being in line with the results of others [6]. On the one hand a number of potential separate tests could be performed pre-op to assess certain hemodynamic parameters, but this approach is limited if even feasible. On the other hand is the proposed approach, with its simplicity particularly in the context of clinical workflow, since the arterial pulse information is collected continuously from the finger cuff-based sensing system, providing a data stream of high hemodynamic information content, irrespective of availability of patient history.

The focus of our preliminary study was to develop a predictive model of vasopressor requirements in this specific obstetric population. The ability to predict with advanced warning adverse events (hypotension) in this vulnerable population is an important step in patient care. If specific pre-operative interventions (e.g. additional intravenous fluid) in patients predicted to need substantial vasopressor administration can minimize the need for pharmacologic intervention, it would be of significant clinical value. A recent review article has shown that vasopressor interventions can adversely affect the fetal acid base status [34].

The population of pregnant patients undergoing C/S was chosen primarily because of the high frequency of adverse events requiring vasopressor support in this vulnerable population (92%). This allowed us to predict specific dosing thresholds of phenylephrine required In future work, we also want to assess the ability of our approach to predict hypotension in other surgical procedures where hypotension is a rarer event.

In the context of different clinical applications the sensitivity versus specificity aspects of the presented analyses should be considered. While the NN-based analysis demonstrated slightly better overall discrimination capability, closer examination of the corner regions of Fig. 5 suggests that the discrete feature approach may provide advantages were specificity is more critical. Increased perfection of a discrimination test is characterized in the ROC curve by an increasingly steep rise as a function of the false positive rate (1-specificity), and it is in that region of the ROC curves shown in Fig. 5 that the discrete feature approach appears to outperform the NN discrimination. In clinical applications where hypotension is a rarer event, the evolution of that aspect of the two discrimination analysis approaches will be or great interest as more data becomes available.

Further refinements and improvements to the predictive approach are possible as the CT system also provides access to heart rate variability, respiration signals and other hemodynamic parameters, such as cardiac output.

The size of the patient population and the classification performance of the parallel approaches support the statistical significance of the presented results, suggesting that it is unlikely that the analysis was optimized for this set of patient data, discounting the zero-effect hypothesis. Further studies will investigate the performance of the approach with scaling and additional physiological variables.

Conclusions

This pilot study has demonstrated that increased coherence in AS variability obtained from the pulse wave analysis of a continuous non-invasive blood pressure device appears to be an effective predictor of hypotension after spinal anesthesia in the obstetrics population undergoing C/S. Autocorrelation spectra were found to be valid biomarkers for this analysis, and it was possible to correlate spectra coherence with specific clinical dosing outcomes. These are significant findings since post-spinal hypotension is a common clinical scenario that has the potential to affect the mother and baby. Next steps are to examine if specific interventions can be used preoperatively to minimize the need for intra-operative vasopressors. We also want to assess the ability of our approach to predict hypotension in other surgical procedures where hypotension is a rarer event.

Abbreviations

C/S: Cesarean section; AS: Arterial stiffness; NIBP: Noninvasive blood pressure; MAP: Mean arterial pressure; CT: CareTaker; PDA: Pulse decomposition analysis; P1: Left ventricular ejection pulse; P2: Renal reflection pulse; P3: Iliac reflection pulse; ROC: Receiver operating characteristic; AUC: Area under curve; PMV: Mean pulse velocity; PWV: Pulse wave velocity; NO: Nitric oxide; NN: Neural network

Acknowledgements

We extend our gratitude to all the patients who were willing to participate in this study.

Authors' contributions

IG and MB helped with study concept and design. IG, BM, and MT helped with enrollment of subjects. IG, MB, BM, and ED helped with writing of the manuscript. IG, MB, JS, and IA helped with data analysis and interpretation. IG, MB, MT, JS, IA, BM, and ED have read and approved the final version of the manuscript.

Author details
[1]Cooper University Hospital, 1 Cooper Plaza, Camden, NJ 08103, USA. [2]Caretaker Medical, Charlottesville, VA, USA. [3]Quahog Research Group, Oakland, CA, USA. [4]University of California – San Francisco, San Francisco, CA, USA.

References

1. Walsh M, Devereaux PJ, Garg AX, Kurz A, Turan A, Rodseth RN, Cywinski J, Thabane L, Sessler DI. Relationship between intraoperative mean arterial pressure and clinical outcomes after noncardiac surgery: toward an empirical definition of hypotension. Anesthesiology. 2013;119(3):507–15.
2. Langesaeter E, Rosseland LA, Stubhaug A. Continuous invasive blood pressure and cardiac output monitoring during cesarean delivery: a randomized, double-blind comparison of low-dose versus high-dose spinal anesthesia with intravenous phenylephrine or placebo infusion. Anesthesiology. 2008;109(5):856–63.
3. Dennis AT, Solnordal CB. Acute pulmonary oedema in pregnant women. Anaesthesia. 2012;67(6):646–59.
4. Mendonca C, Griffiths J, Ateleanu B, Collis RE. Hypotension following combined spinal-epidural anaesthesia for caesarean section. Left lateral position vs. tilted supine position. Anaesthesia. 2003;58(5):428–31.
5. Zieleskiewicz L, Noel A, Duclos G, Haddam M, Delmas A, Bechis C, Loundou A, Blanc J, Mignon A, Bouvet L, et al. Can point-of-care ultrasound predict spinal hypotension during caesarean section? A prospective observational study. Anaesthesia. 2018;73(1):15–22.
6. Davies SJ, Vistisen ST, Jian Z, Hatib F, Scheeren TWL. Ability of an arterial waveform analysis-derived hypotension prediction index to predict future hypotensive events in surgical patients. Anesth Analg. 2020;130(2):352–9.
7. Hatib F, Jian Z, Buddi S, Lee C, Settels J, Sibert K, Rinehart J, Cannesson M. Machine-learning algorithm to predict hypotension based on high-fidelity arterial pressure waveform analysis. Anesthesiology. 2018;129(4):663–74.
8. Kansal A, Mohta M, Sethi AK, Tyagi A, Kumar P. Randomised trial of intravenous infusion of ephedrine or mephentermine for management of hypotension during spinal anaesthesia for caesarean section. Anaesthesia. 2005;60(1):28–34.
9. Muntner P, Shimbo D, Carey RM, Charleston JB, Gaillard T, Misra S, Myers MG, Ogedegbe G, Schwartz JE, Townsend RR, et al. Measurement of blood pressure in humans: a scientific statement from the american heart association. Hypertension (Dallas, Tex : 1979). 2019;73(5):e35–66.
10. Baruch MC: Pulse Decomposition Analysis Techniques. In: The Handbook of Cuffless Blood Pressure Monitoring. edn. Edited by Sola J, Delgado-Gonzalo R; 2019: 75–106.
11. Gratz I, Deal E, Spitz F, Baruch M, Allen IE, Seaman JE, Pukenas E, Jean S. Continuous non-invasive finger cuff CareTaker(R) comparable to invasive intra-arterial pressure in patients undergoing major intra-abdominal surgery. BMC Anesthesiol. 2017;17(1):48.
12. Sung SH, Chen ZY, Tseng TW, Lu DY, Yu WC, Cheng HM, Chen CH. Wave reflections, arterial stiffness, and orthostatic hypotension. Am J Hypertens. 2014;27(12):1446–55.
13. Osman MW, Nath M, Khalil A, Webb DR, Robinson TG, Mousa HA. Longitudinal study to assess changes in arterial stiffness and cardiac output parameters among low-risk pregnant women. Pregnancy Hypertens. 2017; 10:256–61.
14. Kolovetsiou-Kreiner V, Moertl MG, Papousek I, Schmid-Zalaudek K, Lang U, Schlembach D, Cervar-Zivkovic M, Lackner HK. Maternal cardiovascular and endothelial function from first trimester to postpartum. PLoS One. 2018; 13(5):e0197748.
15. Scheeren TWL, Saugel B. Management of Intraoperative Hypotension: prediction, prevention and personalization. In: Vincent JL, editor. Annual Update in Intensive Care and Emergency Medicine. Cham, Switzerland: Springer; 2018.
16. Baruch MC, Warburton DE, Bredin SS, Cote A, Gerdt DW, Adkins CM. Pulse decomposition analysis of the digital arterial pulse during hemorrhage simulation. Nonlinear Biomed Phys. 2011;5(1):1.
17. Callaghan FJ, Babbs CF, Bourland JD, Geddes LA. The relationship between arterial pulse-wave velocity and pulse frequency at different pressures. J Med Eng Technol. 1984;8(1):15–8.
18. Takazawa K, Tanaka N, Fujita M, Matsuoka O, Saiki T, Aikawa M, Tamura S, Ibukiyama C. Assessment of vasoactive agents and vascular aging by the second derivative of photoplethysmogram waveform. Hypertension (Dallas, Tex : 1979). 1998;32(2):365–70.
19. Eyal S, Almog Y, Oz O, Eliash S, Akselrod S. Nonlinear dynamics applied to blood pressure control. Auton Neurosci. 2001;89(1–2):24–30.
20. Hwang JS, Hu TH, Chen LC. An index related to the autocorrelation function of RR intervals for the analysis of heart rate variability. Physiol Meas. 2006; 27(4):339–52.
21. BuSha BF, Banis G. A stochastic and integrative model of breathing. Respir Physiol Neurobiol. 2017;237:51–6.
22. Goksuluk D, Korkmaz S, Zararsiz G, Karaagaoglu AE. easyROC: an interactive web-tool for ROC curve analysis using R language environment. The R Journal. 2016;8(2):213–30.
23. Delacretaz E, de Quay N, Waeber B, Vial Y, Schulz PE, Burnier M, Brunner HR, Bossart H, Schaad NC. Differential nitric oxide synthase activity in human platelets during normal pregnancy and pre-eclampsia. Clin Sci (Lond). 1995; 88(6):607–10.
24. Wilkinson IB, Qasem A, McEniery CM, Webb DJ, Avolio AP, Cockcroft JR. Nitric oxide regulates local arterial distensibility in vivo. Circulation. 2002; 105(2):213–7.
25. Pandey AK, Siwach S, Sangwan V, Sharma S, Das A. Assessment of maternal vascular stiffness indices in three trimesters of normal pregnancy. Indian J Physiol Pharmacol. 2014;58(3):197–205.
26. Wykretowicz M, Krauze T, Guzik P, Piskorski J, Markwitz W, Wykretowicz A, Wysocki H. Arterial stiffness, central hemodynamics and wave reflection in normal pregnancy and control nonpregnant women. Eur J Obstet Gynecol Reprod Biol. 2011;159(1):49–52.
27. McEniery CM, Wallace S, Mackenzie IS, McDonnell B, Yasmin, Newby DE, Cockcroft JR, Wilkinson IB. Endothelial function is associated with pulse pressure, pulse wave velocity, and augmentation index in healthy humans. Hypertension (Dallas, Tex : 1979). 2006;48(4):602–8.
28. Padley JR, Ben-Menachem E. Low pre-operative heart rate variability and complexity are associated with hypotension after anesthesia induction in major abdominal surgery. J Clin Monit Comput. 2018;32(2):245–52.
29. Hanss R, Bein B, Francksen H, Scherkl W, Bauer M, Doerges V, Steinfath M, Scholz J, Tonner PH. Heart rate variability-guided prophylactic treatment of severe hypotension after subarachnoid block for elective cesarean delivery. Anesthesiology. 2006;104(4):635–43.
30. Hanss R, Bein B, Weseloh H, Bauer M, Cavus E, Steinfath M, Scholz J, Tonner PH. Heart rate variability predicts severe hypotension after spinal anesthesia. Anesthesiology. 2006;104(3):537–45.
31. Juri T, Suehiro K, Tsujimoto S, Kuwata S, Mukai A, Tanaka K, Yamada T, Mori T, Nishikawa K. Pre-anesthetic stroke volume variation can predict cardiac output decrease and hypotension during induction of general anesthesia. J Clin Monit Comput. 2018;32(3):415–22.
32. Alecu C, Cuignet-Royer E, Mertes PM, Salvi P, Vespignani H, Lambert M, Bouaziz H, Benetos A. Pre-existing arterial stiffness can predict hypotension during induction of anaesthesia in the elderly. Br J Anaesth. 2010;105(5): 583–8.
33. Kuwata S, Suehiro K, Juri T, Tsujimoto S, Mukai A, Tanaka K, Yamada T, Mori T, Nishikawa K. Pleth variability index can predict spinal anaesthesia-induced hypotension in patients undergoing caesarean delivery. Acta Anaesthesiol Scand. 2018;62(1):75–84.
34. Singh PM, Singh NP, Reschke M, Ngan Kee WD, Palanisamy A, Monks DT. Vasopressor drugs for the prevention and treatment of hypotension during neuraxial anaesthesia for caesarean delivery: a Bayesian network meta-analysis of fetal and maternal outcomes. Br J Anaesth. 2020;124(3):e95–e107.

Efficacy of electrical stimulation on epidural anesthesia for cesarean section

Young Sung Kim, Hyo Sung Kim, Hyerim Jeong, Chung Hun Lee, Mi Kyoung Lee and Sang Sik Choi*

Abstract

Background: Loss of resistance (LOR) technique is a widely used method to identify the epidural space. However, cases of inadequate epidural anesthesia in cesarean section were frequently reported. Also, the success rate of epidural anesthesia with LOR technique varied depending on the proficiency of the practitioner. The purpose of this study was to assess the efficacy and safety of electrical stimulation to identify epidural spaces in cesarean section for novices or clinicians with recent gap in experience.

Methods: Pregnant women scheduled for elective cesarean section were randomly allocated to two groups. Groups were classified based on the methods used for identifying the epidural space: the LOR group (group L) and the LOR with epidural electrical stimulation group (group E). Clinicians with less than 10 epidural cesarean section experiences in the recent year performed epidural anesthesia for cesarean section. In the group E, a RegionalStim® conductive catheter was inserted through the Tuohy needle, and the guidewire passing through the catheter was connected to a peripheral nerve stimulator. The intensity of the stimulation was gradually increased from 0.25 mA to 1.5 mA until paresthesia was elicited and radiated. We assessed the success of epidural anesthesia (complete success, partial success or failure). Other clinical parameters including maternal satisfaction, time required for epidural anesthesia, neonatal Apgar scores, pain scores and adverse events were compared between the two groups.

Results: Except for 6 patients who withdrew consent, 54 patients were enrolled in this study (28 for the group L and 26 for the group E). The demographic data showed no difference between the two groups. There was no adverse event resulted from electrical stimulation. The group E showed higher rate of complete success, sensitivity in finding epidural space and maternal satisfaction compared to the group L (21/26 vs. 15/28, $p = 0.034$, 0.96 vs. 0.68, $p = 0.012$ and 4.04 vs. 3.39, $p = 0.02$, respectively). The other clinical parameters showed no differences between the two groups.

Conclusion: In addition to the conventional LOR technique, identifying epidural spaces using electrical stimulation led to better outcomes without additional risks for novices as well as clinicians with recent gap in experience.

Keywords: Cesarean section, Electrical stimulation, Epidural anesthesia

* Correspondence: clonidine@empal.com
Department of Anesthesiology and Pain Medicine, Korea University Guro Hospital, 148 Gurodong-ro, Guro-gu, Seoul 08308, South Korea

Background

Epidural analgesia and anesthesia are widely used in the obstetrical area. Especially in labor, the usefulness of epidural analgesia is remarkable [1]. Epidural analgesia showed high maternal satisfaction as mothers can walk and move freely with effective labor pain relief [2]. In the cases for cesarean section, epidural anesthesia also demonstrated many advantages than other anesthetic techniques especially for the parturient with congenital heart disease [3]. However, spinal anesthesia appeared to be preferred over epidural anesthesia in the cesarean section [4]. Compared to the epidural analgesia, epidural anesthesia for cesarean section requires more intense anesthesia with wider dermatome levels. When converting epidural labor analgesia into surgical anesthesia for cesarean section, the rate of conversion failure has been reported up to almost 20% [5]. Interestingly, the rate of failed epidural anesthesia conversion was 4.5 times higher for non-specialist anesthesiologists than among obstetric anesthesiologists [6].

In clinical practices, the success rate of epidural anesthesia varied depending on the proficiency of the practitioner [7]. Moreover, from a teaching standpoint, it was difficult to determine immediately whether a resident or novice practitioner had properly performed epidural anesthesia. In the case of spinal anesthesia, the success of the procedure can be predicted mostly by free CSF flow. On the other hand, loss of resistance (LOR) technique, which is widely used for confirmation in epidural anesthesia, is relatively subjective to interpret. Kopacz. et al. [8] reported 60 attempts at epidural anesthesia may be necessary to achieve a 90% success rate. We expected that untrained practitioner would have problems, especially in finding epidural spaces. In addition, proper placement of the epidural catheter may be difficult, particularly when performed by a novice provider.

We have previously shown the utility of electrical stimulation-guided epidural analgesia for vaginal delivery [9]. We thought that electrical stimulation would be also applied to the epidural confirmation for cesarean section. In the present study, we demonstrated the efficacy and the safety of electrical stimulation when confirming epidural spaces in cesarean section. We hypothesized that electrical stimulation-guided epidural anesthesia may help to find a correct epidural space and may result in a higher success rate for novices or clinicians with recent gap in experience.

Methods

Study population

This study was a single-center prospective randomized controlled trial conducted at Korea University Guro Hospital from 2018 to 2019. After obtaining approval from the Korea University Guro Hospital Institutional Review Board (IRB number 2015GR0703), written informed consent was obtained from all subjects participating in the trial. The trial was retrospectively registered at the ClinicalTrials.gov (trial identifier: NCT03443466). The current study was presented in accordance with the Consolidated Standards of Reporting Trials (CONSORT) guidelines. All patients were recruited from the Department of Obstetrics and Gynecology, Korea University Guro Hospital, by the research staff and were enrolled in the study at the hospital before surgery. Written informed consent was obtained from all participants after providing an explanation of the trial.

Patients aged 20 to 42 years, at 36 to 41 weeks' gestation, of American Society of Anesthesiologists (ASA) physical status I to II, and scheduled for cesarean section under epidural anesthesia were included in the study. Patients with severe cognitive impairment, skin infection on the back, history of lidocaine allergy and lumbar surgery, lumbar deformity, and hemostatic disorder were excluded from the study. Those undergoing anticoagulant therapy, having cardiopulmonary compromised status and expecting twin delivery, as well as those who refused to participate were also excluded. Demographic data including age, weight, height, and ASA class were collected from all the patients (Table 1). Patients were randomly allocated to the LOR group (group L) or the LOR + electrical stimulation group (group E), and they were unaware of the group assignment before the surgery. A single independent investigator was responsible for the random allocation sequence generation and the group assignment of patients. Randomization was achieved into 2 blocks using a web-based computer-generated list (www.randomization.com). The subject numbers were kept in opaque, sealed envelopes that were opened in the operating room by an independent anesthesiologist not involved in the study. Both the

Table 1 Demographic data

	Group L (***n*** = 28)	Group E (***n*** = 26)
Age (years)	35.93 ± 2.54	35.15 ± 4.76
Weight (kg)	66.56 ± 8.74	71.18 ± 6.69
Height (cm)	159.48 ± 6.10	160.65 ± 7.67
Body mass index (kg/m^2)	26.17 ± 3.09	27.67 ± 4.00
ASA class (I / II)	7 / 21 (25 / 75)	6 / 20 (23 / 77)
Status of practitioners (R1 / R2 / R3 / R4 / Specialist)	4 / 8 / 2 / 6 / 8	4 / 8 / 2 / 7 / 5

Values are either the mean ± SD or the number of patients (%). Group L used a loss of resistance technique in the epidural cesarean section while group E used electrical epidural stimulation combined with a loss of resistance technique. There was no significant difference between the two groups. ASA class refer to American Society of Anesthesiologists physical status. R1, R2, R3 and R4 refer to first-, second-, third- and fourth-year residents

patients and principal investigator were blinded to group allocation.

Anesthetic protocol

Routine monitoring devices including non-invasive blood pressure measurement, electrocardiogram and pulse oximetry were applied to each patient. We also monitored temperature and urine output during the perioperative period. The baseline values for each measurement were recorded before anesthesia induction. Epidural procedures were performed by anesthesiologists who were novice or with a recent gap in experience (less than 10 experiences for epidural cesarean section in the recent year). A resident who meets the conditions first attempted the procedure. If the residents did not find an epidural space after two attempts, another anesthesiologist who was a specialist performed the procedure. We considered that the practitioners have used one chance to attempt in any of the following circumstances: a) he or she gave up finding an epidural space and changed the injection site, b) the epidural catheter could not be inserted, and c) the leakage of blood or CSF was suspected. They did not know the group assignment for each patient until the test dose administration. The level of their anesthetic experience and status, ranging from first year to fourth year (resident or specialist), were recorded for each case.

After oxygen mask application with 5 L/min of oxygen, for the epidural catheter placement, patients were placed in the left lateral decubitus position. Once a sterile drape was performed, a local infiltration with 1% lidocaine was done at the L2/3 intervertebral level. A midline approach was used with a 17-guage Tuohy needle. Epidural space was then identified using LOR with air. After ensuring no cerebrospinal fluid or blood, 3 ml of 1% lidocaine (30 mg) was administrated as a test dose. In the group E, an epidural catheter (20-gauge, open tip catheter, 800 mm of length, Regional Stim®, Sewoon Medical Co., Ltd., Korea) with a conductive guidewire (Nitinol, 1100 mm of length; 800 mm inside the catheter and 300 mm exposed for connection to the electric nerve stimulator) was inserted 3 cm cephalad beyond the tip of the Tuohy needle right after a test dose administration. The cathode of the electric nerve stimulator (Stimuplex® HNS 12, B. Braun Melsungen, Germany) was connected to the exposed guidewire, and the anode was attached to an electrode on the patient's calf. For stimulation, the electric current was gradually increased from 0 mA to 2 mA, with a frequency of 1 Hz and pulse-width of 300 ms. A minimum required current to elicit paresthesia of a dermatome or motor response of a muscle group including the hip adductors, iliopsoas, gluteus, and hamstrings was recorded for each patient. Usually the current was checked within 3 min, so once epidural space was confirmed by electrical stimulation, the guidewire was removed, and the patient was observed for the remaining time until 3 min past the test dose administration. If there was no adverse sign and intrathecal injection was not suspected, 18 ml of 2% lidocaine was injected via the epidural catheter as a main dose. In the group L, the same process followed the test dose administration except the electrical stimulation. The same guidewire embedded epidural catheter was inserted, and the guidewire was immediately removed. 3 min after the test dose administered, 18 ml of 2% lidocaine was injected via the epidural catheter as a main dose. The patient was thereafter placed on the supine position.

The cold sensory test was performed with an alcohol swab. The additional epidural bolus, 5 ml of 0.75% ropivacaine, was injected through the epidural catheter when the cold sensory blockade did not reach a T7 level in 10 min after the main dose administration or when the patient complained of pain during surgery. After the baby was delivered, 2 ample (20 IU) of oxytocin was mixed to the main fluid for the mother, and the Apgar scores of the baby were assessed at 1 min and 5 min. When hypotension occurred during the perioperative period, ephedrine 4 mg or phenylephrine 50mcg was administered intravenously to keep the systolic blood pressure at − 20 to 20% of the baseline value. Any complications were recorded during the perioperative period.

Study endpoints

The primary outcome was a success rate of epidural anesthesia. We assessed each case as "complete success", "partial success" or "failure". If there were no signs for motor and sensory blockade in 10 min after epidural main dose administration, we regarded it as a "failure" and the anesthesia was converted to general anesthesia. If epidural anesthesia did not reach appropriate range and intensity and if the additional ropivacaine bolus was required, it was regarded as a "partial success". If the anesthesia was maintained enough to proceed with surgery, it was considered as a "complete success". The rate of complete success in epidural anesthesia was calculated as "complete success / complete success + partial success + failure". And the sensitivity in finding the epidural space was calculated as "complete success + partial success / complete success + partial success + failure" in each group. Meanwhile, calculation of the specificity was not available due to methodological limitation.

The secondary outcomes include Apgar scores, presence or absence of hypotension and ephedrine or phenylephrine use during perioperative periods, anesthetic times, fluids, transfusion, urine output, blood loss, pain score 1 h after arrival at PACU, maternal satisfaction, nausea/vomiting and other complications. One- and 5-min Apgar scores were compared to assess the effects of epidural electrical stimulation on the neonate. Anesthesia time was recorded in detail as described below: Time interval between operation room admission and the start of the operation, time A (interval between drape and the test dose administration), time B (time it took to confirm epidural space, place epidural catheter and administer main dose), operation time, time interval between the end of the operation and discharge to the post-anesthesia care unit (PACU). A blinded independent anesthesiologist assessed postoperative pain and other complications in the PACU. Pain was assessed by a visual analogue scale (VAS) score on an 11-point scale, where 0 indicates no pain and 10 refers to unbearable pain. Maternal satisfaction was evaluated by a postpartum interview. It was rated on a scale ranging from 1 to 5, where 1 represents very unsatisfied and 5 represents very satisfied.

Sample size and statistical analysis

A power analysis suggested that a minimum sample size of 26 patients for each group would be required with a significance level of 5% to achieve a power of 90%. It was calculated from our preliminary data: complete success rates of 0.9 for electrical stimulation group and 0.5 for conventional group. To allow for an exclusion rate, the study population was prospectively set at 60 patients.

Statistical analyses were performed with SPSS 22 (IBM, Armonk, NY, USA, Statistical Package for the Social Science 22). The outcomes were assessed based on the intention-to-treat analysis. Data expressed as mean ± standard deviation were tested for normality using the Kolmogorov-Smirnov test and were compared using independent t-tests or Mann-Whitney U tests depending upon the results of the Kolmogorov-Smirnov analysis. Finally, data expressed as the number of patients were compared using chi-square analysis or Fisher's exact test as appropriates. A p-value of < 0.05 was considered significant.

Results

The CONSORT flow diagram is presented in Fig. 1. Total 54 patients were enrolled in this study (28 patients in the group L and 26 patients in the group E) except 6 patients who withdrew consent due to anxiety and family opposition with no particular event prior to the cesarean section.

Demographic data including age, weight, height, body mass index, and ASA class showed no significant differences between the two groups (Table 1). The minimum electric current used to evoke paresthesia or muscle contraction in the group E was 1.06 ± 0.36 mA. Unilateral response was observed in 16 cases (62%) while bilateral response was observed in 10 cases (38%) (Table 2). Unilateral response did not correlate with "partial success" or "failure". Patients with unilateral and bilateral responses exhibited comparable patterns, such that those with unilateral responses reported 13 "complete success" and 3 "partial success" and that those with bilateral responses reported 8 "complete success", 1 "partial success" and 1 "failure". (Table 2).

The rate of "complete success" was significantly higher in the group E (53.6% for group L versus 80.8% for group E) (Table 3). In addition, the sensitivity of LOR + electrical stimulation in finding epidural space in the group E was 0.961 (25/26), whereas the sensitivity of LOR in the group L was 0.679 (19/28) (Table 3). Especially the number of "failure" of group L was much higher than that of group E while the numbers of "partial success" were comparable between the two groups (Table 3).

Maternal satisfaction of group E was significantly higher than that of group L (Table 3). Other secondary outcomes including Apgar scores, presence or absence of hypotension and ephedrine or phenylephrine use, anesthetic times, fluids, transfusion, urine output, blood loss, nausea, and pain score were comparable between the two groups (Tables 3, 4). Overall incidences of hypotension and severe nausea were 59% (32/54) and 5.6% (3/54), respectively (Table 3). No incidence of severe complication or catheter-related complication was reported.

Discussion

In the present study, we showed the usefulness of electric-guided epidural confirmation with LOR technique. In addition to higher maternal satisfaction, there was a significant increase in success rates without increasing any complications.

Compared to epidural anesthesia, spinal anesthesia has several disadvantages including the risks of the extensive block, postdural puncture headache, and abrupt hypotension. Despite these shortcomings, the higher success rate of spinal anesthesia in comparison to that of epidural anesthesia (94% vs 76%) [4] may be the one of the important advantages. Conversely, if success rate of epidural anesthesia improves, the merit of spinal anesthesia diminishes.

After epidural anesthesia have been introduced in 1921, LOR technique and hanging drop technique were independently developed to identify the epidural space in 1932 [1]. And LOR technique is more commonly used especially in the lumbar spine compare to the hanging drop technique because there was a lack of evidence for intrinsic negative pressure in the lumbar epidural spaces [10]. However, the loss of resistance seemed to be more difficult to feel in the parturient. Lechner, et al. [11] reported lower maximum pressure just before loss of resistance and higher pressure in the epidural space in the

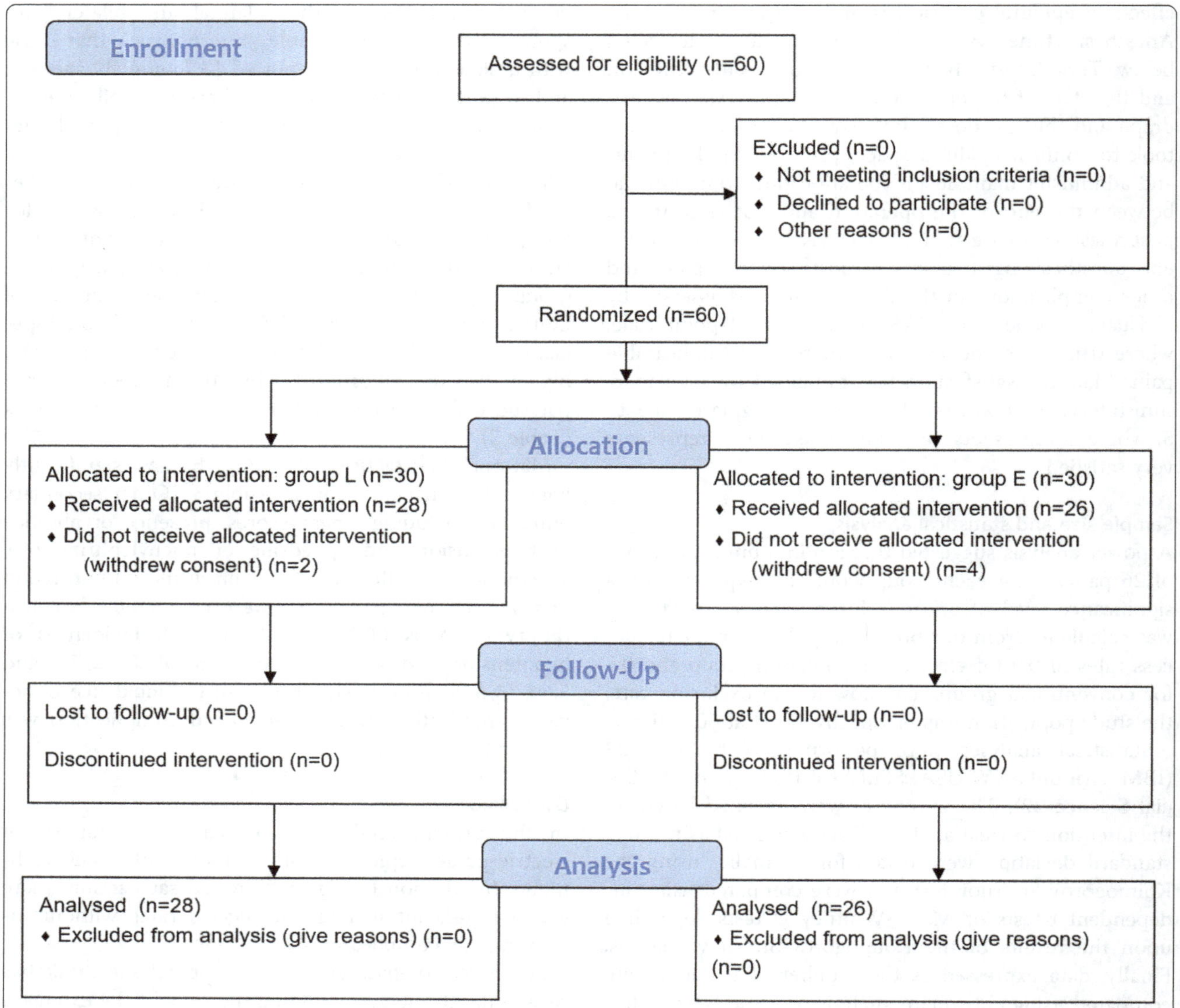

Fig. 1 CONSORT flow diagram. Group L used a loss of resistance technique in the epidural cesarean section while group E used electrical epidural stimulation combined with a loss of resistance technique

parturient, compared to those in the non-parturient probably due to weakened ligament flavum and engorged epidural vein.

There were several other methods to identify the epidural space. C-arm guided epidural confirmation is not used in the obstetrics due to radiation exposure. Sonographic guided epidural confirmation can be considered as an option these days, and the use of ultrasonography is increasing with improvements in ultrasound technology [12]. However, ultrasonography requires relatively expensive equipment. Some other ways to confirm the epidural space include epidural waveform analysis [13] and electrical stimulation that we discuss in the current study.

Tsui et al. [14] first described the use of electrical stimulation to confirm catheter placement in the epidural space. Subsequently, several researchers applied epidural stimulation for catheter placement [15–17]. Previous studies showed favorable results without side effects. However, it was difficult to unify diverse guidelines. In particular, different catheter types required different reference ranges for electric current. Tsui's method, where an epidural catheter was used with a fixed electrode at the distal tip and the electric impulse was conducted through normal saline within the lumen of catheter [14], required a relatively high electric current (1–10 mA at a pulse width of 0.3 ms) to produce motor response [18]. Similar to our catheter, Charghi

Table 2 The outcomes for the electrical stimulation

	N = 26
The minimum electric current (mA)used to evoke paresthesia or muscle contraction	1.06 ± 0.36
The number of cases which required catheter reposition	6 (23)
Cases with unilateral response	16 (62)
Success	13 (81)
Partial success	3 (19)
Failure	0 (0)
Cases with bilateral response	10 (38)
Success	8 (80)
Partial success	1 (10)
Failure	1 (10)

Values are either the mean ± SD or the number of patients (%). A total of 26 patients in the group E were confirmed the responses to electrical stimulation

et al. [19] used a single-port, metal coil-reinforced catheter containing a removable stylet for electric conduction instead of normal saline as a priming solution. Their results were comparable to ours, but the mean stimulatory current threshold was different from Tsui's. Although the absolute value provided in Tsui's criteria was not applicable in different settings, at least it can signal catheter misplacement of intrathecal or epiradicular spaces when the values of the required current needed for electrical response were too low [16, 17].

The success rates of epidural anesthesia are affected by the practitioner's skill. A non-obstetric anesthesiologist's care was regarded as one of the risk factors for epidural failure when provided not only in primary epidural anesthesia for cesarean section but also in conversion of labor epidural analgesia to cesarean delivery anesthesia [6]. There were several ways to define epidural failure, such as conversion to other forms of anesthesia [20], pain during surgery [21], and failure to achieve the predefined degree of nerve block [22]. We saw that failure is due to two reasons: a) failure in finding the epidural space at all and b) mismatched level or unilateralization of drug spreading out on the epidural space. In our study, the number of "failure" in the group E was significantly reduced compared to group L. This finding suggests that the electric confirmation was effective for untrained practitioners in confirming the epidural spaces.

We considered the level of anesthesia and drugs used for epidural anesthesia. To find an insertion point, the Tuffier's line was used as a reference in our study. We regarded the transverse line connecting the tops of the iliac crests as the Tuffier's line. Kim, et al. [23] showed that the mean vertebral level of Tuffier's line in the parturient women was L3-lower vertebral level which was higher than that of non-parturient women (L4-lower vertebral level). Therefore, our target level (L2/3) of epidural injection was the level above the Tuffier's line. However, some cases that deviate from the average in the actual vertebral level were reported [23], so knowing the correct level in advance may improve the results regarding "partial success". Next, there were several concerns about the usefulness of epidural test dose in obstetrics [24]. Local anesthetics may cause unwanted prolonged motor block, but it was not a major problem in the cesarean section. However, epinephrine was not recommended due to its restricted sensitivity [25] and risk exposures regarding high myocardial oxygen consumption and low uterine blood flow [24]. For these reasons, we used lidocaine only as a test dose to exclude an intrathecal injection. We also considered lidocaine as main dose for its fast onset and ropivacaine as

Table 3 Clinical outcomes

	Group L (***n*** = 28)	Group E (***n*** = 26)
Primary outcome (complete success / partial success / failure)	15 / 4 / 9 (54 / 14 / 32)	21 / 4 / 1* (81 / 15 / 4)
Sensitivity in finding the epidural space	0.68	0.96*
Maternal satisfaction	3.39 ± 0.73	4.04 ± 0.72*
Ephedrine or phenylephrine use during operation / PACU	1.23 ± 1.46 / 0.32 ± 0.67	0.89 ± 1.07 / 0.23 ± 0.59
Hypotension (Y / N)	17 / 11 (61 / 39)	15 / 11 (58 / 42)
Nausea (Y / N)	2 / 26 (7 / 93)	1 / 25 (4 / 96)
Pain score (VAS) at discharge in the PACU	1.25 ± 1.40	1.65 ± 1.41
1 min Apgar	8.18 ± 1.16	7.69 ± 1.72
5 min Apgar	9.54 ± 0.58	9.23 ± 0.82

Values are either the mean ± SD or the number of patients (%). Group L used a loss of resistance technique in the epidural cesarean section while group E used electrical epidural stimulation combined with a loss of resistance technique. Sensitivity in finding the epidural space was calculated as "complete success + partial success / complete success + partial success + failure" in each group. The calculation of the specificity was not available due to the methodological limitation. Maternal satisfaction was rated on a scale ranging from 1 (*very unsatisfied*) to 5 (very *satisfied*). Group E showed higher success rate, sensitivity in finding the epidural space and maternal satisfaction compared to group L. The other outcomes were comparable between the two groups. *$p < 0.05$ compared to group L.
Abbreviations: *VAS* Visual analogue scale, *PACU* Post-anesthesia care unit

Table 4 Required time and intake/output in the perioperative periods

	Group L (***n*** = 28)	Group E (***n*** = 26)
Time interval between the admission to the operating room and the start of the operation (min.)	32.37 ± 12.46	27.81 ± 15.92
Time A (interval between drape and test dose administration) (min.)	8.79 ± 3.97	8.81 ± 3.20
Time B (time it took to confirm epidural space, administer main dose and to place epidural catheter) (min.)	4.61 ± 2.50	4.67 ± 2.16
Operation time (min.)	48.93 ± 11.61	50.77 ± 16.82
Time interval between the end of the operation and the discharge to PACU (min.)	6.70 ± 4.11	6.42 ± 3.21
Crystalloid (ml)	1060.37 ± 469.41	1128.08 ± 388.15
Colloid (ml)	37.04 ± 133.44	53.85 ± 152.92
Transfusion (pint)	0.12 ± 0.43	0.08 ± 0.39
Urine output (ml)	249.82 ± 144.49	224.23 ± 115.27
Blood loss (ml)	479.63 ± 138.74	519.92 ± 209.76

Values are the mean ± SD. Group L used a loss of resistance technique in the epidural cesarean section, whereas group E used electrical epidural stimulation combined with a loss of resistance technique. Perioperative time period in each step and intake / output during perioperative periods were comparable between the two groups. *Abbreviation*: *PACU* Post-anesthesia care unit

supplementary dose for anesthetic quality [26]. Because of the simplicity of our regimen (no mixed solution), the risk of drug misadministration by novices appeared to be minimal, and once the epidural has been found, electrical stimulation did not seem to have a significant effect on the partial success rate.

The other outcomes in the study showed the efficiency and the safety of electrical stimulation. In almost all cases, electrical stimulation was performed during the wait time after the test dose administration. Although 6 patients in the group E required catheter repositioning due to lack of response to the electrical stimulation, the delay time was up to 5 min from the average. The difference in Time B, which includes the time for catheter placement, was only 0.06 min between the two groups (Table 4). Therefore, the risk of time consumption was minimized. During the study, no catheter-related adverse event including intrathecal or intravascular injection was reported, and the electrical stimulation did not affect the Apgar score. The most common complication was hypotension, which appeared to be a side effect from the neuraxial block. In addition, the incidence of hypotension and the use of cardiovascular drugs during perioperative period were comparable between the two groups. Most of the hypotensive events were gradually developed, and all were successfully resolved without any sequelae.

Before conducting this study, we tried to stimulate the exact level by identifying the corresponding radiating paresthesia, but the electrical stimulation seemed to have a low spatial resolution. In addition, when the catheter was located to one side, the nerve roots were easily stimulated, and the current value was lowered. There were also individual variations and a wide range of required currents due to possibility of epidural adhesion, epidural vein engorgement or any other anatomical variations. For these reasons, electrical stimulation has a limitation in confirming an appropriate level of anesthesia. Fortunately, most of the unilateral stimulations resulted in bilateral anesthesia. Large doses of local anesthetics seemed to extend to the contralateral side. Therefore, as a straightforward guideline, once a reliable response to the stimulation is detected even in unilateral side, we recommend proceeding to the next step.

There were other limitations as well. First, the usefulness of electrical stimulation may not be evident for the well-trained anesthesiologist. In statistical perspective, the higher success rate in the LOR-only group requires the greater number of sample size to have a significant meaning. Second, the guidewire inside the epidural catheter may increase a risk of incidental intrathecal or vascular puncture in theory. However, this issue has not been reported in this study as well as in Charghis's study [19] which was similar to ours. Third, there was a methodological limitation in allocation concealment (double blind). During the electrical stimulation, the patient and the practitioner may notice the group assignment. However, another blinded independent anesthesiologist assessed the outcomes in the postoperative period to minimize the performance bias. Finally, the use of a test dose could require more electrical current to overcome sensorimotor blockade of lidocaine although the test dose did not appear to have a significant effect in this study.

Despite these limitations, our study suggests several advantages and implications. First was the type of catheter. There was a risk of air lock which disturbs the current flow down the column of saline contained inside the Tsui's catheter [14]. In our study, we used the epidural catheter with a built-in conductive guidewire. Our devices seemed to be simple while reducing the risk described above. The minimum currents of our device were also lower than other electrical epidural stimulation methods. This may reduce the risk of injury from electrical stimulation. Second, the method and the results in the present study may contribute as a guideline and reference values when using our catheter. However, it should be noted that the reference value can be changed in other situations including non-obstetric patients or patients known to have history of lumbar disease or surgery. Third, high maternal satisfaction suggested that electrical stimulation did not appear to be an unpleasant or uncomfortable experience to the patient. In fact, no complaints or problems with electrical stimulation occurred during the study. To our knowledge, this study was the first application of epidural electrical stimulation for cesarean section. Although the method we improved had not changed dramatically, the impact has been substantial. Taken together, at least in the obstetric area, our findings supported the usefulness of electrical stimulation.

We think that our method would be more improved when used in conjunction with ultrasonography because ultrasound guided technique may provide a desired level of anesthesia. In detail, we recommend planning the epidural technique in advance while using ultrasonography to determine the level of vertebral body and the depth and location of epidural space, and then confirming with electrical stimulation. Further studies are required to determine whether the combined use of electrical stimulation and ultrasonography is useful for difficult epidural procedures.

Conclusion

Confirmation of the epidural space using electrical stimulation improved success rate as well as maternal satisfaction without wasting time, fetal distress or any other risks in the cesarean section. It seemed to be effective for inexperienced clinicians and those with recent gap in experience.

Abbreviations

LOR: Loss of resistance; PACU: Post-anesthesia care unit; VAS: Visual analogue scale

Acknowledgements

Not applicable.

Authors' contributions

YSK, CHL and SSC were major contributors in conducting the study and writing the manuscript. HSK and HJ helped to conduct study, recruited patients, performed data acquisition. MKL helped to design the study, analyzed the data and revised the manuscript. All authors gave approval of manuscript that to be submitted.

References

1. Chau A, Tsen LC. Update on modalities and techniques for labor epidural analgesia and anesthesia. Adv Anesth. 2018;36(1):139–62.
2. Sharma RM, Setlur R, Bhargava AK, Vardhan S. Walking epidural : an effective method of labour pain relief. Med J Armed Forces India. 2007;63(1):44–6.
3. Maxwell BG, El-Sayed YY, Riley ET, Carvalho B. Peripartum outcomes and anaesthetic management of parturients with moderate to complex congenital heart disease or pulmonary hypertension. Anaesthesia. 2013; 68(1):52–9.
4. Kinsella SM. A prospective audit of regional anaesthesia failure in 5080 caesarean sections. Anaesthesia. 2008;63(8):822–32.
5. Orbach-Zinger S, Friedman L, Avramovich A, Ilgiaeva N, Orvieto R, Sulkes J, Eidelman LA. Risk factors for failure to extend labor epidural analgesia to epidural anesthesia for cesarean section. Acta Anaesthesiol Scand. 2006; 50(8):1014–8.
6. Bauer ME, Kountanis JA, Tsen LC, Greenfield ML, Mhyre JM. Risk factors for failed conversion of labor epidural analgesia to cesarean delivery anesthesia: a systematic review and meta-analysis of observational trials. Int J Obstet Anesth. 2012;21(4):294–309.
7. Hermanides J, Hollmann MW, Stevens MF, Lirk P. Failed epidural: causes and management. Br J Anaesth. 2012;109(2):144–54.
8. Kopacz DJ, Neal JM, Pollock JE. The regional anesthesia "learning curve" - what is the minimum number of epidural and spinal blocks to reach consistency? Reg Anesth. 1996;21(3):182–90.
9. Lee CH, Choi SS, Lee MK, Kim JE, Chung DI, Lee M. Electric stimulation-guided epidural analgesia for vaginal delivery: a randomized prospective study. PLoS One. 2019;14(1):e0209967.
10. Todorov L, VadeBoncouer T. Etiology and use of the "hanging drop" technique: a review. Pain Res Treat. 2014;2014:146750.
11. Lechner TJM, van Wijk MGF, Jongenelis AAJ, Rybak M, van Niekerk J, Langenberg CJM. The use of a sound-enabled device to measure pressure during insertion of an epidural catheter in women in labour. Anaesthesia. 2011;66(7):568–73.
12. Lee A, Loughrey JPR. The role of ultrasonography in obstetric anesthesia. Best Pract Res Clin Anaesthesiol. 2017;31(1):81–90.
13. Al-Aamri I, Derzi SH, Moore A, Elgueta MF, Moustafa M, Schricker T, Tran DQ. Reliability of pressure waveform analysis to determine correct epidural needle placement in labouring women. Anaesthesia. 2017;72(7):840–4.
14. Tsui BCH, Gupta S, Finucane B. Confirmation of epidural catheter placement using nerve stimulation. Can J Anaesth. 1998;45(7):640–4.
15. Goobie SM, Montgomery CJ, Basu R, McFadzean J, O'Connor GJ, Poskitt K, Tsui BCH. Confirmation of direct epidural catheter placement using nerve stimulation in pediatric anesthesia. Anesth Analg. 2003;97(4):984–8.
16. Jeong JS, Shim JC, Shim JH, Kim DW, Kang MS. Minimum current requirement for confirming the localization of an epiradicular catheter placement. Korean J Anesthesiol. 2012;63(3):238–44.
17. Sutherland MA, Viscomi CM, Dominick TS, Anderson EL. Minimum current requirements for epidural stimulation test confirmation of epidural and intrathecal catheter placement. Reg Anesth Pain Med. 2009;34(6):575–7.
18. Tsui BC, Gupta S, Finucane B. Determination of epidural catheter placement using nerve stimulation in obstetric patients. Reg Anesth Pain Med. 1999; 24(1):17–23.
19. Charghi R, Chan SY, Kardash KJ, Finlayson RJ, Tran DQH. Electrical stimulation of the epidural space using a catheter with a removable stylet. Region Anesth Pain M. 2007;32(2):152–6.
20. Shibli KU, Russell IF. A survey of anaesthetic techniques used for caesarean section in the UK in 1997. Int J Obstet Anesth. 2000;9(3):160–7.
21. Riley ET, Papasin J. Epidural catheter function during labor predicts anesthetic efficacy for subsequent cesarean delivery. Int J Obstet Anesth. 2002;11(2):81–4.
22. Goring-Morris J, Russell IF. A randomised comparison of 0.5% bupivacaine with a lidocaine/epinephrine/fentanyl mixture for epidural top-up for emergency caesarean section after "low dose" epidural for labour. Int J Obstet Anesth. 2006;15(2):109–14.
23. Kim SH, Kim DY, Han JI, Baik HJ, Park HS, Lee GY, Kim JH. Vertebral level of Tuffier's line measured by ultrasonography in parturients in the lateral decubitus position. Korean J Anesthesiol. 2014;67(3):181–5.
24. Massoth C, Wenk M. Epidural test dose in obstetric patients: should we still use it? Curr Opin Anaesthesiol. 2019;32(3):263–7.
25. Norris MC, Fogel ST, Dalman H, Borrenpohl S, Hoppe W, Riley A. Labor epidural analgesia without an intravascular "test dose". Anesthesiology. 1998;88(6):1495–501.
26. Hillyard SG, Bate TE, Corcoran TB, Paech MJ, O'Sullivan G. Extending epidural analgesia for emergency caesarean section: a meta-analysis. Br J Anaesth. 2011;107(5):668–78.

18

Effect of intrathecal lipophilic opioids on the incidence of shivering in women undergoing cesarean delivery after spinal anesthesia

Yamini Subramani[1*†], Mahesh Nagappa[1†], Kamal Kumar[3], Lee-Anne Fochesato[2], Moaz Bin Yunus Chohan[2], Yun Fei Zhu[1], Kevin Armstrong[2] and Sudha (Indu) Singh[1]

Abstract

Background: Shivering is a common side effect in women having cesarean delivery (CD) under spinal anesthesia, which can be bothersome to the patient, and it can also interfere with perioperative monitoring. In several studies, the intrathecal (IT) addition of a lipophilic opioid to local anesthetics has been shown to decrease the incidence of shivering.

Objective: We performed this network meta-analysis to evaluate the effects of intrathecal lipophilic opioids in preventing the incidence of shivering in patients undergoing CD.

Methods: This review was planned according to the PRISMA for Network Meta-Analysis (PRISMA-NMA) guidelines. An English literature search of multiple electronic databases was conducted. We included randomized controlled trials (RCTs) that reported on the incidence of shivering, with study groups receiving either IT fentanyl, sufentanil, or meperidine in women undergoing CD under spinal anesthesia. Quality of the studies was assessed using the modified Oxford scoring system. Using random-effects modeling, dichotomous data were extracted and summarized using odds ratio (OR) with a 95% credible interval (CrI). Statistical analysis was conducted using R studio version 1.0.153 - Inc.

(Continued on next page)

* Correspondence: Yamini.subramani@lhsc.on.ca; yaminisrs@rediffmail.com
†Yamini Subramani and Mahesh Nagappa share the first authorship
[1]Department of Anesthesia and Perioperative Medicine, Schulich School of Medicine, & Dentistry, Western University, London Health Sciences Centre-University Hospital, (LHSC-UH) , London, Ontario, Canada

(Continued from previous page)

Results: Twenty-one studies consisting of 1433 patients (Control group: 590 patients in twenty-one studies; Fentanyl group:199 patients in seven studies; Sufentanil group: 156 patients in five studies; Meperidine group: 488 patients in ten studies) met the inclusion criteria for this systematic review investigating the effect of intrathecal lipophilic opioids in preventing the incidence of shivering in women undergoing cesarean delivery under spinal anesthesia. Methodological validity scores ranged from 3 to 7. The Bayesian mixed network estimate showed the incidence of shivering was significantly lower with IT fentanyl (pooled odds ratio (OR): 0.13; 95% credible interval (CrI): 0.04 to 0.35; $P = 0.0004$) and IT meperidine (OR: 0.12; 95% CrI: 0.05 to 0.29; $P < 0.00001$), but not with IT sufentanil (OR: 0.37; 95% CrI: 0.11 to 1.22; $P = 0.23$). The IT fentanyl group had a significantly lower incidence of intraoperative discomfort [Risk Ratio (RR): 0.19; 95% CI: 0.10–0.35; P < 0.00001], the IT sufentanil group had a significantly higher incidence of pruritus (RR: 6.18; 95% CI: 1.18–32.46; $P = 0.03$) The IT meperidine group had a significantly lower incidence of intraoperative discomfort (2.7% vs. 13.6%; RR: 0.22; 95% CI: 0.09–0.55; $P = 0.001$), but there was a significant increase in nausea and vomiting (IT meperidine group vs. Control group: 42.7% vs. 19.4%; RR: 2.56; 95% CI: 1.14–5.75; $P = 0.02$). Meta-regression analysis based on the opioid dose and quality of the study did not impact the final inference of our result.

Conclusion: IT fentanyl significantly decreased the incidence of shivering in women undergoing CD under spinal anesthesia without increasing maternal adverse events, confirming that routine use in this patient population is a good choice. IT sufentanil did not decrease the incidence of shivering. IT meperidine decreased the incidence and severity of shivering, but its use was also associated with significant nausea and vomiting.

Background

Cesarean delivery is one of the most common operations performed. It is routinely carried out under spinal anesthesia using a combination of local anesthetics and opioids. Intrathecal (IT) addition of a lipophilic opioid to local anesthetic reduces the dose of local anesthetic, shortens the onset of block, markedly improves the quality of anesthesia, prolongs the duration of analgesia and also decreases the incidence of shivering [1].

Up to 85% of patients undergoing cesarean delivery may experience shivering after spinal anaesthesia [2, 3]. The etiology of shivering likely involves multiple mechanisms. Pregnant patients have high circulating concentrations of progesterone which may account for decreased shivering thresholds. The sympathetic blockade associated with spinal anesthesia may impair the thermoregulation causing peripheral vasodilatation. This causes the transfer of heat towards the periphery from core and enhances the heat loss through the skin. In addition, at the central nervous system level, there is increased sweating thresholds and decreased vasoconstriction [4]. The oxygen consumption (upto 600%), carbondioxide production and blood pressure may increase with shivering leading to serious hemodynamic effects in patients with compromised cardiopulmonary function. Shivering may also interfere with non-invasive patient monitoring, disrupting care in the perioperative period [2]. Thus, prevention or treatment of shivering is an important clinical goal.

Common treatment regimens for shivering include increasing the body temperature, physical warming, increasing the operating room temperature, and using various medications such as clonidine, meperidine, fentanyl and morphine [5, 6]. Sufentanil, fentanyl and meperidine, in decreasing order of lipid solubility, are used as adjuvants for spinal anesthesia in patients undergoing cesarean delivery. Several randomized controlled studies investigated the effect of these opioids on the incidence of the shivering. However, inconsistencies in the results impeded meaningful conclusions. Therefore, we performed this systematic review and network meta-analysis (SRNMA) to evaluate the effects of the multiple lipophilic neuraxial opioids on the incidence of shivering in women having cesarean delivery under spinal anesthesia.

Methods

This meta-analysis was planned in accordance with the PRISMA-NMA guidelines (Preferred Reporting Items for Systematic Reviews for Network Meta-Analysis).

Study selection criteria

A systematic search was performed for full reports of randomized controlled trials (RCT) that reported on the incidence of shivering in patients undergoing cesarean delivery under spinal anesthesia with IT lipophilic opioids, such as fentanyl, sufentanil and meperidine. Relevant trials had to report the incidence of shivering in both the intervention and control groups. Any studies without data on control group were excluded from the analysis. The spinal anesthetic technique should have been standardized for both the treatment and control groups and should have included the administration of IT lipophilic opioids.

Literature search

The following databases were systematically searched for relevant studies in English language by an expert librarian: PubMed, Medline, Embase, Cochrane Central Register of Controlled Trials, Web of Science, Scopus and CINAHL. The search was conducted from 1946 to October 2019. Additional studies were identified from the reference list of retrieved reports. MeSH keywords used in the search were "prevention", "incidence", "shivering", "severity", "intrathecal", "spinal", "neuraxial", "fentanyl", "sufentanil", "meperidine", "lipophilic opioids", "obstetric patients", "parturients", "caesarian section", "cesarean delivery." Data from abstracts, letters, retrospective trials, case reports and unpublished data were not considered and were excluded from the analysis.

Study retrieval

Two investigators (YS and KK) independently reviewed the search results in a stepwise manner. Relevant studies were first selected by title review of the search results. Abstracts of the selected studies were screened to determine if the inclusion/exclusion criteria were fulfilled. Then, the full text of the selected manuscript was considered and pertinent information was collected. In case of discrepancies, a senior author (SS) was consulted to resolve the issues.

Data collection

A data collection form was used to collect the following data: (i) study ID; (ii) (ii) drug and dose of IT opioid [fentanyl, sufentanil and meperidine]; (iii) therapeutic allocation and sample size in each group; (iv) primary outcome: outcome measures including the incidence of shivering; (v) secondary outcomes: incidence of side effects such as hypotension, intraoperative discomfort, pruritus, nausea and vomiting.

Study quality assessment

The articles meeting the inclusion criteria were scored independently by two authors (YS and KK) for methodological quality, based on the modified Oxford score to determine the various risks of bias [7]. The key domains assessed were (1) randomization; (2) concealment of allocation; (3) double blinding; (4) flow of patients.

Statistical analysis

Network Meta-analysis (NMA)

We conducted a network meta-analysis to permit comparison of the effect of multiple intrathecal lipophilic opioids across a network of trials within the same or very similar patient population: i.e. direct and indirect data were combined to try to estimate the most effective opioid to prevent the incidence of shivering [8]. Analyses were undertaken using Bayesian random–effects models via Monte Carlo Markov Chain (MCMC) simulations with non-informative prior distributions. Analyses were performed using the R studio version 1.0.153 – Inc.

Crude data (dichotomous data) were extracted from the individual studies and summarized as odds ratios (OR) with 95% credible interval (CrI). The data on the side effects were summarized as the risk ratio (RR) with 95% confidence interval. The data for the individual groups was collected and then pooled across groups using Bayesian random-effects modeling. Continuity correction was done for those cells which had zero as the outcome. Two tailed $P < 0.05$ was considered statistically significant.

For the direct data, the meta-regression and sensitivity analysis of the various subgroups was done to measure the impact of the various doses of IT opioids and quality of the studies on the incidence of shivering. Heterogeneity across studies was investigated for each group by chi-square test and calculating I^2 to estimate the percentage of variation in study estimates that is due to heterogeneity rather than sampling error.

Quality of evidence in the network meta-analysis

The level of confidence in each intrathecal opioid effect, estimated by the network meta-analysis, was assessed using the CINeMA frame work [9] and GRADE approach [10]. The equality of evidence in each opioid effect was assessed for study limitation, indirectness, imprecision, inconsistency (heterogeneity and incoherence) and publication bias. Overall, certainty of the evidence was assessed using the GRADE approach. The study protocol is included in the supplementary file S1.

Results

Twenty-one potentially relevant articles were identified from 115 citations. Twenty-one studies consisting of 1433 patients (Control group: 590 patients in twenty-one studies; Fentanyl group:199 patients in seven studies [11–17]; Sufentanil group: 156 patients in five studies [18–22]; Meperidine group: 488 patients in ten studies [15, 23–31]) contained data regarding the effect of IT opioids on shivering (Flow chart: Fig. 1). One included study by Han et al. 2007 investigated the effect of both, fentanyl and meperidine [15]. Tables 1 and 2 summarise the systematic review of the effects of IT fentanyl, sufentanil and meperidine on shivering in women undergoing cesarean delivery. Out of twenty-one studies, ten studies investigated shivering as the primary outcome [14–16, 21, 24–26, 28–30]. Methodological validity scores determined by modified Oxford score ranged from 3 to 7.

Network meta-analysis (NMA)

The twenty-one studies included in this network meta-analysis investigated the effect of three interventions:

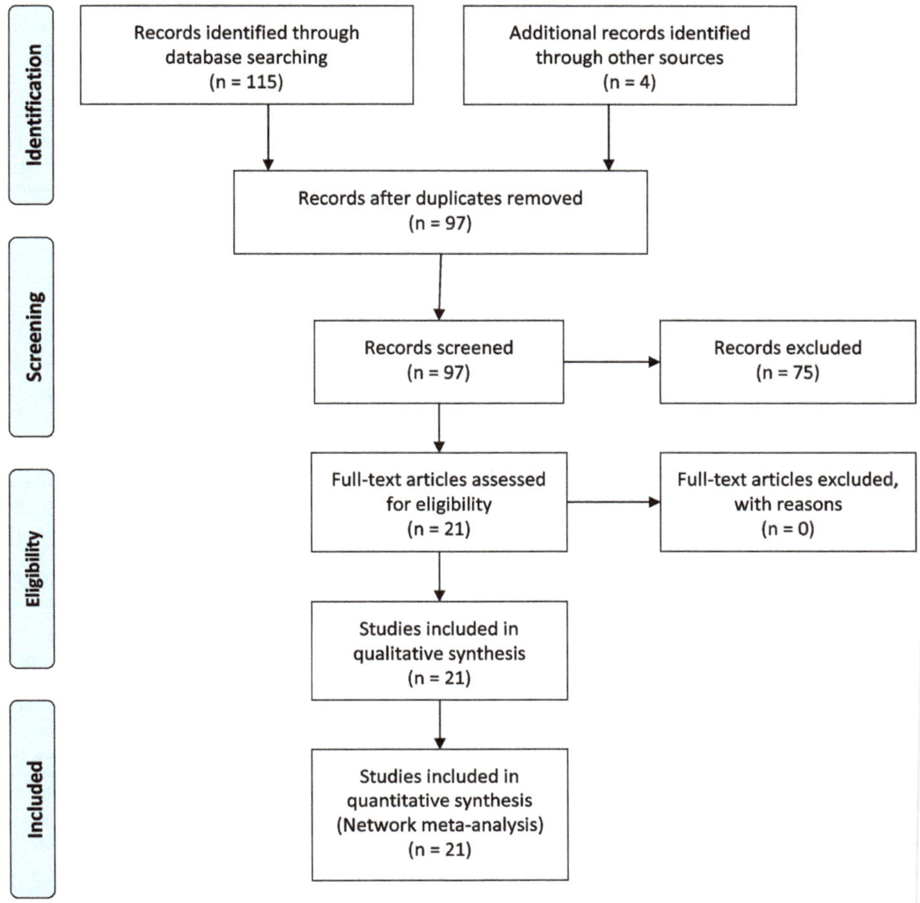

Fig. 1 Flowchart on the literature search

fentanyl (seven studies [11–17]), sufentanil (five studies [18–22]), and meperidine (ten studies [15, 23–31]), with four comparison groups. Six pairwise comparisons and four direct comparisons were conducted. Table 3 summarises the data on the effect of intrathecal opioids on the incidence of shivering. Out of the twenty-one studies comprising 1433 patients, 199 patients received fentanyl [11–17], 156 patients received sufentanil [18–22], 488 patients received meperidine [15, 23–31] and 590 patients were in the control group.

Table 3 provides the effect estimates of direct, indirect and mixed network meta-analysis with quality of evidence rating according to the GRADE approach. Figure 2 displays the network diagram comparing the various intrathecal lipophilic opioids to prevent incidence of shivering in women undergoing cesarean delivery. Supplementary file S2 and S3 show the contribution matrix and league table for comparison of all classes of drugs.

Fentanyl

Data on the incidence of shivering with IT fentanyl (7 RCTs, $n = 199$ patients) were available in all the studies [11–17]. The mixed evidence from the network meta-analysis showed that the incidence of shivering was significantly lower in the IT fentanyl group compared to the control group [IT Fentanyl vs. Control: 22.11% vs. 51.94%; Pooled Odds Ratio (OR): 0.13; 95% Credible Interval (CrI): 0.04 to 0.35; $P = 0.0004$]. The funnel plot and influential analysis on the direct data identified Sadegh et al.2003 as the outlier and contributed the maximum heterogeneity to the end estimate. When this study was excluded and summary estimates were recalculated, the end estimate increased to 0.51(0.36 to 0.71); $P < 0.0001$ and heterogeneity decreased to zero (not shown in the figure). The Begg's test ($P = 0.089$) and Egger regression test ($P = 0.2077$) did not show any evidence of publication bias. Fail-safe N test showed 113 studies required to increase the p value to more than alpha (> 0.05), indicating the absence of publication bias (not shown in the figure). Fentanyl was administered in the dose range of 7.5 to 25 microgram and there was no difference in the outcomes across this dose range (Coefficient − 0.043; 95% CI: − 0.0963 to 0.0103; $P = 0.1139$).

Table 1 Effect of lipophilic opioids on incidence of shivering in women undergoing cesarean delivery after spinal anesthesia: A systematic review of randomized control trials presented in a tabular column

Serial No.	Study reference Study ID year [Country of origin] [Modified Oxford score-R/C/D/F]	Groups Drug & Dosage [Intrathecal administration]	Results
1	[11]Palmer et al. 1995 [USA] [2/0/2/0]	Control Vs. Fentanyl (F) 15 µg	**Group F (14) vs. Control (14)** •Incidence: 0% vs. 14.28% •Severity (Grades 3 and 4): NA **Side Effects:** •Hypotension: 0 vs. 0 •Pruritus: 7.14% vs. 28.57% •Nausea and vomiting: 50% vs 92.85% •Intraoperative discomfort: NA •Respiratory depression: 0 vs. 0
2	[20]Chen et al. 2010 [Germany] [2/0/2/2]	Control Vs. Sufentanil (S) 5 µg	**Group S (32) vs. Control (32)** •Incidence: 0% vs. 38% •Severity (Grades 3 and 4): NA **Side Effects:** •Hypotension: 19% vs. 38% •Pruritus: 31% vs. 0% •Nausea and vomiting: 31% vs. 52% •Intraoperative discomfort: NA •Respiratory depression: 0 vs. 0
3	[22]Abdollahpour et al. 2015 [Iran] [2/0/2/2]	Control Vs. Sufentanil (S) 1.5 µg	**Group S (25) vs. Control (25)** •Incidence: 48% vs. 40% •Severity (Grades 3 and 4): NA **Side Effects:** •Hypotension: 64% vs 84% •Pruritus: NA •Nausea and vomiting: 64% vs. 52% •Intraoperative discomfort: NA •Respiratory depression: NA
4	[15]Han et al. 2007 [Korea] [2/0/2/0]	Control Vs. Fentanyl (F) 12.5 µg	**Group F (20) vs. Control (20)** •Incidence: 30% vs. 65% •Severity (Grades 3 and 4): - 10% vs. 35% **Side Effects:** •Hypotension: NA •Pruritus: NA •Nausea and vomiting: NA •Intraoperative discomfort: NA •Respiratory depression: NA
5	[17]Agrawal et al. 2016 [India] [2/1/0/1]	Control Vs. Fentanyl (F) 25 µg	**Group F (20) vs. Control (20)** •Incidence: 10% vs. 30% •Severity (Grades 3 and 4): NA **Side Effects:** •Hypotension: 75% vs. 75% •Pruritus: 30% vs. 0% •Nausea and vomiting: 15% vs. 70% •Intraoperative discomfort: NA •Respiratory depression: NA
6	[16]Sadegh et al. 2012 [Iran] [2/1/2/2]	Control Vs. Fentanyl (F) 25 µg	**Group F (40) vs. Control (40)** •Incidence: 10% vs. 75% •Severity (Grades 3 and 4): 0 vs. 23% **Side Effects:** •Hypotension: 75% vs. 77.5% •Pruritus: 30% vs. 0% •Nausea and vomiting: 18.95% vs. 67.5% •Intraoperative discomfort: 3% vs. 35% •Respiratory depression: 0 vs. 0

Table 1 Effect of lipophilic opioids on incidence of shivering in women undergoing cesarean delivery after spinal anesthesia: A systematic review of randomized control trials presented in a tabular column *(Continued)*

Serial No.	Study reference Study ID year [Country of origin] [Modified Oxford score-R/C/D/F]	Groups Drug & Dosage [Intrathecal administration]	Results
7	[19]Qian et al. 2009 [China] [2/1/0/2]	Control Vs. Sufentanil (S) 5 µg	**Group S (40) vs. Control (40)** •Incidence: 20% vs. 60% •Severity (Grades 3 and 4): NA **Side Effects:** •Hypotension: 20% vs. 55% •Pruritus: 0 vs. 0 •Nausea and vomiting: 0 vs. 0 •Intraoperative discomfort: NA •Respiratory depression: 0 vs. 0
8	[21]Locks et al. 2012 [Brazil] [2/0/0/2]	Control Vs. Sufentanil (S) 2.5 µg	**Group S (40) vs. Control (40)** •Incidence: 32.5% vs. 62.5% •Severity (Grades 3 and 4): NA **Side Effects:** •Hypotension: NA •Pruritus: NA •Nausea and vomiting: NA •Intraoperative discomfort: NA •Respiratory depression: NA
9	[14]Techanivate et al. 2005 [Thailand] [2/1/2/0]	Control Vs. Fentanyl (F) 20 µg	**Group F (30) vs. Control (30)** •Incidence: 20% vs. 50% •Severity (Grades 3 and 4): 3.33% vs. 13.33% **Side Effects:** •Hypotension: 36.7% vs. 50% •Pruritus: 66.66% vs. 40% •Nausea and vomiting: 33.33% vs. 23.33% •Intraoperative discomfort: 0 vs. 26.7% •Respiratory depression: NA
10	[13]Kang et al. 1998 [Taiwan] [2/0/0/1]	Control Vs. Fentanyl (F) 25 µg	**Group F (15) vs. Control (15)** •Incidence: 0% vs. 33.3% •Severity (Grades 3 and 4): NA **Side Effects:** •Hypotension: 20% vs. 40% •Pruritus: 93.5% vs. 0% •Nausea and vomiting: 60% vs. 66.6% •Intraoperative discomfort: 0 vs. 13.3% •Respiratory depression: 0 vs. 0
11	[12]Chu et al. 1995 [China] [2/0/0/1]	Control Vs. Fentanyl (F) 7.5 µg Fentanyl (F) 10 µg Fentanyl (F) 12.5 µg Fentanyl (F) 15 µg	**Group F 7.5 (15) vs. F 10 (15) vs. F 12.5 (15) vs. F 15 (15) vs. Control (15)** •Incidence: 66.7% vs. 46.6% vs. 33.3% vs. 26.6% vs. 66.7% •Severity (Grades 3 and 4): NA **Side Effects:** •Hypotension: 26.6% vs. 40% vs. 26.6% vs. 26.6% vs. 33.3% •Pruritus: 20% vs. 26.6% vs. 40% vs. 53.3% vs. 0% •Nausea and vomiting: 53.3% vs. 53.3% vs. 46.6% vs. 46.6% vs. 46.6% •Intraoperative discomfort: 41.2% vs. 20% vs. 0% vs. 0% vs. 66.7% •Respiratory depression: 0
12	[18]Lin et al. 1998 [China] [2/0/2/0]	Control Vs. Sufentanil (S) 10 µg	**Group S (19) vs. Control (22)** •Incidence: 21% vs. 4.5% (4 vs. 1) •Severity (Grades 3 and 4): 0 vs. 4.5% (1)

Table 1 Effect of lipophilic opioids on incidence of shivering in women undergoing cesarean delivery after spinal anesthesia: A systematic review of randomized control trials presented in a tabular column *(Continued)*

Serial No.	Study reference Study ID year [Country of origin] [Modified Oxford score-R/C/D/F]	Groups Drug & Dosage [Intrathecal administration]	Results
			Side Effects: •Hypotension: 89.47% vs. 57.89% (17 vs. 11) •Pruritus: 42.1% vs. 4.5% (8 vs. 1) •Nausea and vomiting: 31.57% vs. 57.89% (6 vs. 11) •Intraoperative discomfort: 36.84% vs. 68.42% (7 vs. 13) •Respiratory depression: NA

R/C/D/F: Randomization (2)/Concealment of allocation (1)/Double blinding (2)/Flow of patients (2); NA: Not Available
Modified Oxford Score varies from 0 to 7

Sufentanil

Data on the incidence of shivering with IT sufentanil (5 RCTs, $n = 156$ patients) were available in all the studies [18–22]. The mixed evidence from the network meta-analysis showed that the incidence of the shivering was not significantly lower with IT sufentanil when compared to the control group. (IT Sufentanil vs. Control: 23.71% vs. 45.28%; OR: 0.37; 95% CrI: 0.11 to 1.22; $P = 0.23$). Meta-regression analysis based on the IT sufentanil dose did not change the final inference of the result (Coefficient 0.0919; 95% CI: −0.2495 to 0.4333; $P = 0.5977$).

Meperidine

Data on the incidence of shivering with IT meperidine were available in all the 10 studies [15, 23–31]. The mixed evidence from the network meta-analysis showed that the incidence of shivering was lower in the meperidine group compared to the control group (IT Meperidine vs. Control: 15% vs. 44.2%; OR: 0.12; 95% CrI: 0.05 to 0.29; $P < 0.00001$). For the direct data, the Begg's test ($P = 0.7544$) and Egger regression test ($P = 0.1628$) did not show any evidence of publication bias. Fail-safe N test showed 85 studies required to increase the p value to more than alpha (> 0.05), indicating the absence of publication bias. Meperidine was used in the dose range of 5–35 mg and there was no difference in the outcomes across this dose range (Coefficient − 0.0215; 95% CI: − 0.0649 to 0.0219; $P = 0.3314$). Meta-regression and sensitivity analysis based on the quality of the study for the various subgroups slightly changed the end estimate, but did not change the final inference of our results (Table 4).

Side effects

IT fentanyl

The IT fentanyl group had a significantly lower incidence of intraoperative discomfort (IT Fentanyl vs. Control: 6.89% vs. 34%; Risk Ratio (RR): 0.19; 95% CI: 0.10–0.35; $P < 0.00001$), but there was no significant difference in other maternal adverse events like pruritus (IT Fentanyl vs. Control: 38.14% vs. 18.79%; RR: 2.03; 95% CI: 0.82–5.05; $P = 0.13$), nausea and vomiting (IT Fentanyl vs. Control: 39.10% vs. 58.20%; RR: 0.66; 95% CI: 0.42–1.05; $P = 0.08$) and hypotension (IT Fentanyl vs. Control: 43.57% vs. 54.47%; RR: 0.93; 95% CI: 0.78–1.12; $P = 0.45$).

IT Sufentanil

The IT sufentanil group had a significantly higher incidence of pruritus (IT Sufentanil vs. Control: 20.87% vs. 2.12%; RR: 6.18; 95% CI: 1.18–32.46; $P = 0.03$), but there was no significant difference in other maternal adverse events like hypotension (IT Sufentanil vs. Control: 40.51% vs. 55.46%; RR: 0.74; 95% CI: 0.37–1.47; $P = 0.39$), nausea and vomiting (IT Sufentanil vs. Control: 28.44% vs. 35.29%; RR: 0.83; 95% CI: 0.53–1.29; $P = 0.40$). IT sufentanil did not significantly decrease the intraoperative discomfort compared to the control group (IT Sufentanil vs. Control: 36.84% vs. 59.09%; RR: 0.62; 95% CI: 0.31–1.24; $P = 0.18$).

IT Meperidine

The IT Meperidine group had significantly lower incidence of intraoperative discomfort (IT Meperidine vs. Control: 2.7% vs. 13.6%; RR: 0.22; 95% CI: 0.09–0.55; $P = 0.001$). There was a significant increase in nausea and vomiting (IT Meperidine vs. Control: 42.7% vs. 19.4%; RR: 2.56; 95% CI: 1.14–5.75; $P = 0.02$), but there was no significant difference in other maternal adverse events between the two groups, like hypotension (IT Meperidine vs. Control: 46.9% vs. 41.8%; RR: 0.96; 95% CI: 0.67–1.37; $P = 0.82$) and pruritus (IT Meperidine vs. Control: 18.9% vs. 6%; RR: 0.63; 95% CI: 0.82–3.24; $P = 0.17$).

Quality of the evidence in network estimates

Supplementary files S4 and S5 show the rankogram and various domains examined to assess the quality of evidence in the network meta-analysis. Most of the

Table 2 Effect of Meperidine on incidence of shivering in women undergoing cesarean delivery after spinal anesthesia: A systematic review of randomized control trials presented in a tabular column

Serial No.	Study Reference Study ID year [Country of origin] [Modified Oxford score-R/C/D/F]	Groups Drug, dosage (Intrathecal Administration)	Results
1	[23]Yu et al. 2002 [China] [2/1/2/2]	Control Vs. Meperidine (M) 10 mg	**Group M (20) vs. Control (20)** •Incidence: 15% vs. 40% •Severity (Grades 3 and 4): NA **Side Effects:** •Hypotension: 70% vs. 55% •Pruritus: 0 vs. 0 •Nausea and vomiting: 55% vs. 15% •Intraoperative discomfort: 0% vs. 10% •Respiratory depression: 0 vs. 0
2	[28]Khan et al. 2011 [Iran] [2/0/2/2]	Control Vs. Meperidine (M1) 12.5 mg Meperidine (M2) 25 mg	**Group M1 (24) vs. M2 (24) vs. Control (24)** •Incidence: 20.83% vs. 4.16% vs. 58.33% •Severity (Grades 3 and 4): 0 vs. 0 vs. 16.66% **Side Effects:** •Hypotension: 50% vs. 45.8% vs. 41.7% •Pruritus: 0 vs. 0 vs. 0 •Nausea and vomiting: 25% vs. 75% vs. 4.2% •Intraoperative discomfort: NA •Respiratory depression: 0 vs. 0 vs. 0
3	[31]Atalay et al. 2010 [Turkey] [2/0/2/2]	Control Vs. Meperidine (M1) 25 mg Meperidine (M2) 30 mg Meperidine (M3) 35 mg	**Group M1 (20) vs. M2 (20) vs. M3 (20) Control (20)** •Incidence: 0% vs. 0% vs. 0% vs. 50% •Severity (Grades 3 and 4): NA **Side Effects:** •Hypotension: 20% vs. 30% vs. 55% vs. 65% •Pruritus: 10% vs. 35% vs. 45% vs 0 •Nausea and vomiting: 25% vs. 45% vs. 75% vs. 75% •Intraoperative discomfort: 0 vs. 0 vs. 0 vs. 0 •Respiratory depression: 0 vs. 0 vs. 0 vs. 0
4	[15]Han et al. 2007 [Korea] [2/0/2/0]	Control Vs. Meperidine (M) 12.5 mg	**Group M (20) vs. Control (20)** •Incidence: 20% vs. 65% •Severity (Grades 3 and 4): 5% vs. 35% **Side Effects: NA**
5	[26]Hong et al. 2005 [South Korea] [2/1/2/2]	Control Vs. Meperidine (M) 10 mg	**Group M (30) vs. Control (30)** •Incidence: 3.3% vs. 23.3% •Severity (Grades 3 and 4): 0% vs. 20% **Side Effects: NA**
6	[24]Denis Roy et al. 2004 [Canada] [2/0/2/0]	Control Vs. Meperidine (M) 0.2 mg/kg (15 mg average)	**Group M (20) vs. Control (20)** •Incidence: 45% vs. 85% •Severity (Grades 3 and 4): 10% vs. 45% **Side Effects:** •Hypotension: NA •Pruritus: 0 vs. 0 •Nausea and vomiting: 0 vs. 0 •Intraoperative discomfort: NA •Respiratory depression: 0 vs. 0
7	[29]Rastegarian et al. 2013 [Iran] [2/1/2/2]	Control Vs. Meperidine (M) 0.2 mg/kg (15 mg average)	**Group M (50) vs. Control 50)** •Incidence: 8% vs. 28% •Severity (Grades 3 and 4): 0% vs. 18% **Side Effects:** •Hypotension: 14% vs 12% •Pruritus: 0 vs. 0 •Nausea and vomiting: 18% vs. 0 •Intraoperative discomfort: NA •Respiratory depression: 0 vs. 0
8	[25]Anaraki et al. 2012 [Iran] [2/1/2/2]	Control Vs. Meperidine (M1) 0.2 mg/kg (15 mg average) Meperidine (M2) 0.3 mg/kg (25 mg average) Meperidine (M3) 0.4 mg/kg (30 mg average)	**Group M1 (38) vs. M2 (38) vs. M3 (39) Control (38)** •Incidence: 37.5% vs. 27.5% vs. 15% vs. 47.5% •Severity (Grades 3 and 4): 17.5% vs. 7.5% vs. 2.5% vs. 30% **Side Effects:** •Hypotension: NA •Pruritus: 28.21% vs. 38.46% vs. 48.72% vs. 25.64% •Nausea and vomiting: 15.4% vs. 25.9% vs. 35.8% vs. 8% •Intraoperative discomfort: 4.6% vs. 4.8% vs. 4.3% vs. 17.6%

Table 2 Effect of Meperidine on incidence of shivering in women undergoing cesarean delivery after spinal anesthesia: A systematic review of randomized control trials presented in a tabular column *(Continued)*

Serial No.	Study Reference Study ID year [Country of origin] [Modified Oxford score-R/C/D/F]	Groups Drug, dosage (Intrathecal Administration)	Results
			•Respiratory depression: 0 vs. 0 vs. 0 vs. 0
9	[27]Imarengiaye et al. 2011 [Nigeria] [2/1/2/1]	Control Vs. Meperidine (M) 7.5 mg	**Group M (25) vs. Control (25)** •Incidence: 0% vs. 4% •Severity (Grades 3 and 4): NA **Side Effects:** •Hypotension: 40% vs. 8% •Pruritus: 0 vs. 0 •Nausea and vomiting: 20% vs. 0% •Intraoperative discomfort: 0% vs. 16% •Respiratory depression: 0 vs. 0
10	[30]Shami et al. 2016 [Iran] [2/1/2/2]	Control Vs. Meperidine (M) 5 mg Meperidine (M) 10 mg	**Group M5 (50) vs. Group M10 (50) vs. Control (50)** •Incidence: 13 vs. 3 vs. 25 (26% vs. 6% vs. 3%) •Severity (Grades 3 and 4): 0 vs 0 vs. 1 (2%) **Side Effects:** •Hypotension: 33 vs. 37 vs. 34 (66% vs. 74% vs. 68%) •Pruritus: 3 vs. 13 vs. 0 (6% vs. 26% vs. 0) •Nausea and vomiting: 38 vs. 40 vs. 25 (76% vs. 80% vs. 50%) •Intraoperative discomfort: NA •Respiratory depression: NA

R/C/D/F: Randomization (2)/Concealment of allocation (1)/Double blinding (2)/Flow of patients (2); NA: Not Available
Modified Oxford Score varies from 0 to 7

included studies in the network meta-analysis were randomized double blind controlled studies with no, or some, concerns in the study limitation. To assess the imprecision, effect estimates of the relative treatments lower than 0.95 and greater than 1.05 were considered to be clinically significant. The data were collected from different studies, across different countries, at varying time intervals and the network model showed some degree of incoherence (χ^2 statistics: 0.336; d(f): 2; p value: 0.846). The estimated value of between-study variance for the network meta-analysis is 0.412 indicating some heterogeneity and consistency in the network model. Overall, some of the comparisons were rated down for imprecision, heterogeneity and incoherence (inconsistency), thus the quality of the evidence for the effect estimates was low according to the GRADE approach.

Discussion

In this systematic review evaluating the effects of lipophilic opioids to prevent or reduce shivering in patients having spinal anesthesia for cesarean delivery, fentanyl was found to be more effective than sufentanil and meperidine, however, there was no significant difference between direct or indirect comparison between fentanyl and meperidine. IT fentanyl (7.5–25 mcg) was found to decrease the incidence and severity of shivering as well as to improve the quality of spinal anesthesia in women having CD [32]. Fentanyl is a highly ionized, lipophilic μ-receptor agonist. When it is administered intrathecally, the unionized component is rapidly transferred into the spinal cord. IT fentanyl used with bupivacaine, in doses of 15 microgram has been shown to be effective in prolonging the duration of analgesia, and it also exerts

Table 3 Network meta-analysis: Estimates of direct effect, indirect effect and mixed effect with quality ratings according to GRADE approach, for the incidence of shivering in women undergoing caesarean delivery with intrathecal lipophilic opioids

	Direct evidence		Indirect evidence		Mixed Evidence Bayesian Network meta-analysis	
Comparison	OR (95% CI)	Quality of evidence	OR (95% CI)	Quality of evidence	OR (95% CrI)	Quality of evidence
[e]Meperidine vs. Control	0.17 (0.09–0.31)	Moderate	0.05 (0.00–3.16)	Moderate	0.12 (0.05–0.29)	Moderate[a]
[e]Fentanyl vs. Control	0.16 (0.07–0.35)	Low	0.41 (0.01–16.17)	Low	0.13 (0.04–0.35)	Low[ba]
Meperidine vs. Suphentanil	–	–	0.40 (0.14–1.13)	Low	–	Low[c]
Fentanyl vs. Suphentanil	–	–	0.41 (0.13–1.27)	Low	–	Low[ac]
Suphentanil vs. Control	0.42 (0.18–0.98)	Low	–		–	Low[d]
Fentanyl vs. Meperidine	1.71 (0.25–11.73)	Low	0.87 (0.30–2.50)	Low	1.02 (0.40–2.57)	Low[ac]

OR: Odds ratio; CI: Confidence Interval; CrI: Credible Interval; [a]: rated down for Indirectness; [b]: Contributing direct evidence of low quality; [c]: rated down for major concern in Imprecision; [d]: rated down for Heterogeneity; [e]: Statistically significant results

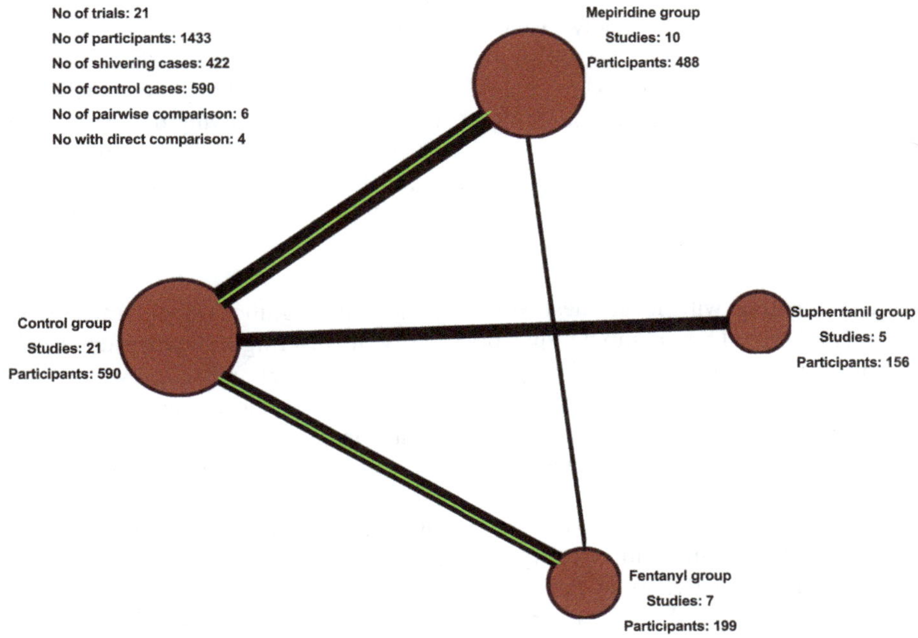

Fig. 2 Network diagram comparing the various classes of drugs. Evidence network of randomized controlled trials comparing the effects of drugs to prevent shivering in women undergoing cesarean delivery with intrathecal lipophilic opioids. The size of the circle is proportional to the number of participants randomized to that treatment. Width of the lines is proportional to the number of trials for that comparison. The green line indicates the statistically significant results between the compared groups

an anti-nausea effect in such small doses. This is probably due to decreased nociceptive stimulation from peritoneal manipulation and uterine exteriorization due to augmented quality of spinal block caused by fentanyl [11]. The reduction of shivering may be attributable to the effect of fentanyl that was added into the subarachnoid space on the thermo-regulator and spinal affect afferent thermal inputs at the spinal cord [33]. It is shown that fentanyl can reduce the intensity and severity of shivering up to 3 h after spinal anesthesia, including the time before delivery of the baby. This reduces the requirement of intravenous medications to treat shivering before delivery, thereby decreasing any harmful effects of medications on the baby [14]. The main detriment of preventing shivering is the fall in body temperature as shivering is a protective autonomic response against hypothermia. However, fentanyl lowered the core temperature for only 2 h, with return to baseline temperature in the third hour, without any harmful effects on the patient [14].

We found that addition of IT fentanyl was associated with lowest incidence of intraoperative discomfort due to increase in the quality of analgesia. The incidence of pruritus with the administration of opioid into the subarachnoid space was reported to be 67% for fentanyl, and 80% for sufentanil [34]. But, several studies have shown that there was no increase in the incidence of pruritus with IT fentanyl doses less than 50 microgram

Table 4 Study Quality assessment: Meta-regression and sensitivity analysis

Subgroups	Quality of study (No. of studies)	Point Estimate	95% CI	I^2	Meta-Regression	
					Coefficient (Standard Error)	**p**-value
Fentanyl	Good (2)	0.24	0.08–0.72	69%	−0.507 (0.393)	0.1969
	Poor - moderate (5)	0.50	0.32–0.79	13%		
Sufentanil	Good (3)	0.40	0.1–1.66	85%	−0.980 (1.113)	0.378
	Poor - moderate (2)	1.23	0.14–10.7	76%		
Low dose Meperidine	Good (7)	0.41	0.27–0.61	26%	−0.125 (0.376)	0.7391
	Poor - moderate (2)	0.46	0.28–0.75	8%		
High dose Meperidine	Good (3)	0.10	0.01–1.0	81%	–	–
	Poor - moderate (0)	-	-	-		

CI: Confidence Interval. Study quality scores were obtained from the modified oxford scoring system. Study was considered good when assigned score was equal or greater than 5 out of 7. *P*-values are based on random-effects model

[35–37]. Also, the pruritus associated with IT fentanyl and sufentanil is transient and resolves rapidly, usually without any need for treatment [11, 21]. The results of our study are supported by similar findings, which compared nine different neuroaxial adjuvants and found fentanyl to be the optimal choice [38].

Sufentanil is highly lipophilic with a higher affinity to opioid receptors, with a less cephalad spread and a much higher analgesic potency when compared with fentanyl or morphine [39–41]. It is well accepted for use in spinal anesthesia together with local anesthetics for caesarean delivery [20]. The combination of hyperbaric ropivacaine 10 mg with sufentanil 5 μg produced effective spinal anaesthesia for caesarean delivery with significantly less hypotension, vomiting and shivering, shorter duration of motor blockade and longer lasting analgesia than hyperbaric ropivacaine15 mg [19]. Our results show, however, that IT sufentanil was not effective in decreasing and severity of shivering in patients undergoing CD. While this finding could be due to the fact that this meta-analysis was limited by the small number of available studies evaluating this outcome, a previous meta-analysis on IT and epidural sufentanil had similar findings, and the authors postulated that the low dose range of IT and epidural sufentanil used (1.5–20 μg) may not be effective in decreasing shivering [42, 43].

Meperidine is an opioid with intermediate lipid solubility and is unique in having local anesthetic properties [44]. It has been used as a sole agent for spinal anesthesia for cesarean delivery [45–47]. It prolongs postoperative analgesia for up to 4 h, which is considerably lower compared to IT morphine, which can provide analgesic effect for up to 24 h [48–50]. An incidence of pruritus of 10.7–32% has been reported with the use of ≥50 mg of IT meperidine, which is much lower than IT morphine [33, 47, 51]. Meperidine is shown to be effective against shivering. While the mechanism of action is not fully understood, the anti-shivering effect of intravenous meperidine is due to its effect on the kappa opioid receptor and decreases the threshold of shivering [26, 52–55]. Possible suggested mechanisms for the anti-shivering effect of meperidine include k-opioid receptor activity, anticholinergic action, biogenic monoamine reuptake inhibition, NMDA receptor antagonism, or stimulation of alpha 2–adrenoceptors, and possibly modulating the heat loss caused by vasodilatation after spinal anesthesia [54, 56–58]. Meperidine slightly increases the threshold for sweating, significantly decreases the threshold for vasoconstriction, and reduces the threshold for shivering [59]. We found that IT meperidine was associated with nausea and vomiting, which limits its clinical efficacy.

Limitations

The doses of IT fentanyl, sufentanil and meperidine differed among the studies, which is a limitation of this systematic review, although the meta-regression ruled out the effect of the varying doses on our primary outcome. Overall, this systematic review and meta-analysis provides the best summary of the effect of the IT lipophilic opioids on shivering after cesarean delivery.

Conclusion

IT fentanyl significantly decreased the incidence and severity of shivering in women undergoing cesarean delivery under spinal anesthesia without increasing maternal adverse events, indicating that its routine use in this patient population should be considered. IT sufentanil did not decrease the incidence or severity of shivering. IT meperidine also decreased the incidence and severity of shivering, but it was associated with significant nausea and vomiting.

Supplementary information

Additional file 1: Supplementary file S1. Study protocol. **Supplementary file S2.** Contribution matrix. **Supplementary file S3.** League table. **Supplementary file S4.** Rankogram with SUCRA. **Supplementary file S5.** Quality of evidence in the network meta-analysis assessed in the following domains: study limitation, imprecision, heterogeneity, incoherence, indirectness, and final report.

Abbreviations

BP: Blood Pressure; CD: Caesarean delivery; Crl: Credible Intervals; IT: Intrathecal; MCMC: Monte Carlo Markov Chain; NMA: Network Meta-analysis; OR: Odds Ratio; PRISMA-NMA: Preferred Reporting Items for Systematic Reviews for Network Meta-Analysis.; RCT: Randomized Controlled Trials; SRNMA: systematic review and network meta-analysis

Acknowledgment

We thank Brie McConnell MLIS (Media and Information Manager, London Health Science Centre, Western University) for her assistance with the literature search.

Authors' contributions

YS: This author helped with study design, conducting the study, data collection, data analysis and writing the manuscript. MN: This author helped with study design, conducting the study, data collection, data analysis and writing the manuscript. KK: This author helped with conducting the study, data analysis and writing the manuscript. LF: This author helped with conducting the study, data analysis and writing the manuscript. MC: This author helped with conducting the study, data analysis and writing the manuscript. YZ: This author helped with writing the manuscript. KA: This author helped with conducting the study, data analysis and writing the manuscript. SS: This author helped with writing the manuscript. The author(s) read and approved the final manuscript.

Author details

[1]Department of Anesthesia and Perioperative Medicine, Schulich School of Medicine, & Dentistry, Western University, London Health Sciences Centre-University Hospital, (LHSC-UH) , London, Ontario, Canada. [2]Department of Anesthesia and Perioperative Medicine, London Health Sciences Centre and St. Joseph's Health Care, Western University, London, Ontario, Canada. [3]Department of Anesthesia and Perioperative Medicine, Schulich School of Medicine, & Dentistry, Western University, London Health Sciences Centre-Victoria Hospital, (LHSC-VH) , London, Ontario, Canada.

References

1. Lee YY, Ngan Kee WD, Muchhal K, Chan CK. Randomized double-blind comparison of ropivacaine-fentanyl and bupivacaine-fentanyl for spinal anaesthesia for urological surgery. Acta Anaesthesiol Scand. 2005;49:1477–82.
2. Kranke P, Eberhart LHJ, Roewer N, Tramèr MR. Postoperative shivering in children: a review on pharmacologic prevention and treatment. Paediatr Drugs. 2003;5:373–83.
3. Kranke P, Eberhart LH, Roewer N, Tramèr MR. Single-dose parenteral pharmacological interventions for the prevention of postoperative shivering: a quantitative systematic review of randomized controlled trials. Anesth Analg. 2004;99:718–27.
4. Sessler DI. Temperature monitoring and perioperative thermoregulation. Anesthesiology. 2008;109:318–38.
5. Alfonsi P, Hongnat JM, Lebrault C, Chauvin M. The effects of pethidine, fentanyl and lignocaine on postanaesthetic shivering. Anaesthesia. 1995;50: 214–7.
6. Horn E-PP, Werner C, Sessler DI, Steinfath M, am Esch JS. Late intraoperative clonidine administration prevents Postanesthetic shivering after Total intravenous or volatile anesthesia. Anesth Analg. 1997;84:613–7.
7. Jadad AR, Moore RAA, Carroll D, Jenkinson C, Reynolds DJJM, Gavaghan DJ, McQuay HJ. Assessing the quality of reports of randomized clinical trials: is blinding necessary? Control Clin Trials. 1996;17:1–12.
8. Bafeta A, Trinquart L, Seror R, Ravaud P. Reporting of results from network meta-analyses: methodological systematic review. BMJ. 2014;348:1741.
9. Salanti G, Del Giovane C, Chaimani A, Caldwell DM, Higgins JPT. Evaluating the Quality of Evidence from a Network Meta-Analysis. PLoS One. 2014;9: e99682.
10. Puhan MA, Schunemann HJ, Murad MH, Li T, Brignardello-Petersen R, Singh JA, Kessels AG, Guyatt GH. A GRADE working group approach for rating the quality of treatment effect estimates from network meta-analysis. BMJ. 2014; 349:g5630.
11. Palmer CM, Voulgaropoulos D, Alves D. Subarachnoid fentanyl augments lidocaine spinal anesthesia for cesarean delivery. Reg Anesth. 1995;20:389–94.
12. Chu CC, Shu SS, Lin SM, Chu NW, Leu YK, Tsai SK, Lee TY. The effect of intrathecal bupivacaine with combined fentanyl in cesarean section. Acta Anaesthesiol Sin. 1995;33:149–54.
13. Kang FC. Subarachnoid fentanyl with diluted small-dose bupivacaine for cesarean section delivery. Acta Anaesthesiol Sin. 1998;36:207–14.
14. Techanivate A, Rodanant O, Tachawattanawisal W, Somsiri T. Intrathecal fentanyl for prevention of shivering in cesarean section. J Med Assoc Thail. 2005;88:1214–21.
15. Han JW, Kang HS, Choi SK, Park SJ, Park HJ, Lim TH. Comparison of the effects of Intrathecal fentanyl and Meperidine on shivering after cesarean delivery under spinal anesthesia. Korean J Anesth. 2007;52:657–62.
16. Sadegh A, Tazeh-Kand NF, Eslami B. Intrathecal fentanyl for prevention of shivering in spinal anesthesia in cesarean section. Med J Islam Repub Iran. 2012;26:85–9.
17. Agrawal A, Asthana V, Sharma J, Gupta V. Efficacy of lipophilic vs lipophobic opioids in addition to hyperbaric bupivacaine for patients undergoing lower segment caeserean section. Anesth Essays Res. 2016;10:420–4.
18. Lin BC. The maternal and fetal effects of the addition of sufentanil to 0.5% spinal bupivacaine for cesarean delivery. Acta Anaesthesiol Sin. 1998;36:143–8.
19. Qian XW, Chen XZ, Li DB. Low-dose ropivacaine-sufentanil spinal anaesthesia for caesarean delivery: a randomised trial. Int J Obstet Anesth. 2008;17:309–14.
20. Chen X, Qian X, Fu F, Lu H, Bein B. Intrathecal sufentanil decreases the median effective dose (ED50) of intrathecal hyperbaric ropivacaine for caesarean delivery. Acta Anaesthesiol Scand. 2010;54:284–90.
21. De Figueiredo Locks G. Incidence of shivering after cesarean section under spinal anesthesia with or without Intrathecal Sufentanil: a randomized study. Rev Bras Anestesiol. 2012;62:676–84.
22. Abdollahpour A, Azadi R, Bandari R, Mirmohammadkhani M, Agrawal A, Asthana V, Sharma JP, Gupta V, Anaraki AN, Mirzaei K, Bogra J, Arora N, Srivastava P, Chen XZ, Qian XW, Fu F, Lu H, Bein B, Chu CC, Shu SS, Lin SM, Chu NW, Leu YK, Tsai SK, Lee TY, de Figueiredo Locks G, Hong JY, Lee IH, Kang FC, Tsai YC, et al. Effects of Adding Midazolam and Sufentanil to Intrathecal Bupivacaine on Analgesia Quality and Postoperative Complications in Elective Cesarean Section. Acta Anaesthesiol Sin. 2012;10: 309–14.
23. Yu S-C, Ngan Kee WD, Kwan ASK. Addition of meperidine to bupivacaine for spinal anaesthesia for caesarean section †. Br J Anaesth. 2002;88:379–83.
24. Roy J-DD, Girard M, Drolet P. Intrathecal Meperidine decreases shivering during cesarean delivery under spinal anesthesia. Anesth Analg. 2004;98: 230–4.
25. Anaraki AN, Mirzaei K. The effect of different intrathecal doses of meperidine on shivering during delivery under spinal anesthesia. Int J Prev Med. 2012;3:706–12.
26. Hong J-Y, Lee IH. Comparison of the effects of intrathecal morphine and pethidine on shivering after caesarean delivery under combined-spinal epidural anaesthesia*. Anaesthesia. 2005;60:1168–72.
27. Imarengiaye CO, Asudo FD, Akpoguado DD, Akhideno II, Omoifo CE, Ogunsakin AT, Akpoduado DD, Akhideno II. Subarachnoid bupivacaine and pethidine for caesarean section: assessment of quality of perioperative analgesia and side effects. Niger Postgrad Med J. 2011;2:18–22.
28. Khan ZH, Zanjani AP, Makarem J, Samadi S. Antishivering effects of two different doses of intrathecal meperidine in caesarean section: a prospective randomised blinded study. Eur J Anaesthesiol. 2011;28:202–6.
29. Rastegarian A, Ghobadifar MA, Kargar H, Mosallanezhad Z. Intrathecal Meperidine plus Lidocaine for prevention of shivering during cesarean section. Korean J Pain. 2013;26:379–86.
30. Shami S, Nasseri K, Shirmohammadi M, Sarshivi F, Ghadami N, Ghaderi E, Pouladi M, Barzanji A. Effect of low dose of intrathecal pethidine on the incidence and intensity of shivering during cesarean section under spinal anesthesia: a randomized, placebo-controlled, double-blind clinical trial. Drug Des Devel Ther. 2016;10:3005–12.
31. Atalay C, Aksoy M, Aksoy A, Dogan N, Kürsad H. Combining Intrathecal bupivacaine and Meperidine during caesarean section to prevent spinal Anaesthesia-induced hypotension and other side-effects. J Int Med Res. 2010;38:1626–36.
32. Uppal V, Retter S, Casey M, Sancheti S, Matheson K, McKeen DM. Efficacy of Intrathecal fentanyl for cesarean delivery: a systematic review and Meta-analysis of randomized controlled trials with trial sequential analysis. Anesth Analg. 2020;130:111–25.
33. Dahl JB, Jeppesen IS, Jørgensen H, Wetterslev J, Møiniche S. Intraoperative and postoperative analgesic efficacy and adverse effects of intrathecal opioids in patients undergoing cesarean section with spinal anesthesia: a qualitative and quantitative systematic review of randomized controlled trials. Anesthesiology. 1999;91:1919–27.
34. Reich A, Szepietowski JC. Opioid-induced pruritus: an update. Clin Exp Dermatol. 2010;35:2–6.
35. Hunt CO, Naulty JS, Bader AM, Hauch MA, Vartikar JV, Datta S, Hertwig LM, Ostheimer GW. Perioperative analgesia with subarachnoid fentanyl–bupivacaine for cesarean delivery. Anesthesiology. 1989;71:535–40.
36. Dahlgren G, Hultstrand C, Jakobsson J, Norman M, Eriksson EW, Martin H. Intrathecal Sufentanil, fentanyl, or placebo added to bupivacaine for cesarean section. Anesth Analg. 1997;85:1288–93.
37. Reuben SS, Dunn SM, Duprat KM, O'Sullivan P. An Intrathecal fentanyl dose-response study in lower extremity revascularization procedures. Anesthesiology. 1994;81:1371–5.
38. Zhang Y-W, Zhang J, Hu J-Q, Wen C-L, Dai S-Y, Yang D-F, Li L-F, Wu Q-B. Neuraxial adjuvants for prevention of perioperative shivering during cesarean section: a network meta-analysis following the PRISMA guidelines. World J Clin cases. 2019;7:2287–301.
39. Leysen JE, Gommeren W, Niemegeers CJE. [3H] sufentanil, a superior ligand for μ-opiate receptors: binding properties and regional distribution in rat brain and spinal cord. Eur J Pharmacol. 1983;87:209–25.
40. Grass JA, Sakima NT, Schmidt R, Michitsch R, Zuckerman RL, Harris AP. A randomized, double-blind, dose-response comparison of epidural fentanyl versus Sufentanil analgesia after cesarean section. Anesth Analg. 1997;85: 365–71.
41. Olofsson C, Nygards E-B, Bjersten A-B, Hessling A. Low-dose bupivacaine with sufentanil prevents hypotension after spinal anesthesia for hip repair in elderly patients. Acta Anaesthesiol Scand. 2004;48:1240–4.
42. Feng LS, Hong G, Yan Z, Qiu LY, Liang LA. Intrathecal Sufentanil does not reduce shivering during Neuraxial anesthesia: a Meta-analysis. Med Sci Monit. 2016;22:258–66.
43. Johnson MD, Sevarino FB, Lema MJ. Cessation of shivering and hypothermia associated with epidural Sufentanil. Anesth Analg. 1989;68:70–1.
44. Ngan Kee WD. Intrathecal pethidine: Pharmacology and clinical applications. Anaesth Intensive Care. 1998;26(2):137–46.

45. Cheun JK, Kim AR. Intrathecal meperidine as the sole agent for cesarean section. J Korean Med Sci. 1989;4:135–9.
46. Kafle SK. Intrathecal meperidine for elective caesarean section: a comparison with lidocaine. Can J Anaesth. 1993;40:718–21.
47. Nguyen Thi TV, Orliaguet G, Ngû TH, Bonnet F, Ngu TH, Bonnet F. Spinal anesthesia with meperidine as the sole agent for cesarean delivery. Reg Anesth. 1994;19:386–9.
48. Abouleish E, Rawal N, Fallon K, Hernandez D, Fallen K, Hernandez D. Combined Intrathecal morphine and bupivacaine for cesarean section. Anesth Analg. 1988;67:370–4.
49. Swart M, Sewell J, Thomas D. Intrathecal morphine for caesarean section: an assessment of pain relief, satisfaction and side-effects. Anaesthesia. 1997;52: 373–7.
50. Palmer CM, Emerson S, Volgoropolous D, Alves D. Dose-response relationship of Intrathecal morphine for Postcesarean analgesia. Anesthesiology. 1999;90:437–44.
51. Kato R, Shimamoto H, Terui K, Yokota K, Miyao H. Delayed respiratory depression associated with 0.15 mg intrathecal morphine for cesarean section: a review of 1915 cases. J Anesth. 2008;22:112–6.
52. Casey WF, Smith CE, Katz JM, O'Loughlin K, Weeks SK. Intravenous meperidine for control of shivering during caesarean section under epidural anaesthesia. Can J Anaesth. 1988;35:128–33.
53. Ikeda T, Sessler DI, Tayefeh F, Negishi C, Turakhia M, Marder D, Bjorksten AR, Larson MD. Meperidine and Alfentanil do not reduce the gain or maximum intensity of shivering. Anesthesiology. 1998;88:858–65.
54. Kurz M, Belani KG, Sessler DI, Kurz A, Larson MD, Schroeder M, Blanchard D. Naloxone, Meperidine, and shivering. Anesthesiology. 1993;79:1193–201.
55. Kang YG, Abouleish E, Caritis S. Prophylactic intravenous ephedrine infusion during spinal anesthesia for cesarean section. Anesth Analg. 1982;61:839–42.
56. Larsen J-J, Hyttel J. 5-HT-uptake inhibition potentiates Antinociception induced by morphine, Pethidine, methadone and Ketobemidone in rats. Acta Pharmacol Toxicol (Copenh). 1985;57:214–8.
57. Takada K, Clark DJ, Davies MF, Tonner PH, Krause TKW, Bertaccini E, Maze M. Meperidine exerts agonist activity at the α 2B-adrenoceptor subtype. Anesthesiology. 2002;96:1420–6.
58. Ebert B, Andersen S, Krogsgaard-Larsen P. Ketobemidone, methadone and pethidine are non-competitive N-methyl-d-aspartate (NMDA) antagonists in the rat cortex and spinal cord. Neurosci Lett. 1995;187:165–8.
59. Kurz A, Ikeda T, Sessler DI, LARSON MD, Bjorksten AR, DECHERT M, Christensen R. Meperidine decreases the shivering threshold twice as much as the vasoconstriction threshold. Anesthesiology. 1997;86:1046–54.

19

Minimally invasive spinal anesthesia for cesarean section in maternal anticoagulation therapy

Dan Huang[†], Linjie Zhu[†], Jie Chen[*] and Jie Zhou[*]

Abstract

Background: Anticoagulant therapy during pregnancy is widely used due to the increasing awareness of maternal hypercoagulability. Few studies have reported the use of minimally invasive spinal anesthesia in these parturients. The objective of this study was to evaluate the safety and feasibility of minimally invasive spinal anesthesia in parturients with anticoagulation therapy undergoing cesarean section.

Methods: This was a randomized, controlled study conducted in 239 parturients using anticoagulants and undergoing selective cesarean section. 37 parturients withdrew, and finally parturients received spinal anesthesia using 27gauge pen type fine spinal needles (experimental group, $n = 110$) and 22gauge traditional spinal needles (control group, $n = 92$). The primary efficacy outcomes included low back pain (LBP) and postdural puncture headache (PDPH) after delivery. Secondary efficacy outcomes included visual analogue scale during subarachnoid puncture (VASdural), difference between visual analogue scale (VAS) during peripheral venipuncture and VASdural (ΔVAS), VAS of back puncture point 24, 48 and 72 h after operation (VASdural-24 h, VASdural-48 h and VASdural-72 h, respectively), maternal satisfaction and hospitalization stay.

Results: No parturient had PDPH and was suspected with spinal or intracranial haematoma in two groups. There was no significant difference in VASlbp-24 h, VASlbp-48 h and VASlbp-72 h ($P = 0.056$; $P = 0.813$; $P = 0.189$, respectively) between two groups. In experimental group, VASdural ($P = 0.017$), ΔVAS ($P = 0.001$) and VASdural-24 h ($P < 0.0001$) were lower, whereas maternal satisfaction was higher ($P = 0.046$). There was no significant difference in VASdural-48 h, VASdural-72 h, urination function, strength recovery and hospitalization stay ($P = 0.069$; $P = 0.667$; $P = 0.105$; $P = 0.133$; $P = 0.754$, respectively) between the two groups.

Conclusions: Minimally invasive spinal anesthesia provided lower VASdural, VASdrual-24 h and a higher maternal satisfaction. Hence, it is considered as a safe, reliable and reasonable option for cesarean section parturients during maternal anticoagulation therapy with normal platelet count and coagulation time.

Keywords: Minimally invasive, Low back pain, Postdural puncture headache, Spinal anesthesia, Cesarean section, Anticoagulants

* Correspondence: 13611906592@163.com; 13601693227@163.com
[†]Dan Huang and Linjie Zhu contributed equally to this work.
Department of Anesthesiology, Renji Hospital, School of Medicine, Shanghai Jiaotong University, Shanghai 200127, China

Background

According to the World Health Organization (WHO) Global Survey on Maternal and Perinatal Health in 2010, Chinese health facilities has the highest cesarean section rate (CSR) (46.2%) in Asia (27.3%) [1], and the CSR had risen far in excess of the optimal 15% recommended by WHO [1, 2]. According to a recent study, the overall annual rate of cesarean deliveries between 2008 and 2014 was increased in China, i.e., up to 34.9% [3]. With the implementation of second child policy, the ratio still remained high. Intravertebral anesthesia is the most commonly used method for parturients undergoing cesarean section. Traditional intravertebral anesthesia may cause postdural puncture headache (PDPH) and low back pain.

PDPH may require epidural blood patching, resulting in prolonged hospital stay and emergency visits after discharge [4, 5]. Previous study has shown that the incidence of PDPH was about 7 to 30% [6]. Decrease of intracranial pressure due to cerebrospinal fluid (CSF) leakage from the subarachnoid space is currently the leading cause of PDPH [5]. The PDPH, which causes significant morbidity in obstetric patients, has higher incidence because of the increased CSF pressure related to pregnancy, dehydration, blood loss, postpartum diuresis, hormonal imbalance, high serum estrogen levels, and increased peridural pressure [7].

Low back pain (LBP) commonly occurs during late pregnancy and also after delivery. Several research studies revealed that at least half of the pregnant women is affected by LBP [8, 9]. Persistence of LBP for 6 months after delivery has been reported in 5 to 40% of patients [10]. A retrospective study of 40,057 women demonstrated that cesarean delivery and epidural anesthesia might increase the risk of subsequent chronic LBP [11]. The paraspinal muscular relaxtion with stretching of spinal ligaments and/or localized tissue trauma are accepted as the pathophysiological factors of LBP after puncture.

The concept of minimally invasive spinal anesthesia has been put forwarded due to its appearance of pen type lumbar puncture needle and unceasing enhancement of piercing technology. It refers to puncturing with 27gauge pen type fine needle to reduce the damage of supraspinous, interspinous and yellow ligament by puncture needle.

However, there are relative contraindications to spinal anesthesia, one of which is the use of anticoagulants. Anticoagulant therapy during pregnancy is widely used due to the increasing awareness of maternal hypercoagulability [12]. The pregnant women are forced to accept general anesthesia in order to avoid epidural hematoma and lose the experience of baby birth moment. Minimally invasive spinal anesthesia happens to solve this problem, reducing the side effects without increasing the risk of spinal anesthesia for maternal anticoagulation therapy.

We therefore performed a randomized, controlled trial in parturients undergoing anticoagulation therapy to evaluate the safety and feasibility of minimally invasive spinal anesthesia. We also investigated the use of 27gauge pen type fine spinal needles and 22 gauge traditional spinal needles for spinal anesthesia on PDPH and LBP in parturients with anticoagulation therapy undergoing cesarean section.

Methods

Research design

This was a prospective randomized controlled study conducted in accordance with the ethics and data protection of Chinese regulations. The protocol was approved by the ethics committee of Renji hospital, School of Medicine, Shanghai Jiaotong University. Written informed consent was obtained from all the parturients before randomization in this prospective, parallel-arm, randomized clinical trial. This trial was a single-site study conducted at the Shanghai Renji hospital. This study was registered at www.ClinicalTrials.gov (NCT02987192).

Participants

Consecutive parturients aged ≥18 years with singleton pregnancy puerpera who were using anticoagulation medications and undergoing selective cesarean section were eligible for inclusion between November 2016 and December 2017. Only parturients with the American Society of Anesthesiologists physical status between I and II were included. Exclusion criteria were as follows: parturients with a history of migraine headache, previous history of PDPH, platelet count lower than 70*10^9, International Normalized Ratio (INR) > 1.5, severe cardiopulmonary insufficiency, infection of skin or subcutaneous tissue at the puncture site, lumbar or spinal cord disease, increased intracranial pressure, weight > 100 kg or < 50 kg and height > 165 cm or < 155 cm.

Randomization

Parturients were randomized in 1:1 ratio to the two study groups by means of a central telephone system to ensure concealed allocation. Randomization was performed using a computer-generated randomization sequence with randomly permuted blocks of 4 or 6. Patient caregivers and investigators collecting the data remained unaware of study-group assignments.

Interventions

Electrocardiogram, blood pressure, pulse oxygen saturation, and heart rate were measured after the parturients entered the operation room. A 20gauge indwelling needle was placed into the peripheral vein. Thromboelastogram, platelet count and coagulation time were detected. All parturients were hydrated with 8 mL/kg body weight Ringer's lactated solution before spinal anesthesia. Spinal anesthesia was performed with a standardized technique. All parturients received spinal anesthesia by an experienced anesthetist. The parturients in the experimental group received spinal anesthesia using 27gauge pen type fine needles (HaiSheng, China), and control group parturients received spinal anesthesia using 22gauge traditional needles (HaiSheng, China). Lumbar puncture was performed in the intervertebral space of L2–3 by placing the parturients in the right lateral decubitus position. The parturients were instructed to remain flexed and not to move their heads during the insertion of the needle. Spinal needle was inserted through the longitudinal dural fiber using a midline approach at L2–3. After verifying the free flow of CSF through the needle tip, 0.75% ropivacaine 2 mL was injected within 5 s.

Two consecutive episodes of hypotension (defined as systolic blood pressure less than 80% of baseline) were treated with a “rescue” intravenous bolus of 100μg phenylephrine and volume expansion. When the skin closure begined, intravenous Patient-Controlled Analgesia (PCA) pump was commenced to infuse 100 mL mixture of sufentanil (0.045μg/kg/h), flurbiprofen (45μg/kg/h), and saline at a rate of 2 mL/h using an analgesia pump (Apon, China). PCA administration was continued until 48 h postoperatively in the two groups.

Outcome measures

The primary efficacy outcomes calculated were LBP and PDPH after puncture. LBP after puncture was defined as the continuous pain and tenderness over the lumbar area around the spinal needle insertion and was recorded using visual analogue scale (VASlbp) on the postoperative days [13]. Pain was defined on a scale of 0 as the absence of pain, and 7–10 as severe pain (disabling; unable to perform daily activities). PDPH was defined according to the International Headache Society Classifications, bifrontal or occipital region headache that remained worse in the upright position and relieved with supine posture and headache within 5 days after dural puncture [14]. Other types of headaches were considered nonspecific and were excluded from the study. The intensity of PDPH was also recorded using visual analogue scale (VASPDPH) on postoperative day 1. Secondary efficacy outcomes included were visual analogue scale during subarachnoid puncture (VASdural), difference between VAS during peripheral venipuncture (VASperipheral) and VASdural (ΔVAS), VAS of back puncture point 24, 48 and 72 h after operation (VAS24h, VAS48h and VAS72h), maternal satisfaction and hospitalization days. The safety outcome was the incidence of hypotension after anesthesia in the operation room. The dosage and withdrawal time of anticoagulants were also recorded.

Sample size calculation

Sample size calculation was based on the data from previous studies. The incidence of PDPH in 22gauge needle was reported as 34% [6] and LBP after caesarean delivery with spinal anesthesia was 31.8% [11], respectively. By assuming a fall by half of the incidences, we calculated that a sample size of 82 parturients per group would be required to achieve a power of 90% with a two-sized α risk of 0.05, which was calculated using PASS software, version 15.0(NSCC, USA).

Statistical analysis

Categorical data were described as frequencies and proportions and were analyzed using Chi-square test. Kolmogorov-Smirnov test was used to examine the normality of distribution of continuous outcomes. Normally distributed continuous variables were described as mean ± standard deviation (SD) and were analyzed using Student’s t test, whereas non-normally distributed continuous variables were presented as median ± interquartile range (IQR) and were performed with the Mann-Whitney U test. Significance was set at 0.05 level. Statistical analyses were performed using GraphPad Prism software, version 6.01(GraphPad Software, Inc. USA).

Results

Demographic, physiologic and surgical characteristics

A total of 239 parturients were randomly assigned to the experimental group ($n = 120$) or control group ($n = 119$). 37 participants withdrew during our study period; 84.5% of 239 parturients were analyzed in our study (Fig. 1). There were 10 withdraws in the experiment group: 1 subject was transferred to the intensive care unit (ICU) immediately post-operatively because of overmuch blood loss during operation, and other 9 subjects met exclusion criteria. 18 subjects in the control group met exclusion criteria and other 9 subjects decided not to participate in the study further after operation without specific reason. Thus, the final numbers of participants were 110 in experiment group and 92 in control group. Both patient characteristics and surgical characteristics were similar in the two groups. Birthweight was also similar between the groups and Apgar score of each neonate at 1 min and 5 min was 10 (Table 1).

Use of anticoagulants and coagulation function

Maternal anticoagulation therapy was shown in Table 2 and Table 3. Daily dosage of low molecular weight heparin (LMWH) was 4100 U. There was no significant difference in the dose and time of anticoagulant between the two groups. Aspirin was the most common anticoagulant medication and alone or duplex anticoagulation medications favored more. There was no significant difference in thromboelastogram, platelet count and coagulation time

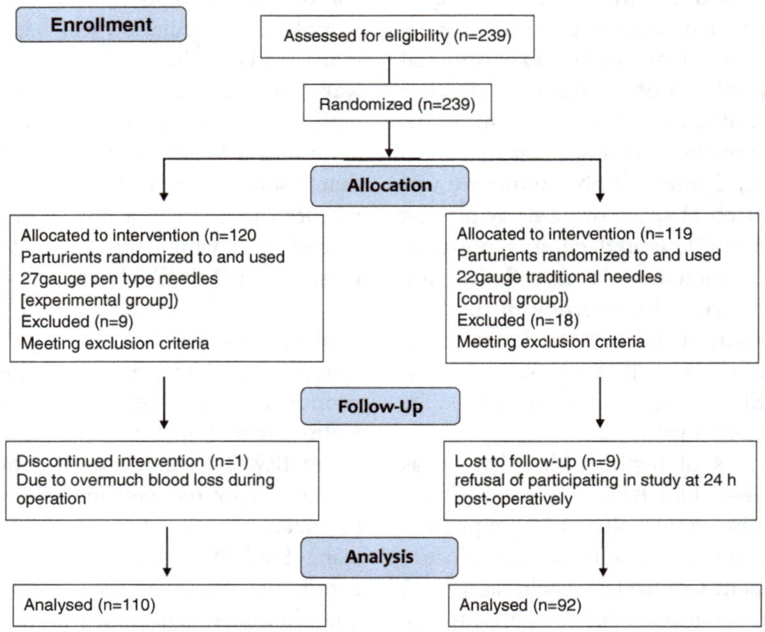

Fig. 1 Flow diagram of a trial comparing low back pain, postdural puncture headache, pain of puncture point, maternal satisfaction and hospitalization days between 22 and 27guage needles

between the two groups. D-Dimer and α angle in the two groups were higher than normal (Table 4). None of the parturients was suspected of spinal or intracranial hematoma.

Primary and secondary efficacy outcomes

In the primary efficacy outcomes, no parturient suffered from PDPH and no significant difference in VASlbp-24 h, VASlbp-48 h and VASlbp-72 h between the two groups was observed ($P = 0.056$; $P = 0.813$; $P = 0.189$, respectively). In the secondary efficacy outcomes, VASdural, ΔVAS and VAS24h in the experimental group were lower than control group (VASdural median 3.0 vs 4.0, $P = 0.017$; ΔVAS median 0.0 vs 1.0, $P = 0.001$; VASdural-24 h median 0.0 vs 1.0, $P < 0.0001$). Maternal satisfaction in experimental group was higher than control group (98.2% vs 91.3%, $P = 0.046$). No significant difference in VASdural-48 h, VASdural-72 h and hospitalization stay was observed between the two groups ($P = 0.069$; $P = 0.667$; $P = 0.754$, respectively).

No differences in the feelings during puncture, puncture time, puncture point bleeding, inserting depth of puncture needle and the time of analgesia block level that reached T6 were observed between the two groups ($P = 0.062$; $P = 0.644$; $P = 0.740$; $P = 0.073$, respectively). Parturients in the two groups had similar incidence of hypotension and received similar volume of vasopressor ($P = 0.123$; $P = 0.073$, respectively). There was no significant

Table 1 Baseline Parturients and Surgical Characteristics

Characteristics	Experimental group ($n = 110$)	Control group ($n = 92$)	*P* value
Age, median (IQR), y	32.0(29.0–35.0)	32.0(28.0–35.0)	.474
Height, median (IQR), cm	160.0(158.0–163.0)	161.0(158.0–165.0)	.527
Body mass index, mean(SD)	26.6(3.7)	26.5(3.3)	.869
Gestational weeks, median (IQR)	38.0(37.0–38.0)	38.0(37.0–38.0)	.643
ASA status I, *n* (%)	50(45.0)	38(41.3)	.572
History of spinal anesthesia, *n* (%)	16(14.5)	12(13.0)	.839
Operation time, median (IQR), min	41.0(33.0–50.0)	41.5(35.0–48.0)	.620
Induction-to-delivery time, median (IQR), min	6.0(5.0–10.0)	7.0(6.0–9.0)	.346
Newborn weight, median (IQR), g	3130.0(2830.0–3375.0)	3150.0(2910.0–3410.0)	.538
Hospital stay, median (IQR), d	3.0(3.0–4.0)	3.0(3.0–3.0)	.754

SD Standard Deviation, *IQR* Interquartile Range, *ASA* American Society of Anesthesiologists

Table 2 Dosage and Withdrawal Time of Anticoagulant

Variables	Experimental group ($n = 110$)	Control group ($n = 92$)	P value
Daily dosage of aspirin, median (IQR), mg	25.0(25.0–50.0)	25.0(25.0–50.0)	.135
Withdrawal time of aspirin, median (IQR), d	4.0(0.3–5)	3.0(1.0–5.0)	.405
Number of aspirin users, n (%)	104(94.5)	88(95.7)	.758
Withdrawal time of LMWH, median (IQR), h	11.0(8.8–13.0)	12.5(11.0–15.0)	.096
Number of LMWH users, n (%)	66(60.0)	44(47.8)	.091
Daily dosage of Salvia miltiorrhiza, median (IQR), g	0.3(0.3–0.6)	0.3(0.3–0.6)	.057
Withdrawal time of Salvia miltiorrhiza, median (IQR), d	1.0(0.0–1.0)	0.0(0.0–2.0)	.686
Number of Salvia miltiorrhiza users, n (%)	14(12.7)	14(15.2)	.684

IQR Interquartile Range, *LMWH* Low Molecular Weight Heparin

difference in urination function, strength recovery and remedy for analgesia after operation between the two groups ($P = 0.105$; $P = 0.133$; $P = 0.344$, respectively) (Table 5).

Discussion

Our research indicated that minimally invasive spinal anesthesia was a reliable and reasonable option for cesarean section in maternal anticoagulation therapy with normal platelet count and coagulation time. Previous literature concluded that the anticoagulant treatment continues to be contraindicated to spinal/epidural anesthesia [15]. Spinal-epidural hematoma during spinal anesthesia was described in 1/200000–250,000. Spinal or intracranial hematoma is a rare but a severe complication [16]. Traumatic puncture was assumed to be the risk factor for the development of this kind of hematoma. Anticoagulant treatments increase the risk of spinal hematoma to 1/40000 in patients undergoing anticoagulation treatment [17]. To prevent spinal hematoma, neuraxial anesthesia is prohibited when the anticoagulant treatment is used as curative dose during delivery. These conclusions refer to the relatively coarse technology and traditional lumbar puncture needle. In our study, there was no significant difference in the puncture point bleeding between the two groups. Defecation function, lower limb strength and sensation of all parturients in our study were normal. We inferred that no parturient was suspected of spinal or intracranial hematoma. Minimally invasive spinal anesthesia in our research was considered as safe and effective approach for maternal anticoagulation

Table 3 Use of Anticoagulants

Types of drugs	Alone medication	Duplex medication	Triple medication	Total, n	%
Aspirin	82	92	18	192	58.2
LMWH	8	84	18	110	33.3
Salvia Miltiorrhiza	2	8	18	28	8.5
Total, n	92	92	18		
%	45.5	45.5	8.9		

LMWH Low Molecular Weight Heparin

due to smaller caliber of puncture needle and lesser damage of intraspinal blood vessel.

No parturient had suffered from PDPH and no significant difference in PDPH using 22 or 27gauge needles was revealed in our observation. Smaller gauge needles were recommended for spinal anesthesia to reduce the incidence of PDPH. Kim et al. reported no significant difference in the cause of PDPH by using 23 and 25 gauge needles in spinal anesthesia [18], which was consistent with our study findings. However, our result differed from the conclusion by Lambert et al. that compared with 26gauge Quincke needle, the incidence of PDPH using a 27gauge Quincke needle was significantly reduced [19]. Previous studies have shown that older people have a lower incidence of PDPH than younger people, which may be related to a decrease in pain perception or pain response in the elderly [20, 21]. Age is likely to be an important factor in the pathogenesis of PDPH. However, it was different with our result as our study subjects only included young women subjects. A successful initial lumbar puncture and avoiding local muscle-ligamentous trauma caused by repeated punctures due to the clinician's technique can be considered the cause of difference.

Our data demonstrated that there was no significant difference in LBP using either 22 or 27gauge needles. Whereas, we found that the procedure of minimally invasive spinal anesthesia provided a lower VAS during subarachnoid puncture, a lower VAS of back puncture point at 24 h after operation and a higher maternal satisfaction. However, the conclusions drawn by previous studies showed discrepancies. Lowery et al. reported that 11% of the oncologic patients were aged between 2 and 17 years, and had LBP after lumbar puncture following the use of a 22gauge cutting Quincke needle [6]. In contrast, Kim M and Yee K, respectively reported no significant difference in pain score in 1–3 days after puncturing with different needles [18, 22]. Our positive result on the advantage of the use of 27gauge puncture needles may be due to the reduction of local muscle-ligamentous trauma associated with needle insertion. It was noteworthy that although effective analgesia, muscular relaxation, immobility,

Table 4 Thromboelastogram, Platelet count and Coagulation Time

Variables	Experimental group (*n* = 110)	Control group (*n* = 92)	*P* value
D-Dimer, median (IQR)	0.7(0.4–0.9)[a]	0.6(0.4–1.0)[a]	.607
FDP, median (IQR)	5.6(3.5–11.0)	6.9(3.8–9.3)	.627
TT, median (IQR)	16.4(12.9–17.4)	14.5(12.5–16.9)	.055
APTT, median (IQR)	26.7(24.8–28.1)	27.6(25.1–29.0)	.097
PT, median (IQR)	10.7(9.4–11.4)	10.1(9.4–11.5)	.512
Fg, median (IQR)	4.3(3.9–4.9)	4.4(3.9–4.9)	.449
INR, median (IQR)	1.0(0.9–1.0)	0.9(0.9–1.0)	.484
PLT^9, median (IQR)	198.0(150.0–259.0)	194.5(175.0–211.0)	.413
Rtime, median (IQR)	6.6(5.9–7.3)	6.9(6.5–7.4)	.090
Ktime, median (IQR)	1.6(1.4–1.8)	1.6(1.5–1.8)	.053
α angle, median (IQR)	73.5(70.7–75.0)[a]	72.6(71.0–73.6)[a]	.054
MA, median (IQR)	69.4(69.1–70.0)	69.6(69.1–70.0)	.088

[a]D-Dimer and α angle in two groups were higher than normal
IQR Interquartile Range, *FDP* Fibrinogen Degradation Product, *TT* Thrombin Time, *APTT* Activated Partial Thromboplastin Time, *PT* Prothrombin Time, *Fg* Fibrinogen, *INR* International Normalized Ratio, *PLT* Platelets, *MA* Maximum Amplitude

Table 5 Primary and Secondary Endpoints

Variables	Experimental group (*n* = 110)	Control group (*n* = 92)	*P*
VASlbp-24 h, median (IQR)	3.0(2.0–4.0)	3.0(3.0–4.0)	.056
VASlbp-48 h, median (IQR)	2.0(1.0–3.0)	2.0(1.0–3.0)	.813
VASlbp-72 h, median (IQR)	1.0(0.0–1.0)	1.0(0.0–1.0)	.189
VASperipheral, median (IQR)	3.0(2.0–5.0)	3.0(3.0–4.0)	.769
VASdural, median (IQR)	3.0(1.0–6.0)	4.0(3.0–6.0)	.017
ΔVAS, median (IQR)	0.0(−1.0–1.0)	1.0(0.0–2.0)	.001
VASdural-24 h, median (IQR)	0.0(0.0–1.0)	1.0(1.0–1.0)	<.0001
VASdural-48 h, median (IQR)	0.0(0.0–0.0)	0.0(0.0–1.0)	.069
VASdural-72 h, median (IQR)	0.0(0.0–0.0)	0.0(0.0–0.0)	.667
maternal satisfaction (satisfaction, %)	108(98.2)	84(91.3)	.046
Puncture time, median (IQR), s	40.0(22.0–60.0)	60.0(30.0–68.0)	.062
Puncture point bleeding (bleeding, %)	10(9.1)	11(12.0)	.644
Inserting depth of puncture needle, median (IQR), cm	5.6(5.5–6.0)	6.0(5.3–6.0)	.740
Time of analgesia block level reached T6, median (IQR), min	6.0(6.0–8.0)	8.0(6.0–8.0)	.073
Incidence of hypotension, *n* (%)	60(54.5)	40(43.4)	.123
Rescue phenylephrine required, median (IQR), μg	100.0(100.0–200.0)	100.0(100.0–175.0)	.073
Rescue intraoperative intravenous anesthesia required, *n* (%)	8(7.3)	10(10.9)	.459
Nausea or vomiting, *n* (%)	12(10.9)	8(8.7)	.644
Postoperative self-urination time, median (IQR), h	18.0(15.0–20.0)	19.0(11.0–21.0)	.105
Recovery of lower limb muscle strength, median (IQR), h	4.0(3.0–5.0)	4.0(4.0–6.0)	.133
First remedy for analgesia, median (IQR), h	5.0(2.0–7.0)	4.0(2.8–7.0)	.344

VASlbp-24 h Visual Analogue Scale of Low Back Pain 24 h after Operation, *VASlbp-48 h* Visual Analogue Scale of Low Back Pain 48 h after Operation, *VASlbp-72 h* Visual Analogue Scale of Low Back Pain 72 h after Operation, *VASperipheral* VAS during Peripheral Venipuncture, *VASdural* Visual Analogue Scale during Subarachnoid Puncture, *ΔVAS* Difference between VASperipheral and VASdural, *VASdural-24 h* VAS of Back Puncture Point 24 h after Operation, *VASdural-48 h* VAS of Back Puncture Point 48 h after Operation, *VASdural-72 h* VAS of Back Puncture Point 72 h after Operation, *IQR* Interquartile Range

and stressed posture resulted in the postural pain primarily, enormous physical and physiological changes during pregnancy and after delivery such as lumbar lordosis, center of gravity rise and fall, and loss of abdominal muscle support that resulted in intense stretch on the lower back should be also considered [11]. Wang CH [23] concluded that postpartum LBP could be related to changes during pregnancy and not related to spinal anesthesia, and this might be the reason for the negative result from our study in LBP using either 22 or 27gauge needles. A cross-sectional study, which is the largest study on pregnancy-related LBP in the literature, also showed that about 1 in 2 women have pregnancy-related LBP in any stage of pregnancy [9].

The risk of venous thromboembolism (VTE) in pregnancy was 5.7/10000 [24]. Guidelines for anticoagulant indications and management have been published by different national and international agencies to prevent venous thromboembolism during pregnancy [25–27]. Although anticoagulation therapy was given, maternal thrombophilias were still increased among these parturients in our research, some of whom had high D-Dimer, normal platelet count and coagulation time. A therapeutic anticoagulation window of 12 h was recommended during delivery when using LMWH as prophylactic [28]. The mean delay between the last injection and the need for anesthesia in our data was more than 12 h. Aspirin was not recommended for drug withdrawal according to the guidelines. Nevertheless, puerperas in our medical center usually underwent a delay of about 6 days before delivery. The use of anticoagulant therapy during pregnancy should be cautious because of the potential for both fetal and maternal complications.

Furthermore, our study showed that aspirin was the most common anticoagulant medication used by pregnant population in our medical center. Aspirin is a preferred anticoagulant and is widely accepted by doctors and parturients in our medical center, occupying the largest proportion of usage. It is suggested that oral low-dose aspirin treatment can prevent the occurrence of preeclampsia, but there are complication of placental infarction [29]. Currently, based on epidemiological evidence, it is recommended to take low-dose aspirin daily as a preventive intervention for high-risk preeclampsia during pregnancy after 12 weeks of gestation [30]. The preference of aspirin usage in our medical center may be due to the prevention of fetal growth restriction and a reversible increase in uterine blood flow [31], whereas evidence on the use of LMWH from randomized control trials in both in vitro and in vivo studies remained inconsistent [32–36]. The use of heparin, including LMWH, was established for the prevention/improvement of thrombophlebitis in the pathological hypercoagulability during pregnancy [37]. Meanwhile, the dosage regimen of coagulant used in our medical center mainly focused on alone and duplex medications rather than triple combination. In women with antiphospholipid (aPL) syndrome with recurrent miscarriages, to improve blood circulation, guidelines recommend an anticoagulant therapy of oral low-dose aspirin combined with intravenous LMWH [37, 38]. Further prospective randomized controlled trials are required to determine the optimal maternal hypercoagulant treatment strategy. Although the beneficial effects of Salvia Miltiorrhiza on anticoagulation, vasodilation, reduction of oxidative stress, and lipid profiles have been put forwarded, studies on Salvia Miltiorrhiza in obstetrics were limited [39]. Morton JS et al. investigated the use of Salvia Miltiorrhiza did not affect placenta- related factors and blood pressure of pregnant women with pregnancy-induced hypertension [40]. Hence, further study on larger sample size is required.

Limitation of the study

Insufficient sample size was the main limitation of our research. Our study did not include twins and obese parturients due to their distinctive body sizes. Because of the difficulty in studying the aim of the study in a prospective way and ethical limits, no magnetic resonance imaging (MRI) was performed on any parturient to check spinal or intracranial hematoma. In addition, since PDPH and LBP were developed till 5 to 7 days after dural puncture, the restricted observation period due to short hospital stay and lack of long-term follow-up information remained as limitations. Besides, our study was a single center study and requires recruitment of more parturients, and monitors for longer follow-up period to obtain confirmatory conclusion and explore the cause and mechanism in future study.

Conclusion

In conclusion, the present study demonstrates that minimally invasive spinal anesthesia provided a lower VAS during subarachnoid puncture, a lower VAS of back puncture point 24 h after operation and a higher maternal satisfaction. Hence, it was considered to be a safe, reliable and reasonable approach for parturients undergoing cesarean section in maternal anticoagulation therapy with normal platelet count and coagulation time. As the date of delivery is difficult to predict, minimally invasive spinal anesthesia could be a potential solution for parturients taking anticoagulants to go through cesarean section successfully by avoiding general anesthesia and get the experience of joy of baby birth moment.

Abbreviations

aPL: Antiphospholipid; CSF: Cerebrospinal fluid; CSR: Cesarean section rate; ICU: Intensive care unit; INR: International normalized ratio; IQR: Interquartile range; LBP: Low back pain; LMWH: Low molecular weight heparin; MRI: Magnetic resonance imaging; PDPH: Postdural puncture headache;

SD: Standard deviation; VASdural: Visual analogue scale during subarachnoid puncture; VASdural-24 h: Visual analogue scale of back puncture point 24 h after operation; VASdural-48 h: Visual analogue scale of back puncture point 48 h after operation; VASdural-72 h: Visual analogue scale of back puncture point 72 h after operation; VASlbp: Visual analogue scale of low back pain; VASPDPH: Visual analogue scale of postdural puncture headache; VASperipheral: Visual analogue scale of during peripheral venipuncture; VASlbp-24 h: Visual analogue scale of low back pain 24 h after operation; VASlbp-48 h: Visual analogue scale of low back pain 48 h after operation; VASlbp-72 h: Visual analogue scale of low back pain 72 h after operation; VTE Venous: Thromboembolism; WHO: World health organization; ΔVAS: Difference between visual analogue scale during peripheral venipuncture and visual analogue scale during subarachnoid puncture

Acknowledgements
All authors thank all the nursing staff, and patients who participated in this study.

Authors' contributions
All authors (DH, LJZ, JC, and JZ) made substantial contributions to the study conception and design, were involved in revising this manuscript critically, approved the final manuscript and agreed to be accountable for all aspects of the work. LJZ collected and analyzed the patient data and DH was a major contributor in writing the manuscript. JC and JZ took part in the coordination of this project. DH applied for funding. DH and LJZ contributed equally to this work.

References

1. Lumbiganon P, Laopaiboon M, Gulmezoglu AM, Souza JP, Taneepanichskul S, Ruyan P, Attygalle DE, Shrestha N, Mori R, Nguyen DH, et al. Method of delivery and pregnancy outcomes in Asia: the WHO global survey on maternal and perinatal health 2007-08. Lancet. 2010;375(9713):490–9.
2. Appropriate technology for birth. Lancet. 1985;2(8452):436–7. https://doi.org/10.1016/S0140-6736(85)92750-3.
3. Li HT, Luo S, Trasande L, Hellerstein S, Kang C, Li JX, Zhang Y, Liu JM, Blustein J. Geographic variations and temporal trends in cesarean delivery rates in China, 2008-2014. JAMA. 2017;317(1):69–76.
4. Angle P, Tang SL, Thompson D, Szalai JP. Expectant management of postdural puncture headache increases hospital length of stay and emergency room visits. Can J Anaesth. 2005;52(4):397–402.
5. Kuczkowski KM. Post-dural puncture headache in the obstetric patient: an old problem. New solutions. Minerva Anestesiol. 2004;70(12):823–30.
6. Lowery S, Oliver A. Incidence of postdural puncture headache and backache following diagnostic/therapeutic lumbar puncture using a 22G cutting spinal needle, and after introduction of a 25G pencil point spinal needle. Paediatr Anaesth. 2008;18(3):230–4.
7. Choi PT, Galinski SE, Takeuchi L, Lucas S, Tamayo C, Jadad AR. PDPH is a common complication of neuraxial blockade in parturients: a meta-analysis of obstetrical studies. Can J Anaesth. 2003;50(5):460–9.
8. Mogren IM, Pohjanen AI. Low back pain and pelvic pain during pregnancy: prevalence and risk factors. Spine (Phila Pa 1976). 2005;30(8):983–91.
9. Sencan S, Ozcan-Eksi EE, Cuce I, Guzel S, Erdem B. Pregnancy-related low back pain in women in Turkey: prevalence and risk factors. Ann Phys Rehabil Med. 2018;61(1):33–7.
10. Turgut F, Turgut M, Cetinsahin M. A prospective study of persistent back pain after pregnancy. Eur J Obstet Gynecol Reprod Biol. 1998;80(1):45–8.
11. Chia YY, Lo Y, Chen YB, Liu CP, Huang WC, Wen CH. Risk of chronic low Back pain among Parturients who undergo cesarean delivery with Neuraxial anesthesia: a Nationwide population-based retrospective cohort study. Medicine (Baltimore). 2016;95(16):e3468.
12. Chow L, Farber MK, Camann WR. Anesthesia in the pregnant patient with hematologic disorders. Hematol Oncol Clin North Am. 2011;25(2):425–43 ix-x.
13. Pan PH, Fragneto R, Moore C, Ross V. Incidence of postdural puncture headache and backache, and success rate of dural puncture: comparison of two spinal needle designs. South Med J. 2004;97(4):359–63.
14. Headache Classification Committee of the International Headache S. The international classification of headache disorders, 3rd edition (beta version). Cephalalgia. 2013;33(9):629–808.
15. Gogarten W, Vandermeulen E, Van Aken H, Kozek S, Llau JV, Samama CM. European Scoeity of a: regional anaesthesia and antithrombotic agents: recommendations of the European society of Anaesthesiology. Eur J Anaesthesiol. 2010;27(12):999–1015.
16. Nathan N, Sol I, Vincelot A, Collet D, Granchamp P, David E. Is a biological assessment necessary to realize an obstetrical epidural anaesthesia in a patient whose interrogation and clinical examination are strictly normal? Ann Fr Anesth Reanim. 2007;26(7–8):705–10.
17. Horlocker TT, Wedel DJ, Rowlingson JC, Enneking FK, Kopp SL, Benzon HT, Brown DL, Heit JA, Mulroy MF, Rosenquist RW, et al. Regional anesthesia in the patient receiving antithrombotic or thrombolytic therapy: American Society of Regional Anesthesia and Pain Medicine evidence-based guidelines (third edition). Reg Anesth Pain Med. 2010;35(1):64–101.
18. Kim M, Yoon H. Comparison of post-dural puncture headache and low back pain between 23 and 25 gauge Quincke spinal needles in patients over 60 years: randomized, double-blind controlled trial. Int J Nurs Stud. 2011;48(11):1315–22.
19. Lambert DH, Hurley RJ, Hertwig L, Datta S. Role of needle gauge and tip configuration in the production of lumbar puncture headache. Reg Anesth. 1997;22(1):66–72.
20. Mylius V, Kunz M, Hennighausen E, Lautenbacher S, Schepelmann K. Effects of ageing on spinal motor and autonomic pain responses. Neurosci Lett. 2008;446(2–3):129–32.
21. Lautenbacher S, Kunz M, Strate P, Nielsen J, Arendt-Nielsen L. Age effects on pain thresholds, temporal summation and spatial summation of heat and pressure pain. Pain. 2005;115(3):410–8.
22. Yee K, Shetty AL, Lai K. ABG needle study: a randomised control study comparing 23G versus 25G needle success and pain scores. Emerg Med J. 2015;32(5):343–7.
23. Wang CH, Cheng KW, Neoh CA, Tang S, Jawan B, Lee JH. Comparison of the incidence of postpartum low back pain in natural childbirth and cesarean section with spinal anesthesia. Acta Anaesthesiol Sin. 1994;32(4):243–6.
24. Parunov LA, Soshitova NP, Ovanesov MV, Panteleev MA, Serebriyskiy II. Epidemiology of venous thromboembolism (VTE) associated with pregnancy. Birth Defects Res C Embryo Today. 2015;105(3):167–84.
25. Benhamou D, Mignon A, Aya G, Brichant JF, Bonnin M, Chauleur C, Deruelle P, Ducloy AS, Edelman P, Rigouzzo A, et al. Prophylaxis of thromboembolic complications in obstetrics and gynaecology. Ann Fr Anesth Reanim. 2005; 24(8):911–20.
26. Bates SM, Greer IA, Middeldorp S, Veenstra DL, Prabulos AM, Vandvik PO. VTE, thrombophilia, antithrombotic therapy, and pregnancy: antithrombotic therapy and prevention of thrombosis, 9th ed: American College of Chest Physicians Evidence-Based Clinical Practice Guidelines. Chest. 2012;141(2 Suppl):e691S–736S.
27. Saar JA, Maack C. European Society of C: [diagnosis and management of acute pulmonary embolism. ESC guidelines 2014]. Herz. 2015;40(8):1048–54.
28. Roueli A, Cesario E, Amsellem J, Agman A, Vauthier-Brouzes D, Nizard J. Is a therapeutic anticoagulation window needed for delivery when using prophylactic low molecular weight heparin during pregnancy? A retrospective monocentric study. Eur J Obstet Gynecol Reprod Biol. 2017; 215:118–23.
29. Suzuki Y, Hattori T, Kajikuri J, Yamamoto T, Suzumori K, Itoh T. Reduced function of endothelial prostacyclin in human omental resistance arteries in pre-eclampsia. J Physiol. 2002;545(Pt 1):269–77.
30. Osikoya O, Jaini PA, Nguyen A, Valdes M, Goulopoulou S. Effects of low-dose aspirin on maternal blood pressure and vascular function in an experimental model of gestational hypertension. Pharmacol Res. 2017;120:267–78.
31. Kang X, Wang T, He L, Xu H, Liu Z, Zhao A. Effect of low-dose aspirin on Midluteal phase uterine artery blood flow in patients with recurrent pregnancy loss. J Ultrasound Med. 2016;35(12):2583–7.
32. Groom KM, David AL. The role of aspirin, heparin, and other interventions in the prevention and treatment of fetal growth restriction. Am J Obstet Gynecol. 2018;218(2S):S829–40.
33. Bose P, Black S, Kadyrov M, Bartz C, Shlebak A, Regan L, Huppertz B. Adverse effects of lupus anticoagulant positive blood sera on placental viability can be prevented by heparin in vitro. Am J Obstet Gynecol. 2004;191(6):2125–31.
34. Di Simone N, Di Nicuolo F, Sanguinetti M, Ferrazzani S, D'Alessio MC, Castellani R, Bompiani A, Caruso A. Low-molecular weight heparin induces in vitro trophoblast invasiveness: role of matrix metalloproteinases and tissue inhibitors. Placenta. 2007;28(4):298–304.
35. Ganapathy R, Whitley GS, Cartwright JE, Dash PR, Thilaganathan B. Effect of heparin and fractionated heparin on trophoblast invasion. Hum Reprod. 2007;22(9):2523–7.
36. Quenby S, Mountfield S, Cartwright JE, Whitley GS, Vince G. Effects of low-molecular-weight and unfractionated heparin on trophoblast function. Obstet Gynecol. 2004;104(2):354–61.

37. Makino A, Suzuki Y, Yamamoto T, Sato T, Kojima K, Suzumori K. Use of aspirin and low-molecular-weight heparin to prevent recurrence of maternal floor infarction in women without evidence of antiphospholipid antibody syndrome. Fetal Diagn Ther. 2004;19(3):261–5.
38. Middeldorp S. Anticoagulation in pregnancy complications. Hematology Am Soc Hematol Educ Program. 2014;2014(1):393–9.
39. Morton JS, Abdalvand A, Jiang Y, Sawamura T, Uwiera RR, Davidge ST. Lectin-like oxidized low-density lipoprotein 1 receptor in a reduced uteroplacental perfusion pressure rat model of preeclampsia. Hypertension. 2012;59(5):1014–20.
40. Morton JS, Quon A, Cheung PY, Sawamura T, Davidge ST. Effect of sodium tanshinone IIA sulfonate treatment in a rat model of preeclampsia. Am J Physiol Regul Integr Comp Physiol. 2015;308(3):R163–72.

20

Objective validation of YouTube™ educational videos for the instruction of regional anesthesia nerve blocks

George L. Tewfik*, Adam N. Work, Steven M. Shulman and Patrick Discepola

Abstract

Background: YouTube™ ("YouTube") is often used as an educational tool to instruct anesthesia providers on regional anesthesia nerve blocks. However, there is no current objective standard to assess the educational quality of these user-uploaded videos. A new approach was used to objectively validate these videos by comparing them to high quality educational sources for the seven most commonly used nerve blocks.

Objective: We sought to evaluate the educational quality of user-uploaded videos when compared to the highest quality anesthesia society websites (NYSORA, ACEP, USRA).

Methods: After reviewing the instructional material available for the seven most frequently conducted nerve blocks on high-quality reference websites, we documented the educational characteristics present including such things as indications, volume, anatomy, etc. Next we reviewed the five most popular videos on YouTube for each block (by views) and documented the presence or absence of these educational characteristics.

Results: Eighteen educational characteristics were documented in the "high-quality" anesthesia society reference material. Correlation was sought between this material and YouTube videos. Although there were varying degrees of correlation between the high quality sources and the videos, rarely did YouTube videos contain as high a percentage of these educational characteristics as the well-established sources. Some videos contained very few of these important educational characteristics.

Conclusion: Although YouTube has been used an educational tool, we recommend that only high quality sources be used to teach or illustrate regional anesthesia nerve blocks.

Background

As one of the most popular open source video content websites available today, YouTube has expanded from being a primarily entertainment website to an instrument for education and information sharing [1–4]. Numerous medical procedures and clinical skills instructional videos can be found quickly, changing the landscape of medical education [2, 4]. Students and providers alike are turning to social media platforms to augment classroom learning and refresh clinical skills [3, 4]. While access to these videos is nearly instantaneous, every piece of content must be used with the awareness that it is often neither peer reviewed nor certified for accuracy [2–4]. However, non-peer reviewed periodicals, websites, conferences and social media have been noted to be sources some healthcare professionals turn to prior to seeking out peer-reviewed material [2]. Nonetheless,

* Correspondence: glt31@njms.rutgers.edu
Department of Anesthesiology, Rutgers, New Jersey Medical School, 185 South Orange Ave., Newark, NJ 07103, USA

many YouTube videos providing misinformation have been reported, leading to potential dangers to patients, and compromising providers' credibility if used as the sole source of information [1, 5, 6].

Previous studies have analyzed instructional content for various specialties, the majority of which used subject matter experts. These are experts in "content analysis", to grade the videos' content based on predefined criteria [7–11]. Most concluded that, while convenient, YouTube content lacked the quality required to safely guide a provider through a specific procedure. Few studies have evaluated the value of regional anesthesia procedures posted to YouTube [9–11].

While others have evaluated large amounts of content posted to YouTube, we asserted that users are most apt to use the first few videos they come across, mostly corresponding to the "top hits," or most viewed. Therefore, our aim was to design a system to objectively evaluate the 5 most viewed instructional videos for some of the most commonly performed regional anesthesia nerve block procedures.

Methods

Study design and setting

This observational retrospective study was conducted in the Department of Anesthesiology at Rutgers- New Jersey Medical School from July to August 2019. Our primary clinical site it University Hospital in Newark, NJ, and serves at New Jersey's only fully public hospital, located in an urban center of nearly 300,000 residents.

Study population and procedure

Four board certified anesthesiologists, each with at least 4 years of post-residency experience practicing regional anesthesia reviewed the content for ultrasound-guided nerve blocks of three well-vetted societies for regional anesthesia: The New York School of Regional Anesthesia (NYSORA)[12], American College of Emergency Physicians (ACEP)[13], and Ultrasound for Regional Anesthesia (USRA)[14] (Table 1). The following seven nerve blocks were reviewed: interscalene, supraclavicular, infraclavicular, axillary, femoral, popliteal and abdominus plane.

Eighteen key characteristics were determined to be present in nearly all of the educational material for these seven blocks. The decision was made to establish these eighteen characteristics as the control against which the Youtube videos would be evaluated (Table 1).

YouTube (www.youtube.com) searches were conducted for each nerve block ("interscalene nerve block", "supraclavicular nerve block", "infraclavicular nerve block", "axillary nerve block", "femoral nerve block" "popliteal nerve block" and "transversus abdominis plane block"). Each search returned between approximately

Table 1 Educational categories for instructional material of regional anesthesia nerve blocks. Column 1 displays the eighteen categories of educational characteristics, whose presence or absence was analyzed in NYSORA, ASRA, USRA and YouTube nerve block instruction. Column 2 is the percentage of instances in which the 35 analyzed YouTube videos (7 blocks with 5 videos each) met each educational characteristic

Indications	62.9%
Transducer position	94.3%
Goal	85.7%
Local anesthetic volume	71.4%
General considerations	94.3%
US anatomy	97.1%
Distribution of anesthesia	71.4%
Equipment	85.7%
Landmarks	97.1%
Patient positioning	91.4%
Technique	100.0%
Atlas picture of anatomy	48.6%
US picture of anatomy	97.1%
Picture of proper transducer placement	94.3%
Picture of proper needle placement	100.0%
Tips for preventing complications	88.6%
Guide for catheter placement	40.0%
References	17.1%

100 and 200 videos. The decision was made to limit evaluation to the top five videos by view count because after the 5th most popular video (by view count) the number of views often dropped off significantly below ~ 100 k views. In addition, it was believed by the researchers that the top five videos by view count would be the most utilized by potential learners, and that many users searching YouTube would not go past the second screen of search results to find an instructional video.

Next, search returns were organized using "filter", then "sort by" and "view count." The five videos for each block with the most views were evaluated. Inclusion criteria included content in the English language and ultrasound guided blocks (vs nerve stimulation only). Videos were excluded if they were not demonstrating an ultrasound guided block, were not in English, or were not relevant to the block/inappropriately titled or labelled. In each of the seven nerve block searches, the top video by view count had between 100,000 and 300,000 views, and the total of views for the top five videos was between 500,000 and 1,000,000 views total. With the significant drop-off for view count following the top five videos, this sample size was considered to be an appropriate representation of the quality of the most-reviewed reference videos.

Each YouTube video was analyzed for the presence or absence of each of these 18 characteristics, and this was recorded for further analysis. Characteristics were recorded as present only if the information contained was correct as determined by the attending anesthesiologists. However, after review, none of the information presented in these 18 categories, when found in the videos, was omitted due to inaccuracies.

Results

The content of the three reference websites (NYSORA, ACEP and USRA) were analyzed for completeness using the categories outlined in Column 1 of Table 1. NYSORA had the most complete instructional content, recording 100% of the categories for each of the seven blocks. ACEP and USRA achieved means of 93.5 and 95.2%, respectively, of categories discussed. The TAP block was omitted for statistical calculations for ACEP, as they did not provide any instructional content for this particular block. "Indications" was the category missed most by USRA, with five out of seven blocks missing this content, while ACEP did not discuss "catheter placement" in any of its instructional videos.

Column 2 of Table 1 demonstrates the percentage of the analyzed YouTube videos (35 total videos from 7 blocks and 5 videos each) which contained each of the 18 educational characteristics, that were established as a control from NYSORA, USRA and ACEP. The least included category in the YouTube videos was "references". Only 6 of the 35 (17.1%) videos evaluated by the research team referenced primary sources. "Guide for catheter placement" (40%) and "Atlas picture of anatomy" (48.6%) were the second and third least referenced categories included in all YouTube videos reviewed.

Table 2 compares and contrasts the differences in percentage of educational characteristics found in educational material between the 3 anesthesia societies (NYSORA, USRA and ACEP) compared to the YouTube videos. This is broken down by each of the individual 7 nerve blocks reviewed for this study. As is evident in the table, none of the reference material for the 7 blocks contains less than 94.4% of the educational categories in the anesthesia society reference material. Compare that to the YouTube videos, which range as low as 68.9% for the popliteal nerve block videos and no higher than 90.0% for the interscalene nerve block instructional videos. (Note: ACEP TAP block was omitted for statistical calculations, as they did not provide any instructional content for this particular block).

Table 2 Percent of educational categories referenced in educational material by nerve block in top 5 YouTube videos as determined by view count

	NYSORA, ACEP, USRA	YouTube
Interscalene	96.3%	90.0%
Supraclavicular	94.4%	82.2%
Infraclavicular	96.3%	86.7%
Axillary	96.3%	80.0%
Femoral	96.3%	73.3%
Popliteal	96.3%	68.9%
TAP	100.0%	77.8%

Overall, the regional anesthesia societies' websites offered very thorough instruction for each nerve block. Figure 1 compares the percentage of educational characteristics present in the traditional online sources (NYSORA, ACEP and USRA) to the average seen in the YouTube videos. As demonstrated herein, in each of the 18 educational characteristics examined, there was a higher percentage of societal reference educational material that contained the material than was present in the YouTube videos analyzed.

Finally, Fig. 2 compares and contrasts the percentage of educational categories referenced in educational material by nerve block. For each of the seven nerve blocks, the educational material provided by NYSORA, ACEP and USRA contained higher percentages of the educational categories than the YouTube videos. Interestingly, the YouTube videos for the four brachial plexus blocks (interscalene, supraclavicular, infraclavicular and axillary) had a higher percentage of educational categories than other classes including lower extremity (femoral and popliteal) and TAP blocks.

Discussion

Social media and internet sources for education are rising influences which have affected the study of medicine, especially in the last decade. These new tools may enhance professional networking and education, organizational promotion, patient care/education and public health programs [1, 5–8, 10, 11].

As the second most popular website in the world [15], with over one billion hours of video watched per day [16], YouTube is an extremely influential resource in entertainment and information gathering for millions of people. Not surprisingly, the site has become a frequently relied upon source of patient medical information gathering, especially by younger physicians, residents and students [17].

Given its popularity and global reach, YouTube has the potential to be an important educational tool for patients, conveying essential health information that could help decrease morbidity and economic burden of preventable diseases [18]. The challenge remains that, while abundant in quantity, the information available is often

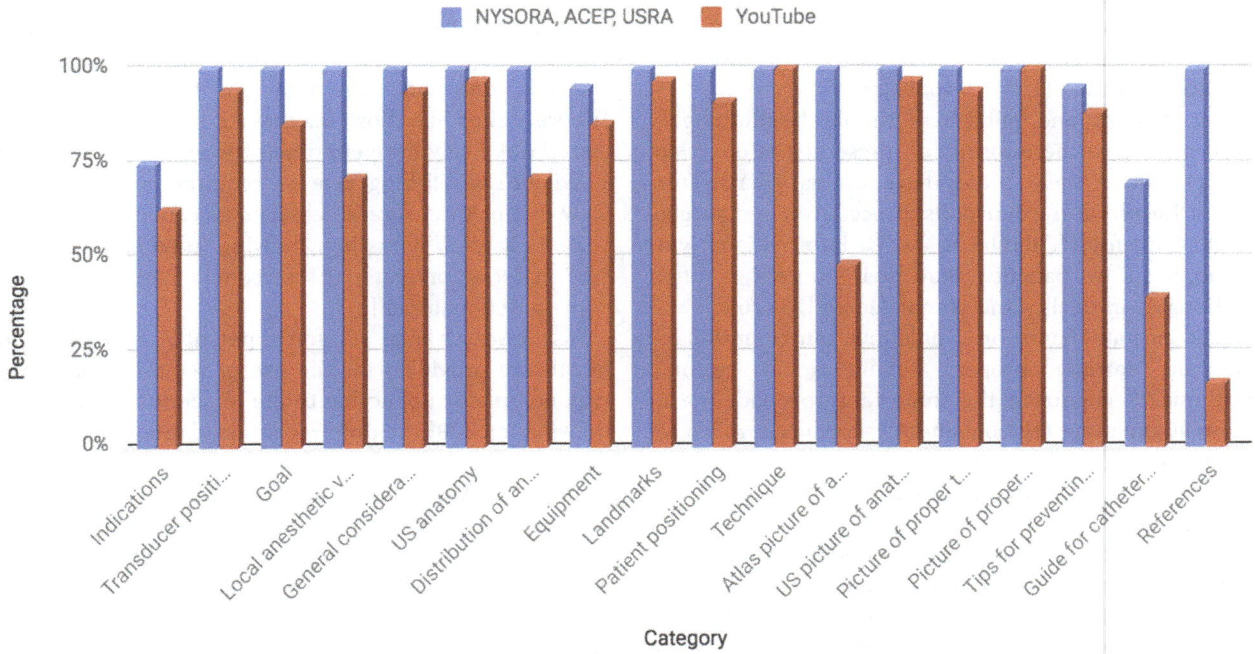

Fig. 1 Comparison of percentage of educational characteristics present in the traditional online sources (NYSORA, ACEP and USRA) compared to the average of the YouTube videos

published by a non-vetted, non-peer reviewed source, and lacks the quality patients require.

There are numerous potential risks for patients and healthcare providers which can be caused by the dissemination of information of poor quality. These may cause damage to professional image, breaching patient privacy, violation of personal/professional boundaries and legal issues [1, 2, 6, 8, 9, 11–16]. Just as importantly, multiple studies evaluating the content of YouTube videos as a source of patient information across different specialties have found them to be of subpar quality and have questioned their usefulness in finding reliable and accurate information [19–22].

Just as YouTube has become a quickly turned to source of medical information for patients, medical students and providers are turning to its content more frequently [3, 4]. With younger generations of medical professionals having access to an exponentially increasing amount of content on YouTube and other social media platforms to augment their learning, caution must

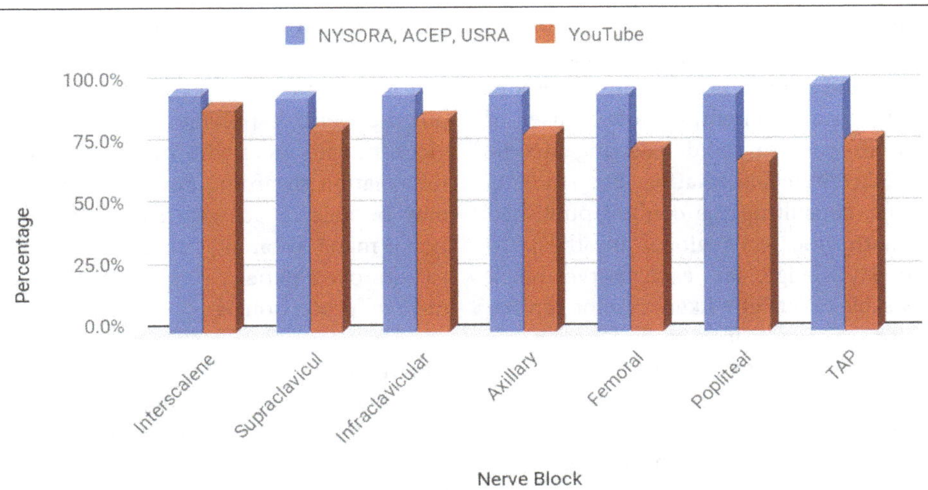

Fig. 2 Percent of educational categories referenced in educational material by nerve block

be taken prior to utilizing these sources. Urgent advocacy is needed for guidelines to prevent the risks presented by these new and alternate avenues of information dissemination and education [1, 7, 11, 16, 17].

Their content and publishers should be thoroughly vetted to ensure the information presented is complete and accurate. Other studies have evaluated YouTube content for physical exam skills, procedures, and surgeries and have found, similar to health informational videos accessed by patients, that their content is often questionable in quality and completeness [23–26].

Visual aids and hands on simulations can be invaluable tools in learning proper techniques in regional anesthesia. Recognizing the important role videos can play in augmenting regional anesthesia education, we set out to evaluate the content of the five most viewed videos for each of 7 ultrasound guided nerve blocks. While a few of the videos were very thorough, touching on nearly 90% of the 18 categories we designated as evaluation criteria, many were lacking a significant amount of information. The overall completeness of the YouTube videos was compared to the content published on the websites of three well respected authorities in regional anesthesia (NYSORA, ACEP and USRA) and noted to be significantly lacking. Figure 2 summarizes these findings, and raises troubling trends.

This study found that even among the five most viewed instructional videos per nerve block that there was a significant variation in completeness. Among all categories evaluated, "references" was missing from nearly 86% of YouTube videos. This is concerning given the fact that the site is an open source platform, allowing anyone to upload content without oversight. Without adequate sourcing of information, one cannot be certain of the accuracy of the information demonstrated to the learner. In contrast, the regional anesthesia society websites cited multiple references for each nerve block in question 100% of the time.

Whereas YouTube has the potential to be an invaluable tool for patients and providers, offering a plethora of extremely easily accessible content, it must be used in the proper manner in order to avoid receiving incomplete, and possibly inaccurate information. For students and young physicians, consulting the content published by the established authorities on regional anesthesia to learn foundational knowledge for each nerve block would be most advisable. YouTube likely cannot replace trusted sources for primary information, such as NYSORA, ACEP and USRA. However, there may be a role in consulting further video content after the provider has knowledge and experience with the procedure to evaluate different techniques or refresh their skills.

Anesthesiologists and physicians must remain resolute when evaluating educational sources for both their own education and disseminating information to patients or colleagues. Although more readily available than only a few years ago, clinical videos of high quality may be available only on sites that are behind a paywall. Whereas sites like those maintained by NYSORA, ACEP and USRA likely have editorial processes of high-quality, YouTube's publishing process requires no editorial review except to ensure an absence of explicit, dangerous, violent, hateful, harassing, bullying, threatening or private material, or material that contains spam, scams or copyrighted material [27].

Past research has set forth potential guidelines for healthcare providers for the use of social media, which may be broadly applicable to the dissemination of online information [28]. Sample recommendations include ensuring content credibility by sharing only information from reputable sources and immediately refuting inaccurate information that a provider encounters [28].

Even more recent research has elucidated the possible effects of social media and internet sources of information as it related to the COVID-19 pandemic [29]. Fake news has been spread easily via social media as it relates to disease origins, manifestations, symptoms and treatments [29]. Social media has spread fake news leading to risky behaviors, such as taking unproven medications such as hydroxychloroquine [29].

When utilizing alternate education sources that are widely accessible, standards and guidelines may need to be established on both a local and national level. Further education may be incorporated for medical students, residents and even practicing anesthesiologists to be able to review, assess and differentiate the sources one uses on the Internet. Digital literacy should not be assumed, and may need to become a part of medical school and/ or residency curricula.

Despite its limitations, however, YouTube will likely grow in influence in medical education. Advantages to publishing on YouTube include the speed of publishing new content and the widespread free access to videos and information. With growing Internet access throughout the world, especially on cell phones and mobile devices, practitioners who may have had limited access to information regarding new techniques and technologies, may be able to access an unending archive of instructional material on sites such as YouTube. This may lead to improved patient care and communication amongst medical professionals.

Conclusion

As one of the most popular websites in the world, YouTube offers a wide range of video content, often including submissions for medical instruction. The proliferation of video content for medical education includes lessons on regional anesthesia nerve blocks.

Although the potential for free, widespread and easily accessible educational material has a very high ceiling, care must be taken to ensure that this video content is of high caliber in order to ensure patient safety and the highest levels of professionalism.

This study sought to develop an objective system by which these free educational materials (in this case YouTube instructional videos for regional anesthesia nerve blocks) could be evaluated, and their quality validated prior to use by the public. Most of the educational videos reviewed on YouTube were of high quality, and contained many of the educational characteristics established from the reference materials. The purpose of this study was not only to compare the quality of videos on YouTube to high-quality reference material, but, more importantly, to attempt to develop an objective system for future evaluation and rating.

One potential solution to ensuring video content of the highest quality may be a rating system or a checklist to ensure certain educational content is present before uploading the material. Some of the videos uploaded to YouTube and evaluated in this study were from sources that produced content of higher quality including RAUKvideos, ThePainSource, Lecturio, Galusweegie, vidRASCI, BK Medical, NYSORA and ImedrxTV. However, without a rating system or system to evaluate the presence or absence of certain educational content, a simple search on YouTube does not elucidate the quality of the content, only the views and relevance based on titles and keywords. Herein we advocate for the implementation and use of an objective system to evaluate this widely-available educational content.

When compared to regional anesthesia societies' website content, the content of the five most viewed instructional videos for each nerve block in question lacked important characteristics in multiple categories. Therefore, YouTube videos should likely not be used as primary sources when initially learning a nerve block; YouTube is not an effective substitute for textbook instruction, nor the high-quality educational material from anesthesia societies that specialize in regional anesthesia. However, these educational videos may be of value to augment already established knowledge for the experienced or learning provider wishing to refresh on skills or explore different techniques.

Abbreviations

NYSORA: The New York School of Regional Anesthesia; ACEP: American College of Emergency Physicians; USRA: Ultrasound for Regional Anesthesia; TAP: transversus abdominis plane

Acknowledgements

Not applicable.

Authors' contributions

GT, AW, SS and PD contributed to the collection and analysis of data, as well as writing and editing the manuscript. Authors have read and approved the manuscript.

References

1. Azer SA, Algrain HA, AlKhelaif RA, AlEshaiwi SM. Evaluation of the educational value of YouTube videos about physical examination of the cardiovascular and respiratory systems. J Med Internet Res. 2013;15(11):e241.
2. Ng FK, Wallace S, Coe B, Owen A, Lynch J, Bonvento B, Firn M, McGrath BA. From smartphone to bed-side: exploring the use of social media to disseminate recommendations from the National Tracheostomy Safety Project to front-line clinical staff. Anaesthesia. 2020;75(2):227–33.
3. Romanov K, Nevgi A. Do medical students watch video clips in eLearning and do these facilitate learning? Med Teach. 2007;29(5):484–8.
4. Yıldırım B, Basaran O, Alatas OD, Yeniceri EN, Alatas OD, Yeniceri EN, Altun I, Tanriverdi O, Dogan V, Acar E, et al. Chest tube insertion techniques on YouTube: is social media a reliable source of learning medical skills? Am J Emerg Med. 2015;33(11):1709–10.
5. Butler DP, Perry F, Shah Z, Leon-Villapalos J. The quality of video information on burn first aid available on YouTube. Burns. 2013;39(5):856–9.
6. Hansen C, Interrante JD, Ailes EC, Frey MT, Broussard CS, Godoshian VJ, Lewis C, Polen KND, Garcia AP, Gilboa SM. Assessment of YouTube videos as a source of information on medication use in pregnancy. Pharmacoepidemiol Drug Saf. 2016;25(1):35–44.
7. Abdulghani HM, Haque S, Ahmad T, Irshad M, Sattar K, Al-Harbi MM, Khamis N. A critical review of obstetric and gynecological physical examination videos available on YouTube: Content analysis and user engagement evaluation. Medicine (Baltimore). 2019;98(30):e16459.
8. Karabay E, Karsiyakali N, Kayar K, Koseoglu H. Hypospadias surgery on YouTube: is it valid? Minerva Pediatr. 2019.
9. Rössler B, Lahner D, Schebesta K, Chiari A, Plöchl W. Medical information on the Internet: Quality assessment of lumbar puncture and neuroaxial block techniques on YouTube. Clin Neurol Neurosurg. 2012;114(6):655–8.
10. Selvi O, Tulgar S, Senturk O, Topcu DI, Ozer Z. YouTube as an informational source for brachial plexus blocks: evaluation of content and educational value. Rev Bras Anestesiol. 2019;69(2):168–76.
11. Tulgar S, Selvi O, Serifsoy TE, Senturk O, Ozer Z. YouTube as an information source of spinal anesthesia, epidural anesthesia and combined spinal and epidural anesthesia. Rev Bras Anestesiol. 2017;67(5):493–9.
12. NYSORA, Inc (New York School of Regional Anesthesia). Techniques. [https://www.nysora.com/techniques]. Accessed 29 Aug 2019.
13. American College of Emergency Physicians, Sonoguide. Ultrasound Guided Nerve Blocks [https://www.acep.org/sonoguide/nerve_block.html]. Accessed 29 Aug 2019.
14. USRA (Ultrasound for Regional Anesthesia). Links for Specific Blocks. [http://www.usra.ca/regional-anesthesia/specific-blocks/home.php]. Accessed 29 Aug 2019.
15. Alexa Internet, Inc. The Top 500 Sites on the Web [http://www.alexa.com/topsites]. Accessed 6 Oct 2019.
16. YouTube. YouTube for press [https://www.youtube.com/intl/en-GB/yt/about/press]. Accessed 6 Oct 2019.
17. Vance K, Howe W, Dellavalle RP. Social internet sites as a source of public health information. Dermatol Clin. 2009;27(2):133–6 vi.
18. Sood A, Sarangi S, Pandey A, Murugiah K. YouTube as a source of information on kidney stone disease. Urology. 2011;77(3):558–62.
19. Ache KA, Wallace LS. Human papillomavirus vaccination coverage on YouTube. Am J Prev Med. 2008;35(4):389–92.
20. Keelan J, Pavri-Garcia V, Tomlinson G, Wilson K. YouTube as a Source of Information on Immunization: A Content Analysis. JAMA. 2007;298(21):2482–4.
21. Nason K, Donnelly A, Duncan HF. YouTube as a patient-information source for root canal treatment. Int Endod J. 2016;49(12):1194–200.
22. Staunton PF, Baker JF, Green J, Devitt A. Online Curves: A Quality Analysis of Scoliosis Videos on YouTube. Spine (Phila Pa 1976). 2015;40(23):1857–61.
23. Camm CF, Sunderland N, Camm AJ. A quality assessment of cardiac auscultation material on YouTube. Clin Cardiol. 2013;36(2):77–81.
24. Fischer J, Geurts J, Valderrabano V, Hügle T. Educational quality of YouTube videos on knee arthrocentesis. J Clin Rheumatol. 2013;19(7):373–6.
25. Ho M, Stothers L, Lazare D, Tsang B, Macnab A. Evaluation of educational content of YouTube videos relating to neurogenic bladder and intermittent catheterization. Can Urol Assoc J. 2015;9(9–10):320–54.

26. Sorensen JA, Pusz MD, Brietzke SE. YouTube as an information source for pediatric adenotonsillectomy and ear tube surgery. Int J Pediatr Otorhinolaryngol. 2014;78(1):65–70.
27. YouTube. YouTube Policies & Safety. https://www.youtube.com/about/policies/#community-guidelines. Accessed 2 June 2020.
28. Ventola CL. Social media and health care professionals: benefits, risks, and best practices. P t. 2014;39(7):491–520.
29. Prévost Jantchou BJA, Valérie Nguyen: Physician Roles and Responsibilities in the Context of a Pandemic in Resource-Limited Areas: Impact of Social Media. Iberoamerican J Med 2020.

Difficulty in diagnosis of delayed spinal epidural hematoma in puerperal women after combined spinal epidural anaesthesia

Alessandro Svelato[1*], Alberto Rutili[2], Caterina Bertelloni[2], Domenico Foti[3], Angela Capizzi[4] and Antonio Ragusa[1]

Abstract

Background: Spinal epidural hematoma is a rare but serious complication of epidural anaesthesia and neurological impairment. Epidural hematoma usually becomes evident within a few hours of the procedure. Delayed clinical presentation of spinal epidural hematoma is even rarer and insidious.

Case presentation: We reported a case of a 44-year-old woman who underwent a caesarean section for a twin pregnancy during which a delayed dorsal spinal epidural hematoma occurred. Symptoms were reported 5 days after surgery and 72 h after removal of the epidural catheter. An MRI scan showed a dorsal epidural hematoma. The patient was moved to the Neurosurgical Department and underwent decompression surgery.

Conclusion: The possibility of the delayed onset of a spinal epidural hematoma in a pregnant woman who undergoes epidural anaesthesia in labour must always be taken into consideration. In order to achieve the best clinical result, we stress the importance of a timely diagnosis and prompt surgical treatment.

Keywords: Spinal epidural hematoma, Obstetric, Labour, Epidural, Diagnosis, Case report

Background

Spinal Epidural Hematoma (SEH), a rare but potentially devastating complication, is a symptomatic bleeding within the spine where blood accumulates outside the dura, mostly caused by traumatic or iatrogenic (spinal surgeries, obstetrical birth trauma, lumbar puncture, spinal manipulations, and epidural procedures) events [1]. SEH can cause rare but potentially catastrophic compression of neural tissue by direct injury or ischemia, with an incidence ranging from 1:2600 to 1:220.000 [2–6]. Parturients can also be predisposed to the development of an epidural hematoma, due to a decreased number or function of platelets (i.e., with pre-eclampsia or hemolysis, elevated liver enzymes, low platelet count [HELLP] syndrome) or anticoagulant use, even if pregnancy is a prothrombotic, hypercoagulable state [2].

* Correspondence: alessandrosvelato@virgilio.it
[1]Department of Obstetrics and Gynecology, Massa Carrara General Hospital, Via Enrico Mattei, 54100 Massa Carrara, Italy

In this manuscript we report a case of difficult diagnosis concerning a delayed epidural hematoma, due to combined spinal epidural (CSE) anaesthesia in a caesarean delivery.

Case presentation

A 44 year-old pregnant nulliparous, weight 70 Kg, height 172 cm, BMI 23.7, at 34 weeks of a twin gestation, obtained by “in vitro” fertilization, was admitted to the General Hospital of Massa, complaining spreading pricking and lower limb edema. The patient suffered from unstable insulin-dependent type I diabetes and sciatica. Considering 4 days of immobilization in bed, low molecular weight heparin (Dalteparin© 2500 UI one per day) was administered [7]. The patient underwent a planned caesarean section under double-space CSE anaesthesia, using a 25-gauge atraumatic spinal needle at level L3-L4 and an 18-gauge Thuoy needle at T12-L1 (B. Braun Perifix® epidural set), placed during a single attempt. Preoperative coagulation parameters were within normal range (Platelet count 120.000 per microliter of blood; Prothrombin time 12 s, Partial thromboplastin time 30 s, fibrinogen 540 mg/dL, INR 0.90). Renal function was normal. The operation was carried out routinely and multimodal pain therapy was started (Patient Controlled Epidural Anaesthesia - PCEA - with chirocaine 0,15% plus sufentanil 0,5 mcg/ml, 4 ml/h; i.v. ketorolac 30 mg/day and oral tramadol 30 mg plus acetaminophen 1000 mg/3 times/day). Four hours after the operation, the urinary catheter was removed, the patient began to stand up and to take care of the newborns. Dalteparin 2500 U/die was continued. PCEA was discontinued 2 days after the operation and the epidural catheter was removed on the 3rd day, 12 h after the last Dalteparin administration. Pain control was optimal. The following day, the patient remained hospitalized without any complications and the two babies were admitted in neonatology.

At 06.00 a.m. of the 6th post-operative day, more than 70 h after the removal of the epidural catheter, the patient complained of acute and severe low-back pain, radiating to the right inferior limb, and paresthesia; there was no motor impairment and she was treated with analgesic drugs without any improvement. After an abdominal ultrasound, urinary retention was observed and a bladder catheter was inserted (residual volume: 1100 ml). A right lower limb motor deficit was observed at 11:50 a.m. and methylprednisolone was administered. Since no improvement in the patient's clinical picture was seen, urgent neurological consultation was requested 8 h after the onset of symptoms (02.00 p.m.). A dorsal MRI scan showed the presence of a T12-L1 posterior SEH, predominantly on the right side, with significant mass-effect and spinal cord signal alteration in the conus medullaris region (Figs. 1 and 2). The patient was transferred to the Neurosurgical Department for decompression laminectomy and removal of the hematoma and the operation began at 07.00 p.m.. Immediately after surgery, the patient partially recovered her sensory disorder and motor functions. Five days after surgery she began intensive rehabilitation.

In the last follow-up examination (36 months later), while mostly improved, motor, sensory and sphincter deficits persisted in varying degrees. The last MRI confirmed signs of permanent ischemic injury at level T12-L1.

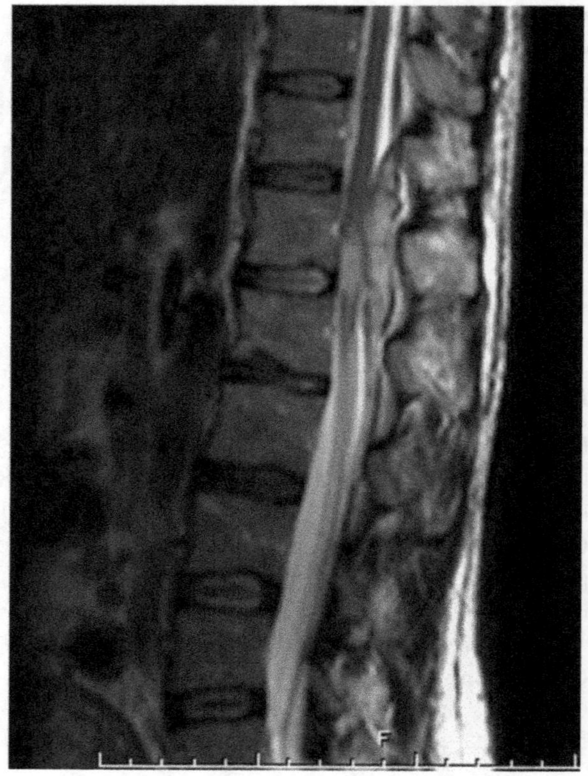

Fig. 1 Sagittal T2-weighted MRI shows hyperintense collection in the posterior spinal epidural space at level D12-L1 and spinal cord signal alteration

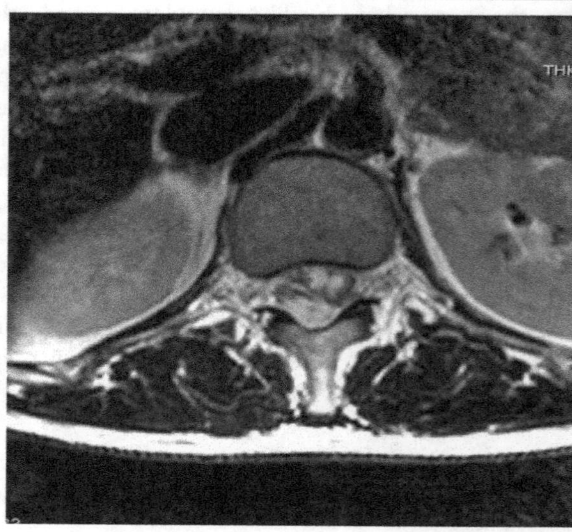

Fig. 2 Axial T2-weighted MRI shows hematoma compressing spinal cord from the right side

Discussion and conclusion

Neuraxial techniques are used to provide analgesia for labour [8, 9] and anaesthesia for surgical delivery. Therefore, complications associated with neuraxial techniques are sometimes seen even in pregnant patients.

We have described a case of SEH, one of the more severe complications.

In our case, the acute and severe low-back pain, radiating to the right inferior limb, and paresthesia were the first signs reported by the patient. The physicians focused their attention only on the medical history of the patient's sciatica, without first ruling out the more dangerous possible diagnosis, even if less frequent. Moreover, they also ignored the risk factors present. There are many risk factors for SEH, but is know that the most important are spinal/epidural procedures in combination with anticoagulant use [2, 3]. We used a double-space CSE anaesthesia, because a caesarean section is a major surgery, along with the concerns of potential surgical complications and longer operating time. If an epidural catheter is available, our protocol for postoperative pain management considers the possibility to prolong epidural analgesia for 48 h, in line with SIAARTI guidelines [10–12]. Moreover, our hospital is a Baby Friendly Hospital, which means that is at the forefront in the promotion of breastfeeding. In this view, postoperative pain control is of primary importance, with the aim of promoting skin to skin contact and the start of breastfeeding. Anticoagulation is also a risk factor for SEH, however the doses of drugs with effects on coagulation that we used, were very low (Deltaparina 2500 UI once daily and ketorolac 30 mg/die for 2 days) in consideration of the patient's weight (70 Kg) [7].

A delay in diagnostic imaging can lead to devastating outcomes, and is an error, since neurological symptoms and back pain can be attributed to epidural infusion and a prolonged effect of the local anaesthetic, or to a musculoskeletal origin [13].

Another element that made the diagnosis difficult was the appearance of the symptoms 3 days after the removal of the epidural catheter. This lag time is possible [14].

The second sign was urinary retention, followed by motor impairment. This case evolution is typical of a SEH [1]. In 30% of cases there is an acute onset of complete paralysis with bowel or bladder disturbances, while in 16% of cases, as well as in our case, the onset is less typical with incomplete paralysis [1, 3]. The presence of motor deficit is an indication for surgery [15]. In the case of sensory symptoms without motor deficit, surgery does not seem to improve outcomes and a wait-and-see approach, with meticulous follow up, seems to be the best option [15]. In the case of motor deficit, as well as in our case, decompression laminectomy within 12 h results in the best surgical outcome [3, 15, 16]. Nevertheless, literature reports cases of good outcome also in the case of surgery performed after 24 h from the onset of symptoms [15].

In conclusion, we should always suspect a delayed onset of SEH in a patient who undergoes epidural anaesthesia or other similar neuraxial procedures. We stress the importance of an early diagnosis of this serious complication and of prompt surgical treatment to maximize neurological improvement. Table 1 lists the most common "red flags" to notice and pitfalls to avoid for a prompt diagnosis.

Table 1 Red flags and pitfalls in the diagnosis of spinal epidural hematoma

Red flags in the diagnosis of spinal epidural hematoma
1) Considering only the most frequent diagnosis, without excluding serious but infrequent diagnoses
2) Persistent motor block
3) Bowel/bladder dysfunction
4) Other symptom (usually back or leg pain)
Pitfalls in the diagnosis of spinal epidural hematoma
1) Ignoring the risk factors
2) Administering treatment before making the diagnosis
3) Not performing surgery only because too much time has passed since the appearance of the symptoms (> 12 h)

After this case we performed an audit that involved all staff members and we have introduced some actions of improvement. For example, we have changed the number of patient evaluation from 1 per day to 2 per day. We have organized a review day about SEH with the aim to inform all staff members about the onset of symptoms and early diagnosis of this condition.

The most important lesson to be learned from our case is thinking that SEH exists and is a potential complication of epidural anaesthesia, so we must always take this complication into consideration in the case of neurological symptoms appearance.

Significant back pain and/or lower limb pain, even if nonspecific symptoms, and in the absence of motor impairment, should alert all staff members to request an urgent neurological, neuroradiological and neurosurgical consultation, even in the late stages of patient hospitalization.

Abbreviations
CSE: Combined spinal epidural; PCEA: Patient Controlled Epidural Anaesthesia; SEH: Spinal Epidural Hematoma

Acknowledgements
Not applicable.

Authors' contributions
AS, AC and AR contributed to writing and reviewing this manuscript. AR and CB contributed to performing anaesthesia. DF contributed to performing the neurosurgical operation. AS, AR and AC contributed to the collection of data. AS, AR, CB, DF and AR contributed to reviewing the manuscript. All authors have read and approved the final manuscript.

Author details
[1]Department of Obstetrics and Gynecology, Massa Carrara General Hospital, Via Enrico Mattei, 54100 Massa Carrara, Italy. [2]Department of Anaesthesia, Massa Carrara General Hospital, Massa Carrara, Italy. [3]Department of Neurosurgery, S. Chiara Hospital, Pisa, Italy. [4]Department of Obstetrics and Gynecology, Imperia General Hospital, Imperia, Italy.

References
1. Shaban A, Moritani T, Al Kasab S, Sheharyar A, Limaye KS, Adams HP Jr. Spinal cord hemorrhage. J Stroke Cerebrovasc Dis. 2018;27(6):1435–46.
2. Hoefnagel A, Yu A, Kaminski A. Anesthetic complications in pregnancy. Crit Care Clin. 2016;32(1):1–28.

3. Kreppel D, Antoniadis G, Seeling W. Spinal hematoma: a literature survey with meta-analysis of 613 patients. Neurosurg Rev. 2003;26(1):1–49.
4. Bateman BT, Mhyre JM, Ehrenfeld J, Kheterpal S, Abbey KR, Argalious M, Berman MF, Jacques PS, Levy W, Loeb RG, Paganelli W, Smith KW, Wethington KL, Wax D, Pace NL, Tremper K, Sandberg WS. The risk and outcome of epidural hematomas after perioperative and obstetric epidural catheterization: a report from the multicenter perioperative outcomes group research consortium. Anesth Analg. 2013;116(6):1380–5.
5. D'Angelo R, Smiley RM, Riley ET, Segal S. Serious complications related to obstetric anesthesia: the serious complication repository project of the Society for Obstetric Anesthesia and Perinatology. Anesthesiology. 2014; 120(6):1505–12.
6. Ruppen W, Derry S, McQuay H, Moore RA. Incidence of epidural hematoma, infection, and neurologic injury in obstetric patients with epidural analgesia/anesthesia. Anesthesiology. 2006;105(2):394–9.
7. Leffert L, Butwick A, Carvalho B, Arendt K, Bates SM, Friedman A, Horlocker T, Houle T, Landau R, Dubois H, Fernando R, Houle T, Kopp S, Montgomery D, Pellegrini J, Smiley R, Toledo P. Members of the SOAP VTE taskforce. The Society for Obstetric Anesthesia and Perinatology consensus statement on the anesthetic Management of Pregnant and Postpartum Women Receiving Thromboprophylaxis or higher dose anticoagulants. Anesth Analg. 2018; 126(3):928–44
8. Ragusa a, Gizzo S, Noventa M, Ferrazzi E, Deiana S, Svelato a. prevention of primary caesarean delivery: comprehensive management of dystocia in nulliparous patients at term. Arch Gynecol Obstet. 2016;294(4):753–61.
9. Svelato A, Di Tommaso M, Spinoso R, Ragusa A. The reduction of first cesarean sections: a cultural issue. Acta Obstet Gynecol Scand. 2016;95(11):1319.
10. Gogarten W, Vandermeulen E, Van Aken H, Kozek S, Llau JV, Samama CM. Regional anaesthesia and antithrombotic agents: recommendations of the European Society of Anaesthesiology. Eur J Anaesthesiol. 2010;27(12):999–1015.
11. Bertini L, Savoia G, De Nicola A, Ivani G, Gravino E, Albani A, Alemanno F, Barbati A, Borghi B, Borrometi F, Casati A, Celleno D, Ciaschi A, Corcione A, De Negri P, Di Benedetto P, Evangelista M, Fanelli G, Grossi P, Loreto M, Margaria E, Mastronardi P, Mattia C, Nicosia F, Nolli M, Rutili A, Santangelo E, Sucre J, Tagariello V, Varrassi G, Paoletti F, Tufano R. SIAARTI. SIAARTI guidelines for safety in locoregional anaesthesia. Minerva Anestesiol. 2006;72(9):689–722.
12. Savoia G, Alampi D, Amantea B, Ambrosio F, Arcioni R, Berti M, Bettelli G, Bertini L, Bosco M, Casati A, Castelletti I, Carassiti M, Coluzzi F, Costantini A, Danelli G, Evangelista M, Finco G, Gatti A, Gravino E, Launo C, Loreto M, Mediati R, Mokini Z, Mondello E, Palermo S, Paoletti F, Paolicchi A, Petrini F, Piacevoli Q, Rizza A, Sabato AF, Santangelo E, Troglio E, Mattia C. SIAARTI study group. Postoperative pain treatment SIAARTI recommendations 2010. Short version. Minerva Anestesiol. 2010;76(8):657–67.
13. Maddali P, Moisi M, Page J, Chamiraju P, Fisahn C, Oskouian R, Tubbs RS. Anatomical complications of epidural anesthesia: a comprehensive review. Clin Anat. 2017;30(3):342–6.
14. Guffey PJ, McKay WR, McKay RE. Case report: epidural hematoma nine days after removal of a labor epidural catheter. Anesth Analg. 2010;111(4):992–5.
15. Lagerkranser M, Lindquist C. Neuraxial blocks and spinal haematoma: review of 166 cases published 1994 - 2015. Part 2: diagnosis, treatment, and outcome. Scand J Pain. 2017;15:130–6.
16. Lawton MT, Porter RW, Heiserman JE, Jacobowitz R, Sonntag VKH, Dickman CA. Surgical management of spinal epidural hematoma: relationship between surgical timing and neurological outcome. J Neurosurg. 1995;83(1):1–7.

Sciatic obturator femoral technique versus spinal anaesthesia in patients undergoing surgery for fixation of open tibial fractures using Ilizarov external fixator

Hoda Shokri[1*] and Amr A. Kasem[2]

Abstract

Background: Peripheral nerve block is preferable for lower extremity surgery because it sufficiently blocks pain pathways at different levels providing excellent anaesthesia at the site of surgery. We designed this study to compare the efficacy and safety of SOFT block (sciatic-obturator-femoral technique) compared with spinal anaesthesia in patients undergoing surgery for fixation of open tibial fractures using Ilizarov external fixator.

Methods: One hundred and seven patients ASA I, II scheduled for fixation of open tibial fractures using Ilizarov external fixator. The patients were randomly allocated to receive either spinal anaesthesia or SOFT block. In spinal anaesthesia group, patients received spinal anaesthesia with hyperbaric bupivacaine 0.5% (7. 5-10mg). In SOFT group, patients received SOFT block with bupivacaine 0.25%. Primary endpoint included the duration of analgesia. The secondary endpoints included patient satisfaction scores, visual analogue scores, incidence of adverse events as vomiting, systemic toxicity from local anaesthetic drug and time to first effect of the techniques.

Results: The duration of SOFT block and time to first analgesic dose in SOFT group was significantly longer ($p <$ 0.001). There was no significant difference between the study groups regarding satisfaction scores, the incidence of cardiovascular collapse, seizures and paraesthesia. Pain scores were significantly lower in SOFT group at 3,6,12 h postoperative ($p < 0.001$). The time to the first effect was significantly longer in SOFT group ($p < 0.001$).

Conclusion: SOFT is a feasible technique of local anaesthesia for control of postoperative pain with unremarkable adverse events compared with spinal anaesthesia, in patients undergoing fixation of tibial fractures using Ilizarov external fixator.

Keywords: Spinal anesthesia, SOFT block, Ilizarov, Analgesia

* Correspondence: Drhoda10@yahoo.com
[1]Assistant Professor of Anaesthesiology, Ain Shams University, Cairo, Egypt

Background

Peripheral nerve block is a popular pain control tool for the lower limb procedures because it lowers the pain scores, reduces opioid requirements and improves patient's satisfaction [1]. On the contrary to different anesthetic techniques, as spinal or general anesthesia, properly performed peripheral nerve blocks are associated with uneventful recovery, brilliantly treat postoperative pain inflicting early hospital discharge [2]. Extra blessings of peripheral nerve blocks are that they can be used in patients receiving anti-coagulants or tormented by lumbo-sacral unwellness and also neuroaxial anaesthesia can be done without airway instrumentation as well [3].

Recently, there is a big interest in regional anesthesia particularly peripheral nerve blockade [3] Research in this field has advanced a lot thanks to the availability of brilliant equipments used in different procedures. Femoral nerve block alone or combined with another peripheral nerve block is used for total knee replacement surgical procedures and has successfully treated postoperative pain bypassing any adverse events as cardiovascular or respiratory problems [4].

SOFT is a recent single-puncture block, it has shown better quality than the earlier approaches of blocking the sciatic, femoral, and obturator nerves and it takes less than 20 mins to perform [5].

We designed this prospective study to compare the efficacy and safety of SOFT compared with spinal anaesthesia in patients undergoing surgery for fixation of open tibial fractures using Ilizarov external fixator.

Methods

After the approval of ethics committee of Ain Shams University, number FMASU R 10 / 2018, this study was registered in ClinicalTrials.gov: NCT03450798 and carried out according to the Consolidated Standards of Reporting Trials (CONSORT) 2010 statement [6].This prospective randomized double blinded parallel group study was conducted over 107 consecutive patients aged from 3 5- 57 years old, American Association of Anesthesiologists(ASA) I and II, scheduled for elective surgery for fixation of open tibial fractures using Ilizarov external fixator. This study was carried out at Ain Shams University hospitals from February 2018 to January 2019. Initially written informed consent was signed by all patients.

Patients unable to communicate with the investigators or hospital staff, morbidly obese patients (body mass index> 40 kg/m^2), patients undergoing bilateral surgery, patients with coagulopathies, renal insufficiency (creatinine> 1.5 mg/dl), ASA III-IV, urgent procedures, contraindications to regional anesthesia, patients with unstable vital signs and patients with head or chest trauma were excluded from the study.

Pre-anaesthetic check, full history and routine investigations were done before the surgery.

After an intravenous (IV) cannula was secured, and midazolam 0.05 mg/kg IV was given to all patients before transfer to the operating room. Standard monitoring devices as electrocardiography, non- invasive blood pressure and pulse oximetry were placed. Then, patients were randomly allocated by sealed envelope technique done according to the randomisation schedule, prepared and opened by a resident not involved in any part of the study to receive either spinal anesthesia or SOFT block, the clinician in charge of data collection and patients' follow-up was blinded to the patients' grouping. A single experienced operator had performed all blocks and spinal anaesthesia and assessed their success did not participate in the study and was blinded to its nature. In spinal group, patients received spinal anaesthesia with hyperbaric bupivacaine (AstraZeneca, UK) 0.5% (7.5-10 mg) which was administered via a 25-G spinal needle at L4-L5 or L3-L4 while the patient positioned in the sitting position under complete aseptic conditions.

In SOFT group, patients received SOFT block where patients were positioned in supine position under complete aseptic conditions, a linear US probe (GE LOGIQe, Wauwatosa, Wisconsin, USA) was placed on the inguinal crease to clearly show the femoral nerve and vessels as shown in Fig. 1. After subcutaneous local anaesthetic wheal using bupivacaine 0.5% was made, a 12-cm stimulating block needle was introduced using an in-plane technique medial to the femoral vein and advanced 1-3 cm below and parallel to the skin. Then, it was redirected toward the fibres of the femoral nerve, where 15 mL of bupivacaine 0.25% was injected. To block the obturator nerve, the probe was shifted medially, superior to the needle and directed cranially to identify the pectineus muscle. The needle was then withdrawn to the subcutaneous tissue and redirected using an out-of-plane technique toward the deep surface of the pectineus without muscle twitches then 10 mL of bupivacaine (AstraZeneca, UK) 0.25% was injected slowly to ensure better spread of the local anaesthetic (LA) as shown in Fig. 2 [4]. To locate the sciatic nerve, the curvilinear probe was handled medial to the femoral vessels, inferior to the needle, and tilted to get the clearest image of the sciatic nerve. The needle was inserted then withdrawn subcutaneously and directed by an in-plane technique toward the sciatic nerve deep to the inferior border of the quadratus femoris muscle as shown in Fig. 3. Then 20 mL of bupivacaine 0.25% was injected after needle had elicited tibial twitches using 1 mA current. The techniques were evaluated every 5 min after completion of the technique for 20 min till successful block was achieved then surgical incision was allowed. Midazolam 2 mg doses (Dormicum 5 mg/ml; Roche

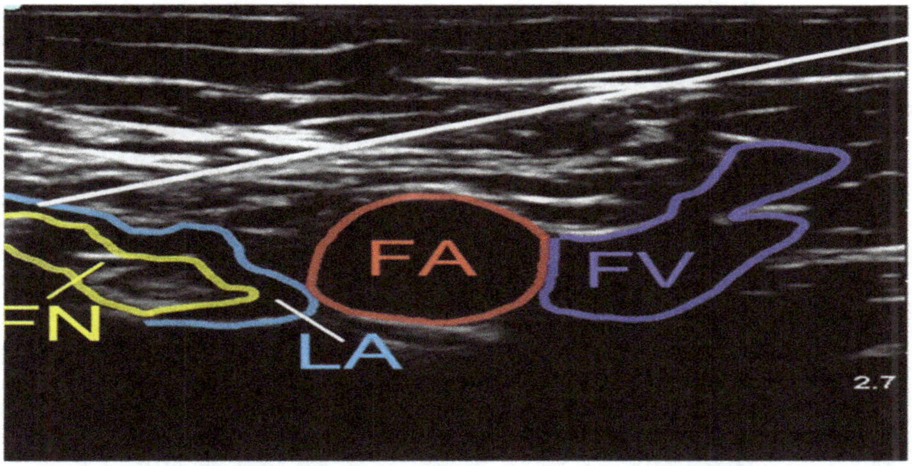

Fig. 1 Ultrasound images obtained during femoral nerve block. Ultrasound image of the needle path to block the femoral nerve. The needle (white line) as shown pierces the fascia iliaca lateral to the femoral nerve (FN) marked by yellow arrow and the needle tip is advanced along the deep border of the nerve. FA, femoral artery

Basel, Swizerland), 50 µg fentanyl (fentanyl 50 µg/ml, 2 ml; (ADVANZ Pharma, UK) and 15 mg ketamine (Ketalar, 50 mg/ml, 10 ml; Pfizer, Sandwich, UK) were given when sedo-analgesia was required. Successful SOFT was confirmed by patient's inability to extend a fully flexed knee, to flex the foot and to adduct an abducted hip respectively. Baseline heart rate and blood pressure values were monitored every 5 min after block performance till the end of surgery. Hypotension was defined as a decrease in systolic arterial blood pressure by 20% or more from baseline values, and it was initially treated with 200 ml IV infusion of Ringer's lactate solution; if this proved to be ineffective, an IV bolus of phenylephrine (40–50 mcg) was given. Bradycardia was defined as heart rate drops by more than 20% from the baseline values, and it was treated with 0.5 mg IV atropine.

At the end of the procedure, patients were transferred to the post-anaesthesia care unit where they were

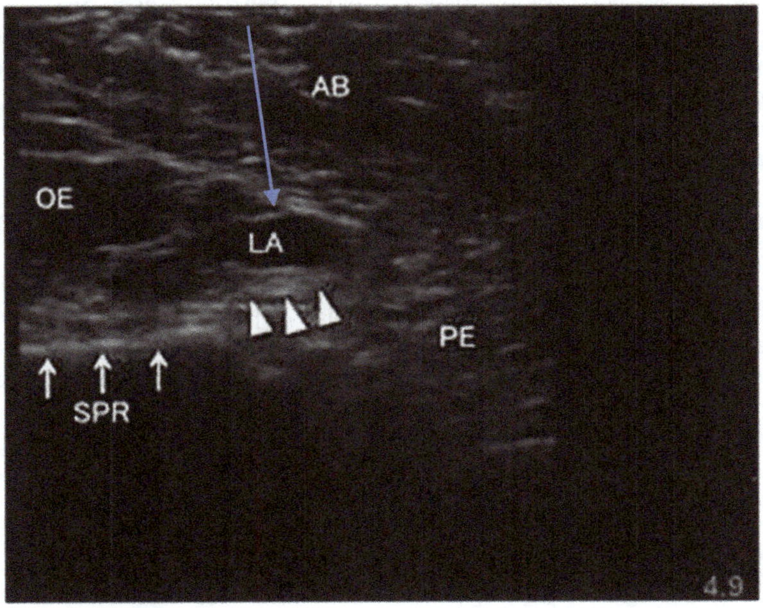

Fig. 2 Ultrasound images obtained during obturator nerve block. The probe was shifted medially and directed cranially. A hyperechoic thick fascia between the pectineus and obturator externus muscles (open triangles) is the target plane. The needle (blue arrow) was moved toward the fascial plane deep to the pectineus (PE) muscle using an out of plane method. LA: local anaesthetic; AB: anterior branch of obturator nerve; SPR: superior pubic ramus (arrows); OE: obturator externus

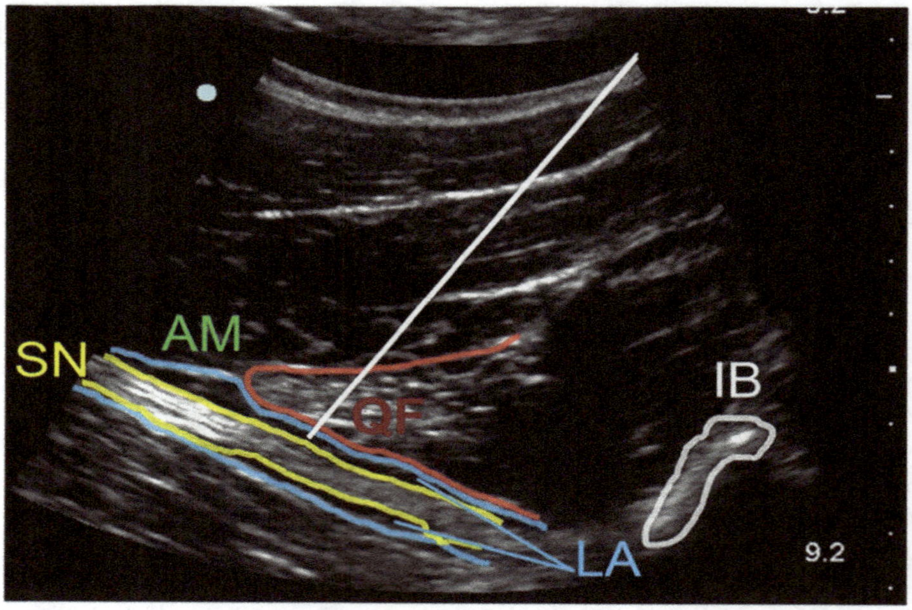

Fig. 3 Ultrasound images obtained during sciatic nerve block. The curved probe is put vertically, inferior to the needle, to see the sciatic nerve (SN) clearly. The needle (white line) was directed by an in-plane technique toward the sciatic nerve deep to the inferior border of the quadratus femoris muscle to block the sciatic nerve deep to the quadratus femoris (QF) muscle. AM = adductor magnus; IB = ischium bone; LA = localanaesthetic injected; P = pectineus; QF = quadratus femoris

followed up 24 h after surgery by an experienced nurse and an end point assessor of the outcomes who were blinded to the nature of study and not part of it. Patient's satisfaction was assessed using 4-point Likert scale through which we can assess the effectiveness of the block or spinal anaesthesia [7] (1 = very dissatisfied, 2 = unsatisfied, 3 = satisfied, 4= very satisfied) and potential complications. Visual analogue score scale was used for assessment of postoperative pain. It is a numerical rating scale where patients were taught to use this score to report the degree of postoperative pain from '0' to '10' with '0' = no pain and '10' = the worst imaginable pain. The same postoperative pain management protocol was followed for all patients. If pain score ≥ 4, patients were given fentanyl 50 μg i.v. bolus as a primary rescue analgesic which can be repeated after 1 h until pain score < 4. In addition to intravenous infusion of acetaminophen 15 mg/kg 6 hourly was administered as a secondary rescue analgesic.

Primary endpoint

Included duration of analgesia: the time to the first analgesic requirement.

Secondary endpoints

Included patient satisfaction scores, visual analogue scores, the incidence of adverse events as episodes of vomiting which was treated by metoclopramide 10 mg i.v. bolus, time to first effect of the technique, systemic toxicity of local anesthetics as seizures, cardiovascular collapse and persistent paraesthesia observed within 48 h of the block.

In case of failure of the block (persistence of pain sensation that requires completion of the procedure using either spinal or general anaesthesia) or incidence of seizures resulting from local anesthetic toxicity, general anaesthesia was given so those patients were excluded from the study.

In case of, cardiovascular collapse, the patients were treated with intravenous fluids and vasopressors.

Sample size calculation

Using Power Calculations and Sample Size software (PASS; NCSS, LLC, East Kaysville, UT, USA) revealed that 120 patients, 60 per arm, were needed after considering a 10% drop out (power of 80%; alpha error at 5%). These calculations were based on a previous study [8] that showed that.

the time to first rescue analgesic requirement (duration of analgesia) for combined sciatic and femoral block group was 336 ± 18 min.

Statistical analysis

The data were analysed using IBM SPSS Statistics for Windows (Version 23.0. Armonk, NY: IBM Corp). Normally distributed numerical data were presented as mean and SD, and skewed data were presented as median and interquartile range. Qualitative data were presented as number and percentage or ratio. Normally distributed numerical data were compared using the unpaired *t*-test. Skewed numerical data were compared using the Mann–Whitney test and categorical data were compared using Fisher's exact test. *P*-value < 0.05 was considered statistically significant.

Results

A group of 120 patients were recruited for the study (Fig. 4), out of which 107 patients were randomised then analysed (50 patients received SOFT block and 57 received spinal anaesthesia). The research team decided to exclude patients from the study either because of clinical condition or violation of the protocol. Thirteen patients were excluded from the study because of patient's withdrawal of consent (7), bilateral surgery (3), patients with unstable vital signs (3).

Demographic data, ASA status, comorbidities, and surgical data were comparable between the two study groups (Table 1).

The intention-to-treat analysis of the primary outcome revealed that the duration of analgesia in patients receiving SOFT block was (9.43 ± 2.7 h) compared with those receiving spinal anaesthesia which was (3.15 ± 1.83 min) ($p < 0.001$) (Table 2). Satisfaction scores were comparable between the study groups ($p = 0.562$) (Table 2). Non- significant difference between the study groups regarding the incidence of vomiting ($p = 0.543$) (Table 2). Only one patient of SOFT group had seizures. (Table 2). Non- significant difference between the study groups regarding the incidence of cardiovascular collapse ($p = 0.591$) and paraesthesia ($p = 0.309$) (Table 2).

The time to the first effect of SOFT was significantly longer in comparison to spinal anaesthesia ($p < 0.001$) (Table 2). Regarding visual analogue pain scores, there was no significant difference between the study groups at 1 h, 18 h, 24 h postoperative (Table 3). Visual analogue pain scores were remarkably lower in SOFT group compared with spinal group at 3 h (CI: 2.57 1-2.869),6 h (CI: 2.929–3.271) and 12 h (CI: 1.664–2.136) postoperatively (Table 3).

Discussion

SOFT is a novel efficient nerve block that is found to accomplish excellent analgesia, its success rate is similar to the earlier discussed multiple nerve block techniques without significant side-effects [5]. However, it needs to be performed by well- trained skilled anaesthetist because of its complexity, so it is not a popular technique as spinal anaesthesia [3]. Good understanding of the regional anatomy and surgical technique is mandatory for the success of the nerve block [9].

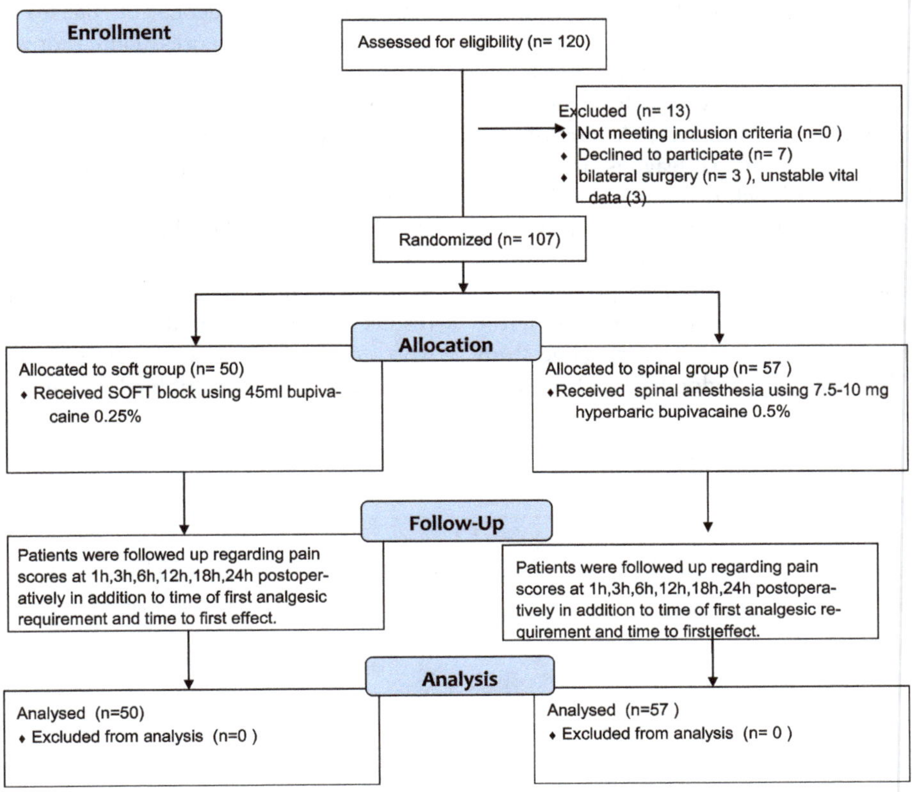

Fig. 4. Study flow chart

Table 1 Demographic data

Demographic data	SOFT group (*n* = 50)	Spinal group (*n* = 57)	P-value
Sex			
Female	26(52%)	35(61%)	0.100
Age(years)	41.53 ± 6.84	43.1 ± 5.18	0.159
ASA			
I	29(58%)	42(74%)	0.559
II	21(42%)	15(26%)	
Surgical procedure duration(min)	207.62 ± 26.78	210.44 ± 32.98	0.608

All data were presented as percentage except age and procedural duration were presented as mean ± SD

This study is the first to compare the efficacy of SOFT with spinal anaesthesia in patients scheduled for elective surgery for fixation of open tibial fractures using Ilizarov external fixator.

The results of our study showed that SOFT block resulted in longer duration of analgesia, and better patient satisfaction scores and lower pain scores postoperatively with less incidence of adverse events as back pain and headache compared with spinal anaesthesia in patients undergoing lower limb surgery.

After literature review, it was found that few studies are consistent with our findings and confirm the analgesic efficacy and safety of this block. For example, a prospective study by Taha et al. was undertaken on 50 patients undergoing knee surgeries. The success rate was 90% of the patients resulting in complete anaesthesia. The median [IQR] patient pain scores on a numeric rating scale of 1–10 was 2, and the median [IQR] performance time was 5.5 min [5]. Moreover, A randomised controlled study by Felix and his colleagues using combined sciatic-femoral nerve block or low-dose spinal anaesthesia used for patients posted for knee arthroscopy. They reported that satisfaction scores in both groups were similar. Sciatic-femoral nerve blocks provided significantly lower pain scores particularly in the first 6 postoperative hours ($p < 0.002$) [10]. A prospective study by Sermin and his friends randomised 60 patients undergoing hallux valgus repair into spinal and popliteal groups. Complications as hypotension and bradycardia of 6and 3% were encountered in spinal anaesthesia group respectively. Regarding popliteal nerve block, there was minimal incidence of complications. Visual analogue scores were significantly lower in popliteal group compared with spinal group. Time of first rescue analgesic requirement was significantly longer in popliteal group [11]. These studies support the findings in our study.

A prospective study by Akcan et al. performed on 30 patients undergoing knee arthroplasty who were randomised into spinal or femoral-sciatic nerve block group. It concluded that spinal anaesthesia group showed significantly higher incidence of nausea and hypotension, lower satisfaction scores. Pain scores were significantly lower in ultrasound guided femoral- sciatic nerve block group [12].

Similarly, a randomised trial by Mc Namee and his collegues included 60 patients undergoing knee replacement surgery using femoral sciatic in addition to obturator block concluded that the duration of analgesia was significantly prolonged (433.06 min) with no incidence of any systemic of neurologic complications [13]. Our results are in agreement with the findings of Kim et al. who compared sciatic, femoral, and lateral cutaneous nerve blocks with combined spinal epidural anaesthesia

Table 2 Comparison of the duration of analgesia, satisfaction scores and postoperative complications between the study groups

	SOFT group (*n* = 50)	Spinal group (*n* = 57)	*P*-value
Time to first analgesic requirement (hours)	9.43 ± 2.7	3.15 ± 1.83	< 0.001*
Time to first effect(min)	22.3 ± 2.07	8.03 ± 1.7	< 0.001*
Patient satisfaction scores	3.24 ± 0.64	3.3 ± 0.48	0.562
Postoperative complications			
Vomiting	5(10%)	7(12%)	0.543
Seizures	1(2%)	0(0.0%)	0.315
Cardiovascular collapse	7(14%)	9(16%)	0.591
Paraesthesia	3(6%)	1(2%)	0.309

All data were presented as percentage except the duration of block and satisfaction scores were presented as mean ± SD * *highly significant

Table 3 Comparison of visual analogue scores between the study groups

Pain scores	SOFTgroup (*n* = 50)	Spinalgroup (*n* = 57)	*P* value	95% CI
1 h	1.12 ± 0.57	1.27 ± 0.45	0.131	0.046–0.346
3 h	1.35 ± 0.36	4.07 ± 0.41	< 0.001[a]	2.571–2.869
6 h	2.13 ± 0.52	5.23 ± 0.37	< 0.001[a]	2.929–3.271
12 h	5.19 ± 0.53	7.09 ± 0.68	< 0.001[a]	1.664–2.136
18 h	3.3 ± 0.5	3.37 ± 0.53	0.485	0.128–0.268
24 h	2.17 ± 0.48	2.24 ± 0.67	0.541	0.156–0.296

[a] means highly significant

in 84 patients scheduled for knee arthroscopy as regard intraoperative patient satisfaction and the duration of postoperative analgesia. Kim noticed that the satisfaction scores were higher in sciatic femoral and lateral cutaneous nerve block group [14].

Similar to our results, Spasiano et al. investigated the efficacy of combined sciatic and femoral blocks in 32 patients undergoing knee arthroscopy. They suggested that femoral sciatic nerve block is an interesting alternative to spinal anaesthesia because the incidence of postoperative complications was negligible [3].

Performance of multiple nerve blocks requires large doses of bupivacaine so we have to be alert about the risk of LA toxicity which causes convulsions at plasma level 4 μg/ml. For this reason, enantiomer LA with lower concentration has to be used [15] and we found that it theoretically provides adequate anaesthesia for this type of surgical procedure. Some studies aimed to reducing the number of nerves blocked to decrease the risk of toxicity but it may cause inadequate anaesthesia to perform the required surgical procedures [16].

Limitations

Our study is subjected to a number of limitations including: Initially, we did not compare the success or failure rate of each block as all patients completed the study successfully (100% success rate) or the time of performance of each block. Moreover, inadequate earlier studies discussing the analgesic advantages of SOFT block as it is a novel technique so further randomised controlled studies need to be performed to prove these effects. In addition, few studies compare the efficacy of peripheral block techniques for the lower limb surgeries as an alternative to extradural or general anaesthesia, and most of them were case reports. Also, we didn't use SOFT for anaesthetic management for surgical procedures of urgent context or prolonged duration. Additional studies are needed to calculate the optimal dose of LA used in combined nerve blocks depending on the nature and duration of the surgical procedure.

Conclusions

Our results showed that SOFT block is a feasible technique of local anaesthesia for control of postoperative pain with unremarkable adverse events compared with spinal anaesthesia, in patients undergoing fixation of open tibial fractures using Ilizarov external fixator.

Abbreviations

ASA: American society of anesthesiologists; LA: Local anaesthetic; PASS: Power calculations and sample size software; SOFT: Sciatic obturator femoral technique

Acknowledgements

Not applicable.

Authors' contributions

HS: Conception and design, editing of manuscript, data collection and analysis and revision of the manuscript. AK: Editing of manuscript, data collection and analysis and revision of the manuscript. All authors have read and approved the final manuscript.

Author details

[1]Assistant Professor of Anaesthesiology, Ain Shams University, Cairo, Egypt. [2]Lecturer of Anaesthesiology, Ain Shams University, Cairo, Egypt.

References

1. Lumb AB. Anesthesia for vascular surgery on extremities. Anesth Intensive Care Med. 2004 June;5:207–2 10.
2. Mansour A. Femoral Nerve Block versus Spinal Anesthesia for Lower Limb Peripheral Vascular Surgery. AJAIC. 2006;(9) No. 1.
3. Spasiano A, Flore I, Pesamosca A, Della RG. Comparison between spinal anaesthesia and sciatic-femoral block for arthroscopic knee surgery. Minerva Anestesiol. 2007;73:13–21. 17159764.
4. Sato K, Sai S, Shirai N, Adachi T. Ultrasound guided Obturator versus sciatic nerve block in addition to continuous femoral nerve block for analgesia after Total knee Arthroplasty. Jpn Clin Med. 2011;2:29–34.
5. Taha AM, Darwich N. SOFT block (Sciatic, Obturator and Femoral nerve block Technique): a single-puncture, sole anesthetic for knee surgery. Can J Anesth/J Can Anesth. 2017;64:1279–81.
6. Schulz KF, Altman DG, Moher D. CONSORT 2010 statement: updated guidelines for reporting parallel group randomised trials. BMC Med. 2010;8:18.
7. Jamieson S. Likert scales: how to (Ab) Use them. Med Educ. 2004;38:1217.
8. Sansone V, De Ponti A, Fanelli G , Agostoni M. Combined sciatic and femoral block for knee arthroscopy: 4 years experience. Arch Orthop Trauma 1999; 119: 163–169.
9. Mitchell ME. Regional anesthesia for hip surgery. Tech Reg Anesth Pain Manag. 1999;3:94–106.
10. Monte FR, Zarate E, Grueso R, Giraldo JC. Comparison of spinal anesthesia with combined sciatic-femoral nerve block for outpatient knee arthroscopy. J Clin Anesth. 2008;20:415–20.
11. Karaasaln S, Tuncel Z, Semsek E, Turan M, Karamen Y. Comparison between ultrasound guided popliteal sciatic nerve block and spinal anesthesia for hallux valgus repair. Foot & Ankle Int. 2016;37(1):85–9.
12. Akkay A, Yasar U, Demirhan A, Engin K.Ultrasound-guided femoral and

sciatic nerve blocks combined with sedoanalgesia versus spinal anesthesia in total knee arthroplasty. Korean J Anesthesiol 2014 67(2): 90–95 http://dx.doi.org/https://doi.org/10.4097/kjae.2014.67.2.90.
13. Mc Namee DA, Parks L, Milligan TR. Post-operative analgesia following total knee replacement: an evaluation of the addition of an obturator nerve block to combined femoral and sciatic nerve block. Acta Anaesthesiol Scand. 2002 Jan;46(1):95–9.
14. Kim JH, Cho MR, Kim SO, Kim JE, Lee DK, Roh WS. A comparison of femoral/sciatic nerve block with lateral femoral cutaneous nerve block and combined spinal epidural anesthesia for total knee replacement arthroplasty. Korean J Anesthesiol. 2012;62:448–53. 22679542.
15. Taha AM, Ghoneim MA. Hip hemiarthroplasty using major lower limb nerve blocks: a preliminary report of a case series. Saudi J Anaesth. 2014;8:355–8.
16. Taha AM, Abd-Elmaksoud AA. Arthroscopic medial meniscus trimming or repair under nerve blocks: Which nerves should be blocked? Saudi J Anaesth. 2016 Jul-Sep;10(3):283–7. https://doi.org/10.4103/1658-354X.174912.

Dural sac cross-sectional area is a highly effective parameter for spinal anesthesia in geriatric patients undergoing transurethral resection of the prostate

Wei Bing Wang*, Ai Jiao Sun, Hong Ping Yu, Jing Chun Dong and Huang Xu

Abstract

Background: Spinal anesthesia is optimal choice for transurethral resection of the prostate (TURP), but the sensory block should not cross the T10 level. With advancing age, the sensory blockade level increases after spinal injection in some patients with spinal canal stenosis. We optimize the dose of spinal anesthesia according to the decreased ratio of the dural sac cross-sectional area (DSCSA), the purpose of this study is to hypothesis that if DSCSA is an effective parameter to modify the dosage of spinal anesthetics to achieve a T10 blockade in geriatric patients undergoing TURP.

Methods: Sixty geriatric patients schedule for TURP surgery were enrolled in this study. All subjects were randomized divided into two groups, the ultrasound (group U) and the control (group C) groups, patient receive either a dose of 2 ml of 0.5% isobaric bupivacaine in group C, or a modified dose of 0.5% isobaric bupivacaine in group U. We measured the sagittal anteroposterior diameter (D) of the dural sac at the L3–4 level with ultrasound, and calculated the approximate DSCSA (A) according to the following formula: $A = \pi(D/2)^2$, ($\pi = 3.14$). The modified dosage of bupivacaine was adjusted according to the decreased ratio of the DSCSA.

Results: The cephalad spread of the sensory blockade level was significantly lower ($P < 0.001$) in group U (T10, range T7–T12) compared with group C (T3, range T2–T9). The dosage of bupivacaine was significantly decreased in group U compared with group C ($P < 0.001$). The regression times of the two segments were delay in group U compared with group C ($P < 0.001$). The maximal decrease in MAP was significantly higher in the group C than in group U after spinal injection ($P < 0.001$), without any modifications HR in either group. Eight patients in group C and two patients in group U required ephedrine ($P = 0.038$).

(Continued on next page)

* Correspondence: w2bwang@sina.com
Department of Anesthesiology, The Affiliated AnQing Hospitals of Anhui Medical University, 352th, Renming Road, AnQing 246003, AnHui province, China

(Continued from previous page)

Conclusions: The DSCSA is a highly effective parameter for spinal anesthesia in geriatric patients undergoing TURP, a modified dose of local anesthetic is a critical factor for controlling the sensory level.

Keywords: Transurethral resection of the prostate, Geriatric, Spinal anesthesia, Bupivacaine, Dural sac cross-sectional area

Background

Benign prostatic hyperplasia has a high incidence rate about 60% among males aged more than 60 years [1]; whereas the rate is up to 90% among patients around 80 years [2]. The high comorbidity rate also directly affecting perioperative morbidity and mortality after TURP [3, 4].

Because of the pain signal from bladder distension travels along the T11 to L2 sympathetic fibers. The stretch sensation of the bladder is carried by the S2 to S4 parasympathetic fibers. Considering this innervation, the height of the regional blockade level up to T10 is sufficient for TURP operation. A higher level of blockade may mask the pain upon perforation of the prostatic capsule. Intrathecal anesthesia is optimal choice for TURP, but the height should not cross the T10 level. The factors such as concentration and volume are the major factors affecting the distribution of local anesthetics after spinal injection [5].

Hypotension is the major risk after the spinal injection. The systemic vascular resistance may decrease by 25% in elderly patients, whereas it may decrease only by 15–18% in normovolemic healthy patients [6]. Because the functional of critical organ and compensate ability for stresses are decreased, it is harmful for geriatric patients to inject more local anesthetics [7]. Thus, it is important to optimize the dosage of spinal anesthetics for geriatric patients.

Spinal anesthesia can reduce the stress response relate to surgery [8], and recognize the TUR syndrome early. The patient can complain of shoulder or periumbilical pain with spinal anesthesia level is less than T10 [9]. It is necessary to diagnosis and effective management the TUR syndrome timely [10]. In a case report, the authors emphasize that it is very important to diagnosis and treatment the TURP syndrome early, the patient have not been found developed hyponatremia until decreased to 90 mmol l^{-1} under general anesthesia during a TURP procedure [11]. The patients can clearly describe the early features of TUR syndrome when patient is conscious, so spinal anesthesia is therefore desirable to facilitate early recognition [10].

The major challenges of spinal anesthesia for geriatric patient are the changes of anatomical and physiological. Some of anatomical irregularities and physiological changes such as reduction in the number of neurons, especially spinal canal stenosis, etc. always associated with increasing age. The blockade level increases after epidural anesthesia and spinal anesthesia [12, 13].

Previous study shown that the depth of intrathecal spaces can accurate prediction by ultrasound imaging [14]. A > 30% reduction in the DSCSA and sagittal anteroposterior diameter has been observed in patients with lumbar spinal stenosis [15]. The DSCSA is a more sensitive measurement parameter to predict lumbar central canal spinal stenosis [16]. Thus, measuring the sagittal anteroposterior diameter of the dural sac with ultrasound can evaluate the degree of lumbar central canal spinal stenosis.

Optimal blockade levels by intrathecal anesthesia is favorable for TURP operation for adequate blockade of the stimulation of bladder traction and less hypotension and bradycardia by too high thoracic block. For geriatric patients, sensory blockade up to T10 is favorable for adequate anesthesia with less hypotension and bradycardia. Most anesthesiologists may reduce the dosage of intrathecal anesthetics to prevent too high blockade by experience. However, as lumbar central canal spinal stenosis is more frequently found in geriatric patients, we hypothesized that local anesthetics would spread more cephalad with a limited space. With goal to achieve T10 sensory blockade in patients receiving TURP operation, we modified the dose of bupivacaine according to the decreased ratio of the DSCSA. By comparing with controlled groups receiving 10 mg of 0.5% isobaric bupivacaine, we analysis the levels of sensory blockade, and the changes of mean arterial blood pressure (MAP) and heart rate (HR).

The purpose of present study is to determine the hypothesis that if DSCSA is an effective parameter to modify the dosage of spinal anesthetics to achieve a T10 blockade in geriatric patients undergoing TURP.

Methods

Design

We conducted a prospective, double blinded, randomized study to measure the sagittal anteroposterior diameter of the dural sac by ultrasound for geriatric patients aged more than70 years undergoing TURP with spinal anesthesia, and then calculated the DSCSA, optimizing the dosage of local anesthetic according to the decreased ratio of the DSCSA.

Subjects and setting

Sixty geriatric patients schedule for TURP surgery were enrolled in this study. The medical ethical committees of The Affiliated AnQing Hospital of Anhui Medical University approved this study on 26, December, 2017, and the study was registered in the Chinese Clinical Trial Registry (Registration number: ChiCTR1800015566). The informed consent were written by all patients.

The exclusion criteria of this study as following: local infection at the puncture site, administrated with anticoagulants, intracranial hypertension, and patients who did not to accept spinal anesthesia. Relative contraindications included some neurologic diseases (e.g. multiple sclerosis), lower limbs pain, and so on.

Study protocol

All subjects were randomized divided into two groups, the ultrasound (group U, $n = 30$) and the control (group C, $n = 30$) groups, according to the random number table generator by computer (prepared by AJS).

All patients transported to the operating room, where they were subjected to standard monitoring electrocardiography (ECG), and pulse oximetry (SPO_2). The MAP and HR were monitored throughout the operation also.

All intrachecal anesthesia operation was performed by the same anesthesiologist (an associate chief physician of anesthesiology). Epidural puncture was located at the L 3–4 intervertebral space, the spinal needle was inserted into the subarachnoid space after successfully epidural puncture, 2 ml of 0.5% isobaric bupivacaine was injected in group C, and group U received a modified dose according to the DSCSA measured by ultrasound when cerebrospinal fluid (CSF) appeared in the needle hub. Then, the spinal needle was withdrawn.

Measurements

MAP and HR were measured every 2.5 min during surgery in the first 30 min after spinal injection and, then every 15 min until the end of the study.

The cephalad sensory level was measured via a cold alcohol cotton swab every 5 min until 30 min after the spinal injection and, then every 15 min until regression below L4. Ten minutes after the spinal injection, if the sensory blockade level was below T10, remifentanil 0.1–0.2 $\mu g\ kg^{-1}\ min^{-1}$ was treated intravenous continuous infusion to maintain a sufficient analgesia level.

The motor block level was measured by modified Bromage scale every 5 min until 30 min after the spinal injection and, then every 15 min until complete motor recovery occurred. Modified Bromage scale: 0: able to move the hip, knee, ankle, and toes; 1: able to move the knee, ankle, and toes; 2: able to move the ankle and toes; 3: only able to move the toes; and 4: unable to move the hip, knee, ankle, and toes.

The local anesthetics was prepared by an anesthesia assistant (HPY), and she did not assessed all patients. Another anesthesiologist (JCD or HX) assessed the cephalad sensory level and measured the Bromage scale, who remained blinded to the local anesthetics.

If the systolic blood pressure decrease more than 30% compare with the baseline, intravenous 5 to 10 mg ephedrine was treated, and a HR of less than 45 beats min^{-1}, intravenous 0.5 mg atropine was treated.

We assessed and recorded the variables, the maximal sensory level, sensory level regression by 2 dermatomes, and complete motor block recovery.

Image analysis

A previous study indicated that 10 mg of 0.5% intrathecal bupivacaine provided a sufficient level of sensory blockade for elderly patients undergoing TURP [17]. Lim YS et al. [16] showed that the average DSCSA was $151.67 \pm 53.59\ mm^2$ in the control group (without lumbar central canal spinal stenosis) and $80.04 \pm 35.36\ mm^2$ in the lumbar central canal spinal stenosis group. Thus, we hypothesized that the dosage would be more excessive for some geriatric patients with lumbar central canal spinal stenosis, and that would be a greater cephalad spread of local anesthetics. We measured the sagittal anteroposterior diameter (D) of the dural sac at L3–4 with ultrasound, and calculated the approximate DSCSA (A) according to the formula: $A = \pi(D/2)^2$, ($\pi = 3.14$). For example, to determine the DSCSA (Fig. 1), the diameter (the distance between AC and PC) of the dural sac was measured. The diameter shown in the picture A was 14.3 mm, and the DSCSA was 160.5 mm^2. However, another diameter shown in the picture B was 9.0 mm, and the DSCSA was 63.6 mm^2.

Modified dose of bupivacaine

We confirmed that the primary DSCSA was 150 mm^2 and that the primary dose of bupivacaine was 10 mg. The modified dose of bupivacaine was adjusted according to the decreased ratio of the DSCSA compared with the primary DSCSA of 150 mm^2. For example, if we measured the D of the dural sac to be 10 mm, then, A = 78.5 mm^2, and the decreased in the ratio of DSCSA was 48% ((150–78.5)/150 = 0.48), thus, the modified dose of bupivacaine was decreased by 48%, so 5.2(10–10*0.48 = 5.2) mg bupivacaine was spinally injected.

Statistical analysis

We using G*Power software to estimate the sample size. Taking into consideration the results of previous studies, we set an alpha as 0.05 and a power as 0.8, the result of

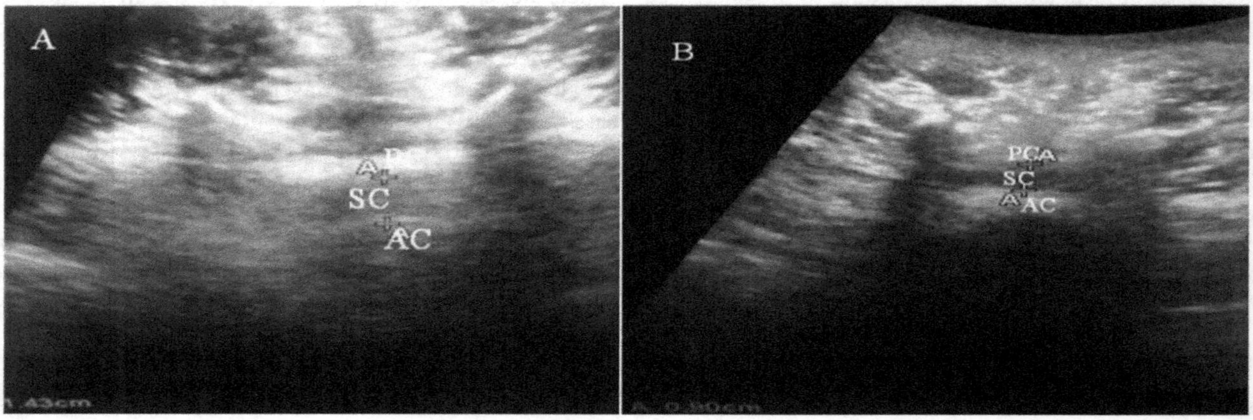

Fig. 1 SC = spinal canal, AC = anterior complexus, including the posterior longitudinal ligament and vertebral ligament, PC = posterior complexus, including the ligamentum flavum and endorhachis

software shown that at least 26 patients in each group, therefore, 30 patients in each group was a sufficient sample size.

The various parameters were statistically analysed using the SPSS 17.0 (SPSS Inc., Chicago, IL, USA). Continuous data were evaluated with independent samples t-test, sensory level with Mann-Whitney U test, and frequency data with Chi square test. $P < 0.05$ was considered statistically significant.

Results

The patients flow diagram of this study is shown in Fig. 2. Seventy patients were assessed for eligibility for this study, four patients refused to participate this study and six patients did not meet the inclusion criteria, and finally 60 patients were randomly divided into two groups, 30 patients in each group.

Demographic characteristics (age, weight, height), ASA classification, duration of surgery, dosage of bupivacaine

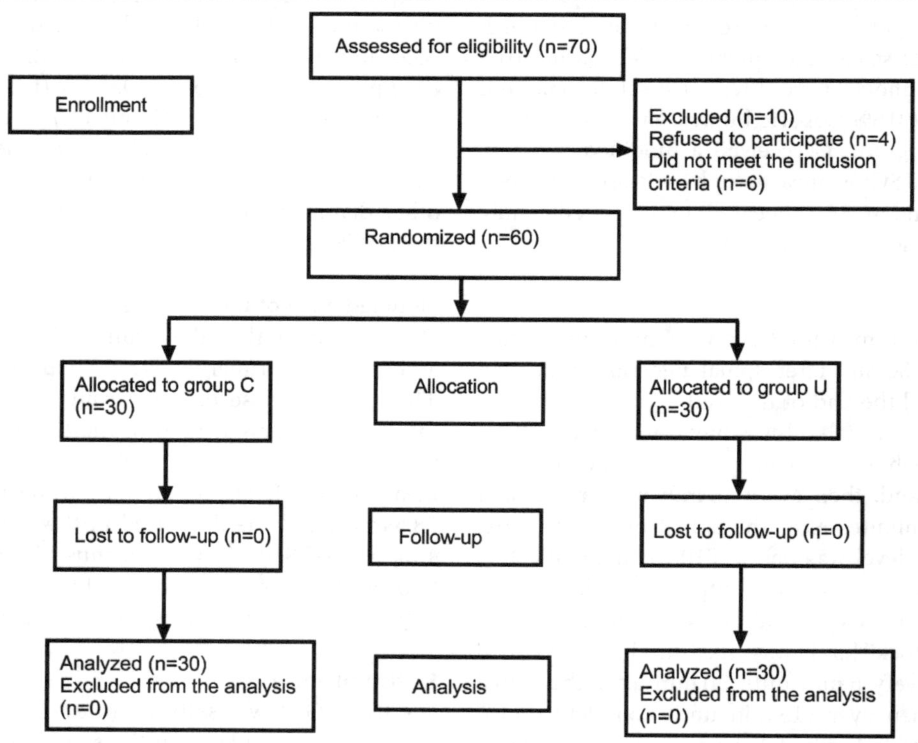

Fig. 2 CONSORT flow diagram

and DSCSA were compared in two groups (Table 1). The dosage of bupivacaine was significantly decreased ($P < 0.001$) in group U compared with group C.

The main data of the spinal anesthesia were collected and shown in Table 2. The evolution of the sensory blockade level were shown in Fig. 3. The cephalad spread of the sensory blockade level was significantly lower ($P < 0.001$) in group U (T10, range T7–T12) compared with group C (T3, range T2–T9). The regression times of the two segments were delay in group U than in group C ($P < 0.001$, Table 2).

Figure 4a and b represents the evolution of the MAP and HR in the first 30 min of the study, respectively. The maximal decrease in MAP was significantly higher in the group C than in group U after spinal injection ($P <$ 0.001, Table 3). Eight patients in group C and two patients in group U required ephedrine ($P = 0.038$, Table 3).

Discussion

The purpose of this study was to determinate the relationship between the DSCSA and the dose of local anesthetic. Two groups with the same demographic date were compared but injected with different doses of bupivacaine to show the highest spreads level up to T3 in group C and T10 in group U, (Table 2.). The results confirm our hypothesis, a higher cephalad spread would occur without a modified dose in group C, and a higher cephalad spread would not occur with a modified dose according to the DSCSA in group U.

A questionnaire based on Japanese population for predicting lumbar stenosis, the results shown that the incidence increased with age, with an incidence of 1.7–2.2% between ages 40 and 49, and of 10.3–11.2% between ages 70 and 79 [18]. In our study, the dosage of bupivacaine was significantly lower in group U than in group C ($P < 0.001$, Table 1.). This finding may be related to the lumbar stenosis in some geriatric patients. Low dose of local anesthetic is the important reason to limit the higher cephalad spread.

Table 1 Demographic characteristics, ASA status, duration of surgery, dose of anesthetics and DSCSA (Mean ± SD)

	Group C ($n = 30$)	Group U ($n = 30$)	*P*-value
Age (years)	78.3 ± 5.8	77.4 ± 5.5	0.555
Height (cm)	169.0 ± 6.9	169.6 ± 7.2	0.771
Weight (kg)	65.9 ± 8.9	66.0 ± 8.6	0.977
ASA(I / II / III)	16/10/ 4	18 /9/ 3	0.855
Duration of surgery (min)	92.4 ± 17.8	86.2 ± 19.3	0.354
DSCSA(mm^2)	106.8 ± 8.2	102.5 ± 7.6	0.924
Dose of bupivacaine (mg)	10.0 ± 0.0	6.7 ± 1.6	< 0.001

ASA American Society of Anesthesiologists, *DSCSA* dural sac cross-sectional area

Table 2 Main data of the spinal block

	Group C ($n = 30$)	Group U ($n = 30$)	*P*-value
Maximal sensory level	T3(T2-T9)	T10(T7-T12)	< 0.001
Onset time to maximal sensory block (min)	25.2 ± 10.4	26.3 ± 12.2	0.636
Regression by 2 segments (min)	102.0 ± 28.2	156.1 ± 42.3	< 0.001
Total motor recovery (min)	186.2 ± 58.0	175.1 ± 44.2	0.620

Degenerative spondylosis is a significant etiology of lumbar spinal stenosis. Wear-and-tear changes and trauma, among other factors, such as lumbar disc herniation, ligamentum flavum hypertrophy, osteoporosis, posterior longitudinal ligament ossification, the spinal venous plexus proliferation, and congenital stenosis, which in turn will cause spinal stenosis, occur with aging [19]. Therefore, the traditional dose of local anesthetics may be excessively for patients with lumbar spinal stenosis. It is unclear whether this is the case for patient with lumbar spinal stenosis, so it is important for anesthesiologists to control the sensory level for each patient. The greater the cephalad spread is, the higher the incidence of hypotension and bradycardia.

The MAP was significantly decreased in group C compared with group U (Table 3.). Previous studies [20] shown the same results as our finding, and it may be related to widely sympathetic block caused by excessive bupivacaine with the higher cephalic sensory level in group C, so it needs more ephedrine to maintain the MAP in group C than in group U ($P = 0.038$, Table 3).

The regression times of the two segments were significantly longer in group U than in group C ($P < 0.001$, Table 2). The spread and eliminate of local anesthetics after spinal injection could be explained by its pharmacokinetics. The arachnoidal and dural was determinate the eliminate of local anesthetics, and it's concentration gradient was determinate by vascular absorption in epidural venous plexus. Simultaneously, the subarachnoid space venous plexus also absorbed local anesthetics. If the blockade level is high accordingly the dosage of bupivacaine to block a segment is low. It require a greater meningeal surface to eliminate local anesthetics if the block level is spread greater.

Patients undergoing TURP are generally older and have various comorbidities [4]. It is important to restrict the blockade level to maintain the hemodynamic instability after spinal injection. Although there are many factors that determines the sensory level, including the dosage of local anesthetic and not by the block position, anesthetic volume, or concentration [21–23]. Therefore, the dosage of spinal injection should be decreased in

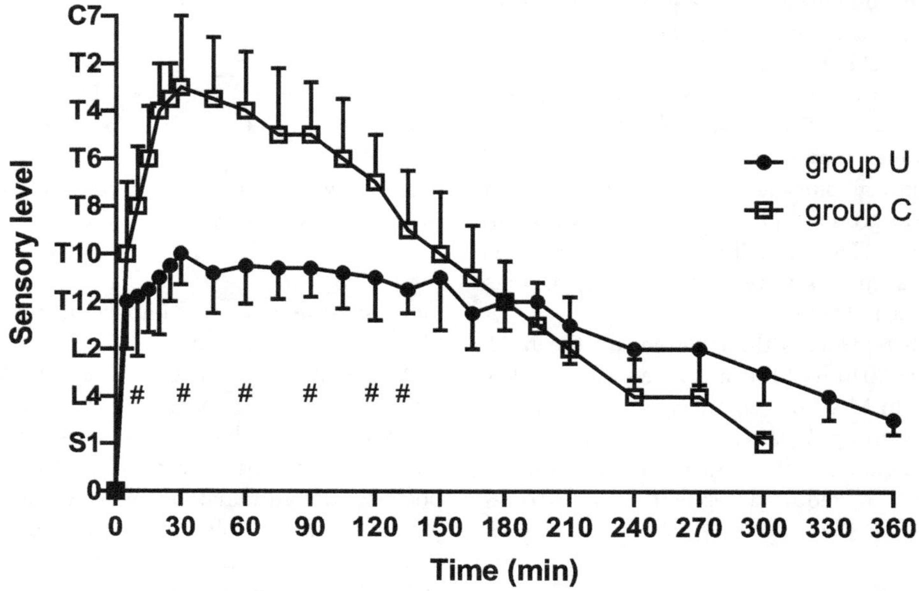

Fig. 3 Evolution of the sensory level over time in two groups, the sensory level were higher from 10 to 135 min after spinal injection in group C than in group U, #$P < 0.001$

order to restrict the blockade level. Most anesthesiologists think that decreased the dosage of spinal injection may induce insufficient spinal block. There were many studies to balance between the low dose of spinal injection and insufficient spinal block, the coadministration of additives such as opioids or dexmedetomidine was together with spinal injection to improve the block quality [17, 24]. However, the complications such as bradycardia, hypotension, vomiting, nausea, pruritus and excessive sedation were emerged after the coadministration [25–27]. Compare with the normal population, the DSCSA was a 30% decrease in patients aged more than 70(Table 1), so we suggest a 30% reduction of bupivacaine for patients aged more than 70, especially measure DSCSA for each patient around 80 before performing spinal anesthesia. The benefits of DSCSA-adjusted dosage for intrathecal anesthesia includes less hypotensive episodes and less ephedrine to treat them.

In addition, a higher cephalad blockade level is not required for TURP surgery, and a T10 is sufficient sensory level. The sympathetic such as pelvic plexus and hypogastric plexus, and parasympathetic such as S_3 and S_4 dominate prostate and bladder. Because of the urethral internal sphincter and external sphincter are dominated by the pelvic plexus and the pudendal nerve respectively, both of the nerves were block, and then the urethral sphincter would be adequately relaxed and the endoscope could pass smoothly. A previous study shown that T12–L1 sensory block was sufficient for TURP to avoid discomfort due to irrigation-induced bladder distension, but there were more many patients required analgesics during the postoperative period [3]. In our study, only one patient who showed abdominal discomfort with sensory level regression to <T10 because the duration of surgery exceeded 2 h in group U, remifentanil 0.1μg kg^{-1} min^{-1} was treated intravenous continuous infusion for abdominal discomfort during the operation, 20 min after, the surgery was finished.

The most anatomical change in geriatric patients is lumbar central canal spinal stenosis. The most frequently applied criteria are the measurement of the anteroposterior diameter of the cross-sectional area of the dural sac and of the osseous spinal canal for lumbar central canal spinal stenosis [28]. Thus, the analysis of the DSCSA is very important for anesthesiologists to evaluate the degree of lumbar central canal spinal stenosis in each patient. Currently, the optimal cut-off value of 111.09 mm^2 for the DSCSA has a high sensitivity (80.0%) and specificity (80.8%) for predicting lumbar central canal spinal stenosis [14]. This optimal cut-off value is less than that of some patients without lumbar central canal spinal stenosis. Therefore, greater cephalad spread results from an excessive dose without regulation according to the DSCSA in group C.

There were several limitations of the current study. Unlike magnetic resonance imaging (MRI), ultrasound cannot be used to accurately discriminate the AC from PC, thus, some errors may arise in the sagittal anteroposterior diameter of the dural sac. Second, the DSCSA is not a normal circle, so, the DSCSA we calculated according to the formula is only an approximate value. Third, the research population included a small number

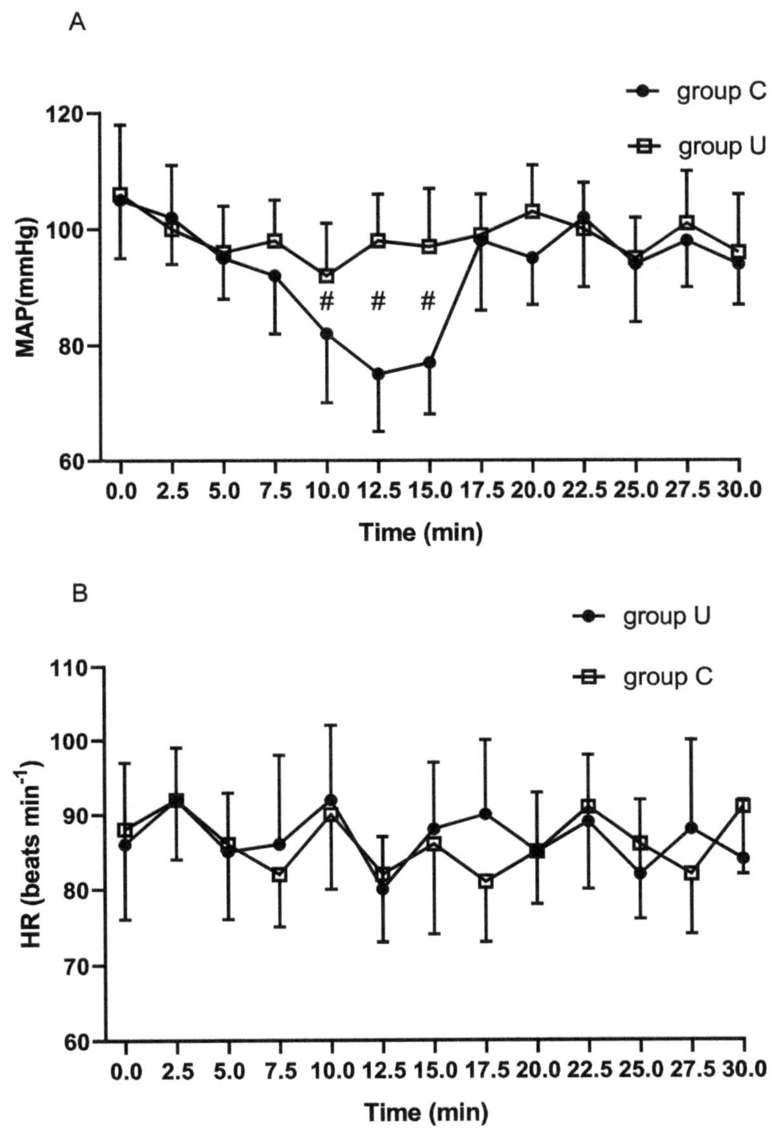

Fig. 4 a The changes of the MAP over the first 30 min after spinal injection in two groups, the MAP were significent decreased at the time of 10 min, 12.5 min and 15 min in group C than in group U, $^{\#}P< 0.001$. **b** The changes of the HR over the first 30 min after spinal injection in two groups, there were no significent different at each time in two groups

Table 3 Hemodynamic characteristics

	Group C ($n = 30$)	Group U ($n = 30$)	P-value
Baseline MAP (mmHg)	105.3 ± 10.2	106.0 ± 12.0	0.865
Baseline HR (beats min^{-1})	82.3 ± 10.2	86.0 ± 9.2	0.726
Maximal decrease in MAP (% of baseline value)	26.2 ± 13.3	12.2 ± 10.1	< 0.001
Number of patients receiving ephedrine	8	2	0.038

MAP mean arterial pressure, *HR* heart rate

of lumbar central canal spinal stenosis patients. The demographic characteristics, such as weight, height and degree of obesity still various.

Despite these limitations, the results are important for spinal anesthesia in geriatric patients to compare the DSCSA and the dose of local anesthetics.

Conclusions

The DSCSA is a highly effective parameter for spinal anesthesia in geriatric patients undergoing TURP, a modified dose of local anesthetic is a critical factor for controlling the sensory level.

Abbreviations

TURP: Transurethral resection of the prostate; DSCSA: Dural sac cross-sectional area; MAP: Mean arterial blood pressure; HR: Heart rate; CSF: Cerebro-spinal fluid; NIBP: Noninvasive blood pressure; ECG: Electrocardiography; SpO_2: Peripheral capillary oxygen saturation; MRI: Magnetic resonance imaging

Acknowledgements

The authors sincerely thank all staff members in the Department of anesthesia and operating room of The Affiliated AnQing Hospitals of Anhui Medical University. The authors sincerely thank AiJiao Sun, M. D for his contributions to the randomization design and his assistance with the study. The authors acknowledge Dr. HongPing Yu, who performed data extraction, and Dr. JingChun Dong and Dr. Huang Xu, who helped review the study design and date analysis.

Authors' contributions

WBW and AJS design the study, acquisition of data by HPY and JCD, drafting of the article and critical revision by WBW and HX, and all authors agree with the final version to be submitted and any revisions.

References

1. Arrighi HM, Metter EJ, Guess HA, Fozzard JL. Natural history of benign prostatic hyperplasia and risk of prostatectomy. The Baltimore longitudinal study of aging. Urology. 1991;38(1 Suppl):4–8.
2. Berry SJ, Coffey DS, Walsh PC, Ewing LL. The development of human benign prostatic hyperplasia with age. J Urol. 1984;132:474–9.
3. Kim SY, Cho JE, Hong JY, Koo BN, Kim JM, Kil HK. Comparison of intrathecal fentanyl and sufentanil in low-dose dilute bupivacaine spinal anesthesia for transurethral prostatectomy. Br J Anaesth. 2009;103:750–4.
4. Hong JY, Yang SC, Ahn S, Kil HK. Preoperative comorbidities and relationship of comorbidities with postoperative complications in patients undergoing transurethral prostate resection. J Urol. 2011;185:1374–8.
5. Tuominan M. Bupivacaine spinal anesthesia. Acta Anaesthesiol Scand. 1991;35:1.
6. Rooke GA, Freund PR, Jacobson AF. Hemodynamic response and change in organ blood volume during spinal anesthesia in elderly men with cardiac disease. Anesth Analg. 1997;85:99–105.
7. Cook DJ, Rooke GA. Priorities in perioperative geriatrics. Anesth Analg. 2003; 96(6):1823–36.
8. O'Donnell A, Foo I. Anaesthesia for transurethral resection of the prostate. Contin Educ Anaesth Crit Care Pain. 2009;9:92–6.
9. Lynch M, Anson K. Time to rebrand transurethral resection of the prostate? Curr Opin Urol. 2006;16:20–4.
10. McGowan-Smyth S, Vasdev N, Gowrie-Mohan S. Spinal anesthesia facilitates the early recognition of TUR syndrome. Curr Urol. 2016;9(2):57–61.
11. Demirel I, Ozer AB, Bayar MK, Erhan OL. TURP syndrome and severe hyponatremia under general anaesthesia. BMJ Case Rep. 2012;2012:bcr-2012.
12. Simon MJ, Veering BT, Stienstra R, van Kleef JW, Burm AG. The effects of age on neural blockade and hemodynamic changes after epidural anesthesia with ropivacaine. Anesth Analg. 2002;94:1325–30.
13. Tsui BC, Wagner A, Finucane B. Regional anaesthesia in the elderly: a clinical guide. Drugs Aging. 2004;21:895–910.
14. Chin KJ, Perlas A. Ultrasonography of the lumbar spine for neuraxial and lumbar plexus blocks. Curr Opin Anaesthesiol. 2011;24(5):567–72.
15. Lau YYO, Lee RKL, Griffith JF, Chan CLY, Law SW, Kwok KO. Changes in dural sac caliber with standing MRI improve correlation with symptoms of lumbar spinal stenosis. Eur Spine J. 2017;26(10):2666–75.
16. Lim YS, Mun JU, Seo MS, Sang BH, Bang YS, Kang KN, Koh JW, Kim YU. Dural sac area is a more sensitive parameter for evaluating lumbar spinal stenosis than spinal canal area: a retrospective study. Medicine (Baltimore). 2017; 96(49):e9087.
17. Doger C, Yüksel BE, Canoler O, Ornek D, Emre C, Kahveci K. Effects of intrathecal bupivacaine and bupivacaine plus sufentanil in elderly patients undergoing transurethral resection. Niger J Clin Pract. 2014;17(2):149–53.
18. Yabuki S, Fukumori N, Takegami M, Onishi Y, Otani K, Sekiguchi M, Wakita T, Kikuchi S, Fukuhara S, Konno S. Prevalence of lumbar spinal stenosis, using the diagnostic support tool, and correlated factors in Japan: a population-based study. J Orthop Sci. 2013;18(6):893–900.
19. Wu L, Cruz R. Lumbar Spinal Stenosis. StatPearls [Internet]. Treasure Island (FL): StatPearls Publishing; 2019 Jan-2018 Oct 27.
20. Kooger Infante NE, Van Gessel E, Forster A, Gamulin Z. Extent of hyperbaric spinal anesthesia influences the duration of spinal block. Anesthesiology. 2000;92(5):1319–23.
21. Pitkanen M. Spinal (subarachnoid) blockade. Neural blockade in clinical anesthesia and pain medicine. In: Cousins MJ, Carr DB, Horlocker TT, Bridenbaugh PO, editors. Wolters Kluwer Health, vol. 4. Philadelphia: Lippincott Williams & Wilkins; 2009. p. 221.
22. Ruppen W, Steiner LA, Drewe J, Hauenstein L, Brugger S, Seeberger MD. Bupivacaine concentrations in the lumbar cerebrospinal fluid of patients during spinal anaesthesia. Br J Anaesth. 2009;102:832–8.
23. Veering BT, Immink-Speet TT, Burm AG, Stienstra R, van Kleef JW. Spinal anaesthesia with 0.5% hyperbaric bupivacaine in elderly patients: effects of duration spent in the sitting position. Br J Anaesth. 2001;87:738–42.
24. Chattopadhyay I, Banerjee SS, Jha AK, Basu S. Effects of intrathecal dexmedetomidine as an additive to low-dose bupivacaine in patients undergoing transurethral resection of prostate. Indian J Anaesth. 2017; 61(12):1002–8.
25. Ozbek H, Deniz MN, Erakgun A, Erhan E. Comparison of 75 and 150 μg doses of intrathecal morphine for postoperative analgesia after transurethral resection of the prostate under spinal anesthesia. J Opioid Manag. 2013;9(6): 415–20.
26. Akan B, Yagan O, Bilal B, Erdem D, Gogus N. Comparison of levobupivacaine alone and in combination with fentanyl and sufentanil in patients undergoing transurethral resection of the prostate. J Res Med Sci. 2013; 18(5):378–82.
27. Kaur N, Goneppanavar U, Venkateswaran R, Iyer SS. Comparative effects of buprenorphine and dexmedetomidine as adjuvants to bupivacaine spinal anaesthesia in elderly male patients undergoing transurethral resection of prostrate: a randomized prospective study. Anesth Essays Res. 2017;11(4): 886–91.
28. Macedo LG, Bodnar A, Battie MC. A comparison of two methods to evaluate a narrow spinal canal: routine magnetic resonance imaging versus three-dimensional reconstruction. Spine J. 2016;16:884–8.

24

Effects of combined warmed preoperative forced-air and warmed perioperative intravenous fluids on maternal temperature during cesarean section

Ting-ting Ni[1], Zhen-feng Zhou[2], Bo He[3] and Qing-he Zhou[4*]

Abstract

Background: Preventing the frequent perioperative hypothermia incidents that occur during elective caesarean deliveries would be beneficial. This trial aimed at evaluating the effect of preoperative forced-air warming alongside perioperative intravenous fluid warming in women undergoing cesarean sections under spinal anesthesia.

Methods: We randomly allocated 135 women undergoing elective cesarean deliveries to either the intervention group (preoperative forced-air and intravenous fluid warming, $n = 69$) or the control group (no active warming, $n = 66$). The primary outcome measure was the core temperature change between groups from baseline to the end of the surgical procedure. Secondary outcomes included thermal comfort scores, the incidences of shivering and hypothermia (< 36 °C), the core temperature on arrival at the post-anesthesia care unit, neonatal axillary temperature at birth, and Apgar scores.

Results: Two-way repeated measures ANOVA revealed significantly different core temperature changes (from the pre-spinal temperature to that at the end of the procedure) between groups ($F = 13.022$, $P < 0.001$). The thermal comfort scores were also higher in the intervention group than in the control group ($F = 9.847$, $P = 0.002$). The overall incidence of perioperative hypothermia was significantly lower in the intervention group than in the control group (20.6% vs. 51.6%, $P < 0.0001$).

Conclusions: Warming preoperative forced-air and perioperative intravenous fluids may prevent maternal hypothermia, reduce maternal shivering, and improve maternal thermal comfort for patients undergoing cesarean sections under spinal anesthesia.

Keywords: Cesarean section, Spinal anesthesia, Warming

* Correspondence: jxxmxy@163.com
[4]Department of Anesthesiology, The Affiliated Hospital of Jiaxing University, Jiaxing, Zhejiang Province, China

Background

Neuraxial (spinal, epidural, or combined spinal–epidural techniques) anesthesia is the preferred anesthetic technique for cesarean deliveries. Perioperative hypothermia is a commonly reported side effect of regional anesthesia affecting up to 60% of patients undergoing cesarean deliveries under spinal anesthesia [1–4]. The hypothermia can cause numerous complications including postoperative wound infections, increased blood loss and transfusion requirements, myocardial ischemia, high risk of coagulopathy, shivering, increased hospital stay, and patient discomfort [5–12]. Neonatal outcomes such as birth temperature and Apgar scores have also been linked to maternal temperature [13, 14].

Perioperative hypothermia under spinal anesthesia has different etiologies, but mostly it is caused by spinal anesthesia altering thermoregulation and reducing the threshold for vasoconstriction and shivering [15]. Neuraxial anesthesia decreases the thermoregulatory vasoconstriction below the sensory blockade level, leading to heat loss by redistribution of heat from the core to the periphery [16]. The core-to-peripheral redistribution of body heat is difficult to treat, but it should be preventable by prewarming the periphery compartment [17]. Prewarming increases the heat content in the periphery of the patient and reduces the core-to-peripheral tissue temperature gradient, which otherwise promotes the heat redistribution after spinal anesthesia [18]. Intraoperative forced-air warming has been shown to be uncomfortable for the patient and may affect the early maternal-newborn bonding [3]. Unlike the forced-air warming, warmed intravenous fluids do not disturb the operation during the surgical procedure. Despite the existence of prospective studies on active warming during cesarean delivery, no consensus regarding its efficacy exists. Studies have suggested that single-modality interventions to prevent hypothermia (forced-air or intravenous fluid warmings) result in only marginal or no benefit for patients undergoing cesarean sections [1, 4, 19, 20].

Therefore, we aimed to evaluate the effect of the combined application of 30 min of preoperative warm forced-air and perioperative warm intravenous fluids in women receiving spinal anesthesia for cesarean deliveries and we assumed that combination of warmed preoperative forced-air and warmed perioperative intravenous fluids could prevent maternal hypothermia during cesarean sections under spinal anesthesia.

Methods

Study design

The Ethical Committee of Ningbo NO.7 Hospital approved this study, which follows the tenets of the Declaration of Helsinki, and we pre-registered it at http://www.chictr.org.cn/index.aspx (ChiCTR1800019117). This study adheres the applicable CONSORT guidelines. We enrolled healthy pregnant women undergoing elective cesarean deliveries under spinal anesthesia after obtaining their informed consents. American Society of Anesthesiologists physical status I-II parturients, aged 18 to 40 years, with more than 37-week gestations, singleton pregnancies, and scheduled for cesarean delivery under spinal anesthesia were eligible for enrollment. We excluded women with coagulation abnormalities, thyroid disease, cesarean delivery using epidural or general anesthesia, and baseline temperatures ≥37.5 °C.

Study protocol

After obtaining the signed informed consents, we randomly allocated eligible participants to either the control or the intervention groups. Randomization was computer-generated using Microsoft Excel's random number generator, and we concealed allocations using sequentially numbered opaque sealed envelopes.

All parturients fasted for 8 h before the cesarean section. Once in the preoperative waiting area, the parturients in the intervention group received 30 min of upper body preoperative warming using a forced-air warming device (EQ-5000 230 V, Smiths Medical ASD, Rockland, USA) set to 43 °C and nurses established intravenous accesses. The women in the intervention group received Ringer's lactate solution pre-warmed to 37 °C through a 3MRanger™ Fluid Warmer until the end of the procedure. We monitored the patients during the interventions. We discontinued the intervention in cases in which the parturients experienced adverse side effects related to warming such as diaphoresis or nausea and vomiting, or if the core thermometer was > 37.5 °C.

After prewarming, we immediately transferred the term parturients to the operating room (OR). Participants in the intervention group received 30 min of upper body preoperative warming in the preoperative waiting area, and received IV fluid warming during the observation period (preoperative waiting area, OR and PACU). The women in the control group received usual care consisting of no active warming and they received the intravenous fluid at room temperature throughout the procedure (preoperative waiting area, OR and PACU). We recorded data on vital signs including heart rate, blood pressure, hemoglobin peripheral saturation, and baseline core temperature in the preoperative area. The same operator measured patients' core temperatures using an infrared tympanic thermometer (PRO6000, Braun, Marlborough, MA USA 01752) with disposable covers, and recorded the average value of three measurements. The hospital maintained central control of the temperatures of the preoperative area, OR, and post-anesthesia care unit (PACU), and we obtained the temperature readings from the thermostat.

An anesthesiologist not involved in the study applied all spinal anesthesias at the L3–4 interspace, with 2 mL of 0.5% plain bupivacaine, using a 25-gauge Quincke needle. The surgeon commenced the operations once a sensory blockade above the T4 level was achieved according to the results of pinprick tests. After the operation, all patients were transferred to the PACU covered with a cotton sheet and a blanket.

We obtained values for core temperature, maternal thermal comfort scores, and the incidences of shivering and hypothermia at the following timepoints: T_0 = baseline, T_1 = pre-spinal, T_2 = post-spinal, T_3 = after 15 min in the OR, T_4 = after 30 min in the OR, T_5 = surgery end, T_6 = PACU arrival, T_7 = after 15 min in the PACU, T_8 = after 30 min in the PACU. According to Guidelines [21], we defined maternal hypothermia as a core temperature < 36 °C. We assessed thermal comfort scores using a verbal numerical scale on which we defined 0 as completely unsatisfied with the "thermal comfort" and 100 as completely satisfied. We graded shivering during and after the cesarean section according to the Bedside Shivering Assessment Scale (0, no shivering; 1, shivering localized to the core and neck; 2, shivering including the upper extremities; 3, total body shivering) [22]. The anesthesiologist provided meperidine according to their own criteria. A midwife recorded neonatal axillary temperature, and Apgar scores at 1 and 5 min after birth. Based on our institutional guidelines, if the core temperature was lower than 35.5 °C, rescue warming would performed for the parturients by using a forced-air warming device.

We defined bradycardia as a heart rate < 50 beats/min, and treated it with 0.5 mg of intravenous atropine. When the systemic pressure decreased more than 30% of the baseline pressure or dropped below 90 mmHg, we administered ephedrine (5 mg). Mean arterial pressure and heart rate was measured at baseline, prespinal, postspinal and at the end of the procedure.

We recorded demographic data (age, height, weight, parity, and gravidity) and surgical and anesthetic variables (Preoperative and total volume of intravenous fluids, estimated blood loss, duration of surgery, and the ambient temperatures in the preoperative area, OR, and PACU).

Statistical analyses

The primary outcome measure was the core temperature change between two groups from baseline to the end of the surgical procedure. Secondary outcomes included thermal comfort scores during the operation, the incidence of shivering and hypothermia (< 36 °C), the core temperature on the arrival at the PACU, neonatal axillary temperature at birth, and Apgar scores at 1 and 5 min).

Analysis of covariance for repeated measures was under taken to calculate the sample size. A bonferroni correction for multiple pairwise comparisons was used, giving an adjusted *P* value level of significance ($P < 0.01$). A clinically significant difference in the core temperature between study groups was set at 0.4 °C according to our pilot trial with a standard deviation of 0.5 °C,which was also consistent with Chung et al' s study [23]. A sample size of120 patients, including 20% dropouts, was estimated to provide 90% power for detecting a statistically significant difference between groups at an α level of 0.01.

We expressed normally distributed continuous data as means ± SDs, and compared variables between study groups using the Student t test. Nonparametric data are presented as medians (interquartile ranges), and compared between study groups using the Mann–Whitney U test. We investigated associations among discrete variables using the $\chi 2$ or Fisher exact tests. Two-way repeated measures ANOVA was applied with change from baseline as the dependent variable, and the intervention, time, and the treatment multiplied by time interaction as independent variables. We also used two-way repeated measures ANOVA to assess the core temperature change and the thermal comfort between groups at each timepoint. We performed all statistical analyses using the SPSS software (version 22.0, SPSS, Chicago, IL, USA). We considered *P*-values < 0.05 as statistically significant.

Results

Patients were enrolled in the study between January 2019 and June 2019.We considered 144 patients for eligibility, and excluded 9 before randomization. In the end we randomly allocated 135 patients to one of the two groups (69 women to the intervention group, and 66 to the control group). We had to exclude one patient from the intervention group and two patients from the control group due to failed spinal anesthesia (Fig. 1). The demographic and obstetric characteristics, as well as the surgical and anesthetic values, were did not differ significantly between the two groups. Vital sign parameters such as peripheral oxygen saturation, heart rate, mean arterial pressure measurement at the each point, and the incidence of hypotension and vomiting, ephedrine dose administered also had no difference between two groups during the observation period. The room temperatures in the preoperative area, OR, and PACU were similar for the two groups (Table 1).

Our two-way repeated measures ANOVA analysis revealed a significant difference in the core temperature changes from the T_1 to T_7 timepoints between the two groups ($F = 13.022$, $P < 0.001$), and the group×time interaction difference was also significant ($F = 23.195$, $P < 0.001$). The patients in the intervention group experienced higher perioperative mean temperatures during the procedure than those in the control group (T_1-T_3, $P < 0.001$, T_4-T_7, $P < 0.05$). In the control group, the core

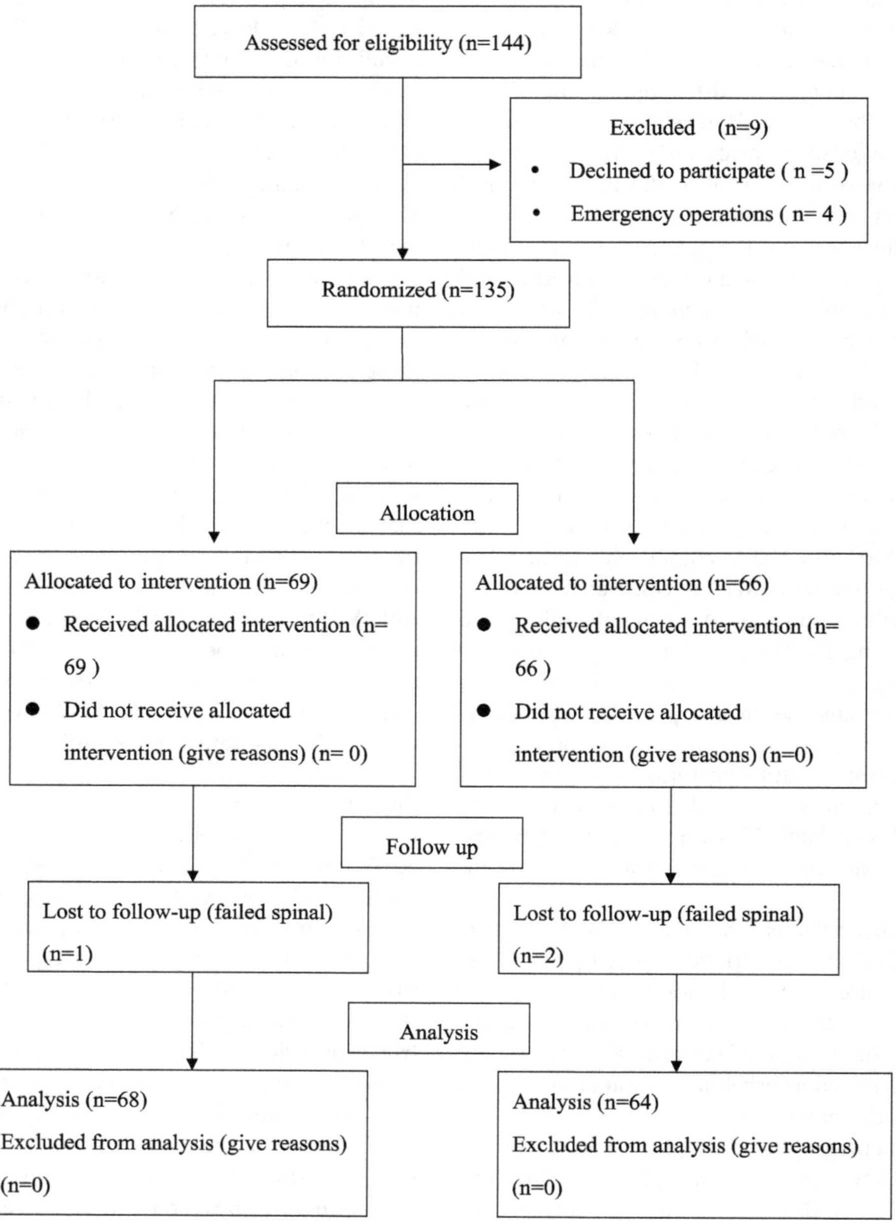

Fig. 1 Flow diagram outlining the enrollment and randomization study procedures

temperature was decreased at all the time points compared to the baseline. We also found a slight decline in the core temperatures from the baseline during the procedure (except $T_1$and T_2) in the intervention group (Fig. 2).

Thermal comfort scores were higher in the intervention group than in the control group ($F = 9.847$, $P = 0.002$), the group × time interaction difference was also significant ($F = 2.750$, $P = 0.008$). The maternal thermal comfort scores differed significantly between two groups from the T_2 to T_6 timepoints (all $P < 0.05$ or $P < 0.001$). In comparisons with the baseline thermal comfort scores, the timepoints in the control group (except T_1) and those in the intervention group (except $T_1$and T_6) all exhibited decreased thermal comfort scores (Fig. 3).

Core temperatures on arrival at the PACU were greater in the intervention group (36.2 ± 0.4 °C) than in the control group (35.5 ± 0.3 °C), $P = 0.007$. The incidences of shivering were 56.3% in the control group and 19.1% in the intervention group during the surgical procedure ($P < 0.001$), and the shivering assessment scores were higher in the control than in the intervention group. The overall

Table 1 Demographic, surgical, and anesthetic characteristics of the study population

	Intervention($n = 68$)	Control($n = 64$)
Age, y	28.5 ± 5.1	27.5 ± 4.6
BMI, kg/m^2	28.1 ± 3.2	28.4 ± 3.4
Gestation, weeks	38.6 ± 1.4	38.7 ± 1.3
Gravidity	2.0 [1.0–3.5]	2.0 [1.0–3.0]
Parity	1.0 [0.0–1.0]	1.0 [0.0–1.0]
ASA I, n(%)	56(82.4%)	52(81.3%)
Hypotension, n(%)	30(44.1%)	28(43.8%)
Ephedrine,mg	13.6 ± 9.7	12.5 ± 8.5
Vomiting, n(%)	7(10.3%)	6(9.4%)
Estimated blood loss, mL	272 ± 70	267 ± 74
Exposed time, min duration,min	50.2 ± 7.7	48.9 ± 8.1
Baseline temperature, °C	36.7 ± 0.4	36.7 ± 0.3
Prespinal temperature, °C	37.0 ± 0.3	36.6 ± 0.3
Preoperative ambient temperature, °C	22.6 ± 0.6	22.9 ± 0.8
OR ambient temperature, °C	23.9 ± 0.7	24.2 ± 0.8
PACU ambient temperature, °C	23.2 ± 0.6	22.8 ± 0.6
Preoperative crystalloid amount, mL crystalloid amount	371 ± 55	363 ± 55
Total crystalloid amount, mL	1291 ± 246	1343 ± 264

Data are expressed as means ± SDs, medians [interquartile ranges], or numbers (%)
Exposed time: including surgery duration, clean up time, and finding sheets time
BMI body mass index, *ASA* American Society of Anesthesiologists, *OR* operating room, *PACU* post-anesthesia care unit

incidence of perioperative hypothermia was significantly lower in the intervention group than in the control group ($P < 0.001$). Neonatal outcomes were similar between the two groups (Table 2).

Discussion

In our study, our intervention with 30 min preoperative forced-air warming and perioperative administration of warmed intravenous fluids reduced the extent of core temperature decline, decreased the incidence of preoperative hypothermia and shivering, and improved maternal comfort in patients undergoing cesarean section with spinal anesthesia as opposed to the outcomes in the control group patients.

The results of our study are similar to those of the study by Chung et al. in which preoperative forced-air warming prevented hypothermia and shivering in patients undergoing elective cesarean delivery with spinal anesthesia [23]. However, in that study the difference in maternal temperatures between groups was evident only at one timepoint (45 min after prewarming). Therefore, the impact of their single intervention was likely smaller than the impact of our combined warming of forced-air and intravenous fluids. The combined active warming modalities applied in our intervention group maintained a significantly higher mean temperature nearly throughout the entire surgical procedure (at the seven timepoints). The intervention group had a significantly higher temperature on arrival at the PACU compared with the control group. Similarly, our study also demonstrated that our combined warming technique can reduce the incidence of perioperative hypothermia significantly (20.6% in the intervention group compared with 56.3% in the control group).

Unlike forced air-warming which warms the patient from the outside, the warming of intravenous fluids prevents hypothermia by offsetting the 0.25°C reduction in body temperature that occurs with each liter of intravenous fluids administered at room temperature [24]. To minimize spinal hypotension, women undergoing caesarean delivery often receive large volumes of intravenous fluid intraoperatively. Thus, fluid warming may be particularly important and effective during caesarean deliveries [25]. These findings agree with those in other studies. Horn et al. found that 15 min of preoperative warming provided additional efficacy when added to warmed intravenous fluids in the setting of epidural anesthesia, resulting in an average 1°Cdifference between control and intervention groups at the end of the operations [13]. Unlike forced air-warming during all the surgical procedure [25], brief period of prewarming, would be more acceptable to awake patients, easy to accommodate and could be combined with intraoperative warming, which is undoubtedly effective once the redistribution period has passed.

The combined technique has the potential to minimize maternal temperature drops. Similarly, in a study by De Bernardiset al, thermal gowns and warmed intravenous fluids decreased the patient temperature drops and the incidence of shivering as compared to the same variables in the control group [26]. In contrast, in Munday et al's study, 20 min of preoperative forced-air warming with intravenous fluid warming did not prevent temperature drops in women undergoing cesarean delivery [27]. However, the OR ambient temperature was lower in that study (21.4 °C). The time between the end of the warming regime and the OR entry was longer than those in our study. In their study, the time interval was smaller than 20 min, but some women may have experienced longer delays. Therefore, their study design may have been less powerful than ours to detect differences between two groups.

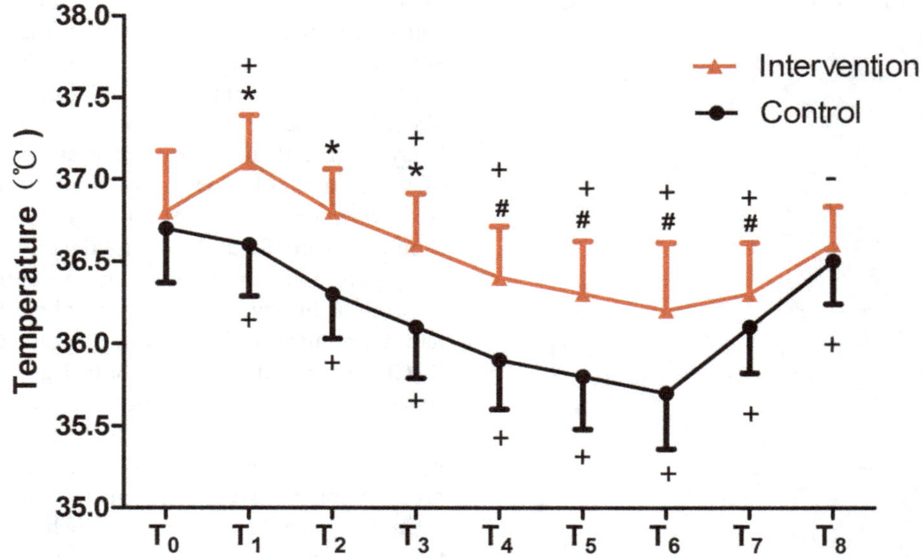

Fig. 2 Core tympanic temperatures during the procedure. Compared with control group, the patients in intervention group experienced higher perioperative mean temperatures during the procedure (T_1-T_3, $P < 0.001$, T_4-T_7, $P < 0.05$). Timepoints: T_0 = baseline, T_1 = pre-spinal, T_2 = post-spinal, T_3 = after 15 min in the OR, T_4 = after 30 min in the OR, T_5 = surgery end, T_6 = PACU arrival, T_7 = after 15 min in the PACU, T_8 = after 30 min in the PACU. OR: operating room; PACU: post-anesthesia care unit. $^{*}P < 0.001$, $^{\#}P < 0.05$ refer to statistically significant differences between the intervention and the control groups. $^{+}P < 0.001$, $^{-}P < 0.05$ refer to comparisons with the baseline (T_0)

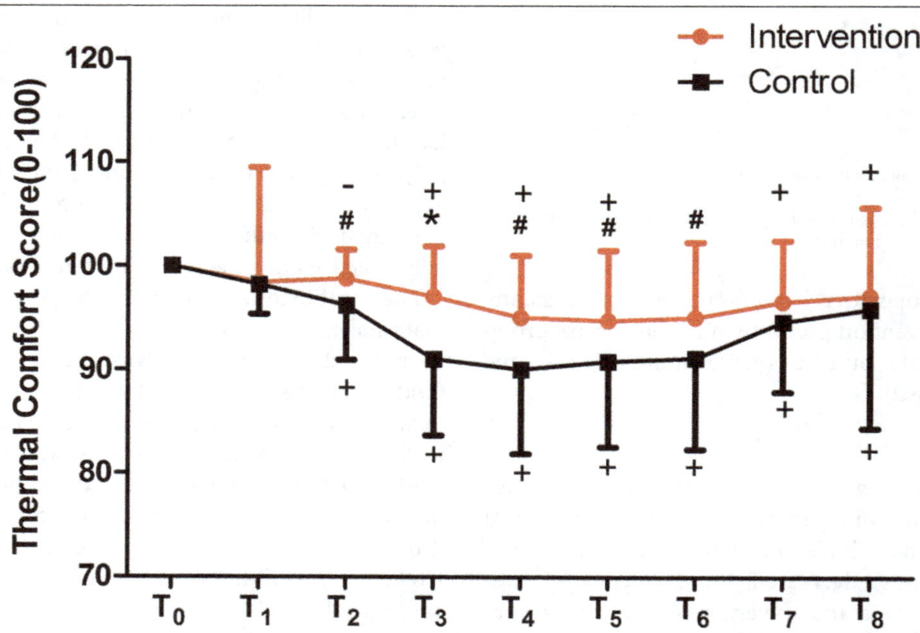

Fig. 3 Maternal comfort scores during the procedure. The maternal thermal comfort scores differed significantly between two groups from the T_2 to T_6 timepoints (all $P < 0.05$ or $P < 0.001$). Timepoints: T_0 = baseline, T_1 = pre-spinal, T_2 = post-spinal, T_3 = after 15 min in the OR, T_4 = after 30 min in the OR, T_5 = surgery end, T_6 = PACU arrival, T_7 = after 15 min in the PACU, T_8 = after 30 min in the PACU. We measured thermal comfort scores using a verbal numerical scale in which 0 was defined as completely unsatisfied with their "thermal comfort" and 100 as completely satisfied. $^{*}P < 0.001$, $^{\#}P < 0.05$ refer to statistically significant difference between the intervention and the control groups. $^{+}P < 0.001$, $^{-}P < 0.05$ refer to comparisons with baseline (T_0)

Table 2 Secondary maternal and neonatal outcomes

	Intervention (n = 68)	Control (n = 64)	*P* value
PACU arrival temperature °C	36.2 ± 0.4	35.5 ± 0.3	0.007
Delivery temperature °C	36.6 ± 0.3	36.0 ± 0.3	< 0.0001
Perioperative shivering	13(19.1%)	36(56.3%)	< 0.0001
Shivering assessment score	0 [0–0]	1 [0–2]	0.01
Perioperative hyperthermia	14(20.6%)	33(51.6%)	< 0.0001
Apgar score			
1 min	9 [9–9]	9 [9–9]	0.21
5 min	10 [10–10]	10 [10–10]	0.43
Neonatal temperature °C	36.3 ± 0.3	36.3 ± 0.4	0.350

Data are expressed as means ± SDs, medians [interquartile ranges], or numbers (%)
Bedside Shivering Assessment Scale: 0 = no shivering; 1 = shivering localized to the core and neck; 2 = shivering including the upper extremities; 3 = total body shivering
OR operating room, *PACU* post-anesthesia care unit

In our study, shivering was significantly less common in the patients who were actively warmed, a finding that may be explained by the significantly higher core temperatures in the combined active warming patients than in the controls. The intensity and incidence of shivering may indicate the severity of hypothermia. Our study showed that the overall incidence of perioperative hypothermia decreased significantly in the intervention group compared to the incidence in the control group. Shivering is both thermogenic accompanied by vasoconstriction or non-thermogenic as that induced by catecholamines resulting from pain or anxiety [28]. A meta-analysis demonstrated that warmed intravenous fluids are effective at reducing the incidence of hypothermia and shivering [29]. In addition, our combined active warming interventions improved the thermal comfort scores of the patients in the intervention group as opposed to the score in the control group. Thermal comfort scores are subjective measures of patient comfort during the perioperative period, and may differ from actual temperature measurements and do not necessarily reflect recorded shivering episodes. Results of studies [20, 30, 31] and a meta-analysis [29] suggest that forced-air warming can improve thermal comfort scores.

We found no significant differences in neonatal outcomes between the two groups, which is not surprising given our small sample size and our limited neonatal outcome measurements. Though our study found that the patients in the intervention group experienced higher temperatures at the time of delivery, but both groups all had normal core temperatures with a difference of 0.6 degrees, which did not affect the neonatal temperature. Further studies specifically powered to evaluate the impact of active warming on neonatal outcomes are still required.

We are aware of the limitations in our study. Our infrared tympanic thermometers lack evidence of their quality and accuracy. However, they are not invasive and provide an acceptable and comfortable measurement to patients. Also, we did not use intrathecal morphine as a spinal anesthetic. However, many institutions prefer to use intrathecal opioids for postoperative analgesia after cesarean delivery, so this may affect the generalizability of our study. A study has shown that intrathecal morphine administration may exacerbate hypothermia [19]. Finally, it was not a blinding clinical trial, and it may increase the bias.

Conclusion

In all, preoperative forced air-warming combined with perioperative intravenous fluid warming may prevent maternal hypothermia, reduce maternal shivering, and improve maternal thermal comfort in those undergoing cesarean section with spinal anesthesia.

Abbreviations

ASA: American Society of Anesthesiologists; BMI: Body mass index; OR: Operating room; PACU: Post-anesthesia care unit

Acknowledgements

None.

Authors' contributions

QHZ: contributed to the design of the work, and writing the manuscript. TTN: contributed to performing all statistical analyses, drafting the manuscript. ZFZ: Suggestions for methods and results sections, tables, and figures.BH: acquisition of data. All authors read and approved the final manuscript.

Author details

[1]Department of Anesthesiology, NO.7 Hospital of Ningbo, Ningbo, Zhejiang Province, China. [2]Department of Anesthesiology, People's Hospital of Zhejiang Provincial (People's Hospital of Hangzhou Medicine College), Hangzhou, Zhejiang Province, China. [3]Department of Gynecology, NO.7 Hospital of Ningbo, Ningbo, Zhejiang Province, China. [4]Department of Anesthesiology, The Affiliated Hospital of Jiaxing University, Jiaxing, Zhejiang Province, China.

References

1. Yokoyama K, Suzuki M, Shimada Y, Matsushima T, Bito H, Sakamoto A. Effect of administration of pre-warmed intravenous fluids on the frequency of hypothermia following spinal anesthesia for cesarean delivery. J Clin Anesth. 2009;21:242–8.
2. Carpenter L, Baysinger CL. Maintaining perioperative normothermia in the patient undergoing cesarean delivery. ObstetGynecolSurv. 2012;67:436–46.
3. Petsas A, Vollmer H, Barnes R. Peri-operative warming in caesarean sections. Anaesthesia. 2009;64:921–2.
4. Butwick AJ, Lipman SS, Carvalho B. Intraoperative forced air-warming during cesarean delivery under spinal anesthesia does not prevent maternal hypothermia. AnesthAnalg. 2007;105:1413–9 table of contents.
5. Rajagopalan S, Mascha E, Na J, Sessler DI. The effects of mild perioperative hypothermia on blood loss and transfusion requirement. Anesthesiology. 2008;108:71–7.

6. Melling AC, Ali B, Scott EM, Leaper DJ. Effects of preoperative warming on the incidence of wound infection after clean surgery: a randomised controlled trial. Lancet. 2001;358:876–80.
7. Kurz A, Sessler DI, Lenhardt R. Perioperative normothermia to reduce the incidence of surgical-wound infection and shorten hospitalization. Study of wound infection and temperature group. N Engl J Med. 1996;334:1209–15.
8. Flores-Maldonado A, Medina-Escobedo CE, Ríos-Rodríguez HM, Fernández-Domínguez R. Mild perioperative hypothermia and the risk of wound infection. Arch Med Res. 2001;32:227–31.
9. Schmied H, Kurz A, Sessler DI, Kozek S, Reiter A. Mild hypothermia increases blood loss and transfusion requirements during total hip arthroplasty. Lancet. 1996;347:289–92.
10. Hart SR, Bordes B, Hart J, Corsino D, Harmon D. Unintended perioperative hypothermia. Ochsner J. 2011;11:259–70.
11. Frank SM, Fleisher LA, Breslow MJ, Higgins MS, Olson KF, Kelly S, et al. Perioperative maintenance of normothermia reduces the incidence of morbid cardiac events. A randomized clinical trial. JAMA. 1997;277:1127–34.
12. Peng RY, Bongard FS. Hypothermia in trauma patients. J Am Coll Surg. 1999; 188:685–96.
13. Horn E-P, Schroeder F, Gottschalk A, Sessler DI, Hiltmeyer N, Standl T, et al. Active warming during cesarean delivery. AnesthAnalg. 2002;94:409–14 table of contents.
14. Suzuki M, Kinoshita T, Kikutani T, Yokoyama K, Inagi T, Sugimoto K, et al. Determining the plasma concentration of ketamine that enhances epiduralbupivacaine-and-morphine-induced analgesia. AnesthAnalg. 2005; 101:777–84.
15. Ozaki M, Kurz A, Sessler DI, Lenhardt R, Schroeder M, Moayeri A, et al. Thermoregulatory thresholds during epidural and spinal anesthesia. Anesthesiology. 1994;81:282–8.
16. Matsukawa T, Sessler DI, Christensen R, Ozaki M, Schroeder M. Heat flow and distribution during epidural anesthesia. Anesthesiology. 1995;83:961–7.
17. Hynson JM, Sessler DI. Intraoperative warming therapies: a comparison of three devices. J Clin Anesth. 1992;4:194–9.
18. Hynson JM, Sessler DI, Moayeri A, McGuire J, Schroeder M. The effects of preinduction warming on temperature and blood pressure during propofol/nitrous oxide anesthesia. Anesthesiology. 1993;79:219–28 discussion 21A-22A.
19. Hui C-K, Huang C-H, Lin C-J, Lau H-P, Chan W-H, Yeh H-M. A randomised double-blind controlled study evaluating the hypothermic effect of 150 microg morphine during spinal anaesthesia for caesarean section. Anaesthesia. 2006;61:29–31.
20. Horn E-P, Bein B, Steinfath M, Ramaker K, Buchloh B, Höcker J. The incidence and prevention of hypothermia in newborn bonding after cesarean delivery: a randomized controlled trial. AnesthAnalg. 2014;118:997–1002.
21. Conforti A, Alviggi C, Mollo A, De Placido G, Magos A. The management of Asherman syndrome: a review of literature. Reprod Biol Endocrinol. 2013;11: 118.
22. Badjatia N, Strongilis E, Gordon E, Prescutti M, Fernandez L, Fernandez A, et al. Metabolic impact of shivering during therapeutic temperature modulation: the bedside shivering assessment scale. Stroke. 2008;39:3242–7.
23. Chung SH, Lee B-S, Yang HJ, Kweon KS, Kim H-H, Song J, et al. Effect of preoperative warming during cesarean section under spinal anesthesia. Korean J Anesthesiol. 2012;62:454–60.
24. Kurz A, Ikeda T, Sessler DI, Larson MD, Bjorksten AR, Dechert M, et al. Meperidine decreases the shivering threshold twice as much as the vasoconstriction threshold. Anesthesiology. 1997;86:1046–54.
25. Cobb B, Cho Y, Hilton G, Ting V, Carvalho B. Active warming utilizing combined IV fluid and forced-air warming decreases hypothermia and improves maternal comfort during cesarean delivery: a randomized control trial. AnesthAnalg. 2016;122:1490–7.
26. de Bernardis RCG, Siaulys MM, Vieira JE, Mathias LAST. Perioperative warming with a thermal gown prevents maternal temperature loss during elective cesarean section. A randomized clinical trial. Braz J Anesthesiol. 2016;66:451–5.
27. Munday J, Osborne S, Yates P, Sturgess D, Jones L, Gosden E. Preoperative warming versus no preoperative warming for maintenance of Normothermia in women receiving Intrathecal morphine for cesarean delivery: a single-blinded, randomized controlled trial. AnesthAnalg. 2018; 126:183–9.
28. Webb PJ, James FM, Wheeler AS. Shivering during epidural analgesia in women in labor. Anesthesiology. 1981;55:706–7.
29. Sultan P, Habib AS, Cho Y, Carvalho B. The effect of patient warming during caesarean delivery on maternal and neonatal outcomes: a meta-analysis. Br J Anaesth. 2015;115:500–10.
30. Woolnough M, Allam J, Hemingway C, Cox M, Yentis SM. Intra-operative fluid warming in elective caesarean section: a blinded randomised controlled trial. Int J ObstetAnesth. 2009;18:346–51.
31. Fallis WM, Hamelin K, Symonds J, Wang X. Maternal and newborn outcomes related to maternal warming during cesarean delivery. J ObstetGynecol Neonatal Nurs. 2006;35:324–31.

Palonosetron versus ondansetron for prevention of nausea and vomiting after total abdominal hysterectomy under spinal anesthesia with intrathecal morphine

Guilherme Oliveira Campos[1,2*], Marcelo de Jesus Martins[3], Gabriel Nascimento Jesus[1,4], Paulo Roberto Rios de Oliveira[5], Caio Nogueira Lessa[5], João Carlos Macêdo Fernandes de Oliveira Junior[1], Lucas Jorge Santana de Castro Alves[6], Rodrigo Leal Alves[1,4] and Norma Sueli Pinheiro Módolo[3]

Abstract

Background: Hysterectomy is a widely performed surgery and neuraxial anesthesia with intrathecal morphine provides superior quality of recovery. Postoperative nausea and vomiting (PONV) is a frequent problem with intrathecal morphine use. Although palonosetron is effective for prevention of PONV after general anesthesia, its efficacy after neuraxial anesthesia has not been established. This study was conducted to compare the use of palonosetron with ondansetron for PONV prophylaxis in patients at a high risk of PONV during total abdominal hysterectomy (TAH) under spinal anesthesia with intrathecal morphine.

Methods: This prospective, randomized double-blind study conducted at São Rafael Hospital involved 140 American Society of Anesthesiologists physical status I or II women who underwent TAH under spinal anesthesia with intrathecal morphine and who had at least 3 risk factors for PONV based on Apfel's simplified score. The patients were randomized into two groups: one received palonosetron whereas the other received ondansetron. All patients received spinal anesthesia with intrathecal morphine, as well as dexamethasone plus palonosetron or ondansetron for PONV prophylaxis. The overall incidence of PONV, incidence of early- and late-onset nausea and vomiting, severity of nausea, and use of rescue antiemetics were recorded.

Results: The overall incidence of PONV was 42.9% in the palonosetron group and 52.9% in the ondansetron group ($p > 0.05$). No significant differences existed in the incidence of early- and late-onset nausea or early-onset vomiting between the two groups. The incidence of late-onset vomiting was significantly lower in the palonosetron group.

Conclusions: Palonosetron exhibited efficacy similar to that of ondansetron for reducing the overall incidence of PONV after TAH under spinal anesthesia with intrathecal morphine; however, palonosetron reduced the incidence of late-onset vomiting significantly better than ondansetron.

Keywords: Antiemetics, Morphine, Ondansetron, Postoperative nausea and vomiting, Spinal anesthesia

* Correspondence: guioliveiracampos@gmail.com
[1]Department of Anesthesiology, São Rafael Hospital, D'Or Institute for Research and Education (IDOR), Salvador, Brazil
[2]Department of Anesthesiology, Cardiopulmonar Hospital, Salvador, Brazil

Background

Postoperative nausea and vomiting (PONV) is a common perioperative complication that is associated with clinical and economic consequences, including wound dehiscence, delayed nutrition, prolonged hospital stay, and reduced patient satisfaction. Despite advances in prevention and treatment, the incidence of PONV remains high, especially in high-risk patients [1].

Total abdominal hysterectomy (TAH) is a surgery that is often performed worldwide, and neuraxial anesthesia with intrathecal morphine has been shown to provide improved quality of recovery because of superior, prolonged pain control after TAH [2]. However, PONV is a frequent complication after TAH due to both the effects of intrathecal morphine and the intrinsic characteristics of the patients [3–7].

Palonosetron is a second generation 5HT-3 receptor antagonist that has a greater binding affinity and a longer plasma half-life than other drugs in the same class [8, 9]. Studies have reported the superiority of palonosetron relative to other 5HT-3 receptor antagonists for the prevention of PONV in patients undergoing general anesthesia. However, little is known regarding the ability of palonosetron to prevent PONV after spinal anesthesia [10–12].

The aim of the current study was to compare the efficacy of palonosetron versus ondansetron, both in combination with dexamethasone, for PONV prophylaxis in patients undergoing TAH under spinal anesthesia with intrathecal morphine.

Methods

This study was approved by the Research Ethics Committee (1.238.882/2015) of São Rafael Hospital, a tertiary care hospital in Salvador, Brazil. The trial was conducted from January to October of 2015, in adherence with the Consolidated Standards of Reporting Trials (CONSORT) guidelines, and was registered with the Brazilian Clinical Trial Registry (RBR-4gnm8n, August 18, 2014).

After they had provided written informed consent, 175 consecutive female patients scheduled to undergo elective TAH were recruited for this prospective, randomized, double-blinded study. The inclusion criteria were age 18 to 65 years, American Society of Anesthesiologists physical status I or II, and at least 3 risk factors for PONV as determined by Apfel's simplified risk score. Exclusion criteria were body mass index > 35, contraindications to spinal anesthesia, use of corticosteroids or antiemetic medications in the 24 h preceding the surgery, and allergy to any medication used in the study protocol.

After enrollment, patients were randomly assigned in a 1:1 ratio to receive either ondansetron or palonosetron. The group assignment was presented in opaque sealed envelopes to a pharmacist who was not involved in the study. Randomization was performed with a block size of 6 using a central web-based system. A nurse who was not involved in the study opened the envelopes and prepared the medications as injectable solutions of either palonosetron 0.075 mg or ondansetron 4 mg, both diluted in normal saline to a total volume of 2 mL, in identical syringes. The study drug was administered intravenously (i.v.) immediately after the spinal block.

Preoperative fasting was initiated at midnight for all patients, and none received premedication. After arrival in the operating room, standard monitoring was applied (electrocardiography, pulse oximetry, and a non-invasive blood pressure cuff) and the subjects received 10 mL/kg of lactated Ringer's solution i.v., 2 mg midazolam i.v., and 50 µg fentanyl i.v.

The patients were then placed in a sitting position, and a spinal block was performed at the L3–L4 or L4–L5 interspace using a 27-gauge Sprotte needle, followed by intrathecal injection of 15 mg hyperbaric bupivacaine and 100 µg preservative-free morphine. An appropriate block level (T6 dermatome) was confirmed prior to skin incision. Patients in both groups received additional titrated doses of midazolam (up to 10 mg i.v.) to maintain a level of sedation between − 1 and − 3 on the Richmond Agitation-Sedation Scale (0 for alert and calm, − 5 for unarousable). Ephedrine 5 mg i.v. was titrated to maintain an arterial blood pressure within 20% of baseline. Atropine 0.5 mg i.v. was given as needed to maintain a heart rate above 50 beats per minute.

Considering the high risk of PONV and ethical issues, all patients received dexamethasone 8 mg i.v. just after placement of the i.v. catheter as part of the PONV prophylaxis regimen. For postoperative analgesia, all patients received a multimodal regimen consisting of ketoprofen 100 mg i.v. every 8 h and metamizole 2 g i.v. every 6 h, beginning in the operating room. Morphine 3 mg i.v. up to every 4 h was used if the patient's pain score was greater than 4 on the visual analog scale (VAS; 0 = no pain, 10 = the worst pain imaginable). Patients were observed in the post-anesthesia care unit for at least 1 h after surgery before they were transferred to the ward.

The incidence of PONV, severity of nausea, and the use of rescue antiemetics were evaluated at 1, 6, 24, and 48 h after surgery. An episode of vomiting was defined as either vomiting (expulsion of stomach contents) or retching (involuntary attempt to vomit that did not expel stomach contents). Severity of nausea was assessed using a VAS ranging from 0 to 10 (0 = no nausea, 10 = worst nausea imaginable). Rescue antiemetics (metoclopramide 10 mg i.v. followed by ondansetron 4 mg i.v. if there was no response to metoclopramide) were administered upon the patient's request or with the onset of vomiting.

A simplified PONV impact scale questionnaire consisting of two questions was administered to all patients just before hospital discharge. A score from 0 to 6 was derived based the patient's answers to the questions and scores above 4 were considered to indicate clinically significant PONV [13]. Patients were also asked to rate their experience regarding the management of PONV on a 4-point scale (poor, average, good, or excellent). Adverse events, such as dizziness and headache, were also investigated and recorded during the 48-h observation period.

The primary outcome measured was the incidence of PONV during the entire observation period. Secondary outcomes included the incidence of either nausea or vomiting, severity of nausea, use of rescue antiemetics, incidence of clinically important PONV, and overall patient satisfaction with the management of PONV. Early-onset nausea and/or vomiting were considered to occur within the first 6 h after surgery, whereas late-onset nausea and/or vomiting were considered to occur between 6 and 48 h after surgery.

In order to calculate the sample size, we conducted a retrospective review of the incidence of PONV in patients who had undergone TAH in the preceding year at São Rafael Hospital. A PONV incidence rate of approximately 60% was observed in patients who received ondansetron and dexamethasone in the operating room. It was estimated that a sample size of 67 patients per group would achieve 80% power for the detection of a 40% reduction in the incidence of PONV in the palonosetron group with an alpha error of 5% [14]. To account for patient dropout, we randomized 70 patients to each group.

The analysis was performed on an intention-to-treat basis using data from all randomized patients who underwent TAH. Dichotomous variables are expressed as relative and absolute frequencies. As the continuous variables in the study did not yield normal distributions, they are expressed as medians and interquartile ranges, as were the ordinal variables. The non-parametric Mann-Whitney test was used to compare data derived from continuous and ordinal variables in the two groups. Dichotomous variables were analyzed using the χ^2 test or Fisher's exact test as appropriate, and $P < 0.05$ was considered statistically significant. Statistical analysis was performed using SPSS for Windows (version 14, SPSS Inc., Chicago, IL, USA).

Results

Of the 175 patients who were initially screened, 140 met the inclusion and exclusion criteria and were randomly assigned to a study group. All patients who underwent randomization completed the trial, and there were 70 patients in each group (Fig. 1). The groups were well matched for age, height, body mass index, clinical comorbidities, smoking status, and preoperative fasting time. There were no significant differences in the duration of anesthesia, volume of infused crystalloid, total dose of midazolam, or use of vasopressors or atropine (Table 1).

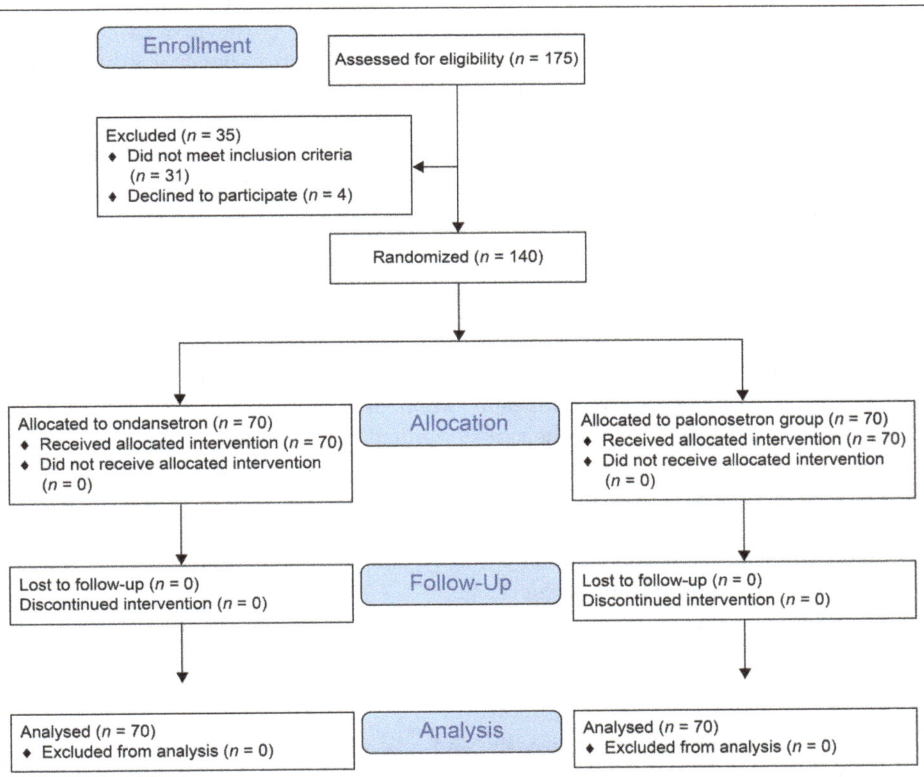

Fig. 1 CONSORT flow diagram

Table 1 Characteristics, anesthetic, and surgical data of patients in the ondansetron and palonosetron groups

	Ondansetron	Palonosetron	*P* value
Age (years)	44 (41/47)	45 (42/48)	0.334
Weight (kg)	68.4 ± 10.7	70.3 ± 12.0	0.317
Height (cm)	158 ± 6	159 ± 5	0.609
Body mass index (kg/m^2)	27.2 ± 3.9	27.7 ± 4.0	0.453
Motion sickness/ previous PONV	7.1%	5.7%	0.730
Smoking	0%	1.4%	1.000
Hypertension	22.8%	27.1%	0.558
Diabetes mellitus	4.2%	1.4%	0.620
Other comorbidities	15.7%	8.5%	0.301
Fasting time (minutes)	770 (660/900)	720 (600/900)	0.508
Use of atropine	1.4%	10.0%	0.063
Use of ephedrine	20.0%	25.7%	0.421
Midazolam total dose (mg)	4.87 ± 1.8	4.8 ± 2.0	0.750
Duration of anesthesia (minutes)	95 (80/111)	90 (80/105)	0.242
Time in post-anesthesia care unit (minutes)	60 (55/66)	60 (55/65)	0.779

Values are presented as median (1st and 3rd quartiles), mean ± SD, or relative frequency (%)
PONV postoperative nausea and vomiting

There were no significant differences in the incidence of PONV during the total, early, or late periods between the two groups. There was also no significant difference in the severity of nausea between the two groups. There was a significantly lower incidence of late-onset vomiting in the palonosetron group than in the ondansetron group; however, there was no significant difference in the overall incidence of vomiting or in the incidence of early-onset vomiting. The need for rescue medication for PONV and the total dose of metoclopramide was similar between the two groups (Table 2).

There were no significant differences in patient satisfaction with the management of PONV between the two groups (Table 3). The incidence of clinically significant PONV was low in both groups, as determined by the simplified PONV impact scale; however, there was no statistically significant difference in the incidence of clinically significant PONV between the two groups (Table 3) [13].

The degree of postoperative pain, the need for rescue i.v. morphine, and the cumulative consumption of rescue i.v. morphine were similar between the two groups (Table 4). No patient had symptoms suggestive of postdural puncture headache. The incidence of adverse effects potentially attributable to serotonin receptor antagonists, such as dizziness and headache, was low in both groups (no statistically significant difference was detected), and adverse effects were considered mild in all cases (data not shown).

Table 2 Frequencies of PONV and use of rescue medication in the ondansetron and palonosetron groups

	Ondansetron	Palonosetron	*P* value
PONV	52.9%	42.9%	0.236
Nausea	51.4%	42.9%	0.310
Early-onset nausea	27.1%	21.4%	0.430
Late-onset nausea	35.7%	30.0%	0.472
Vomiting	35.7%	22.9%	0.095
Early-onset vomiting	20.0%	14.3%	0.370
Late vomiting*	27.1%	11.4%	0.018
Use of rescue medication	30.0%	27.1%	0.708
Cumulative dose of metoclopramide (mg)*	0 (0/10)	0 (0/10)	0.840

Early-onset regarded as ≤6 h after surgery and late-onset regarded as 6–48 h after surgery
PONV postoperative nausea and vomiting
#Presented as median (1st and 3rd quartiles)
*$P < 0.05$

Discussion

Several clinical trials have studied the efficacy of palonosetron in the management of PONV, and almost all of them have reported a beneficial role of palonosetron when compared to placebo or other 5HT-3 receptor antagonists [8, 9, 15–18]. Two very recent meta-analyses showed reductions in the incidence of PONV when palonosetron was compared with ondansetron in patients who underwent general anesthesia [11, 12]. To our knowledge, the current study is the first to compare palonosetron with ondansetron in patients at a high risk of PONV who received neuraxial anesthesia with intrathecal morphine.

In the current study, there was no statistically significant reduction in the overall incidence of PONV in patients who received palonosetron versus those who received ondansetron, which suggests that the prophylactic effect of palonosetron on PONV is similar to that of other 5HT-3 receptor antagonists in patients undergoing neuraxial anesthesia. However, we observed a significant reduction in the incidence of late-onset vomiting with palonosetron, which could be attributable to the longer duration of action of palonosetron. Thus, palonosetron may better attenuate the prolonged adverse effects of intrathecal morphine than shorter acting 5HT-3 receptor antagonists.

Table 3 Frequency of moderate/severe nausea, clinically significant PONV, and low patient satisfaction with PONV control

	Ondansetron	Palonosetron	*P* value
Moderate/severe nausea (VAS ≥ 5)	44.2%	35.7%	0.301
Clinically significant PONV ([a]score ≥ 5)	5.7%	2.8%	0.681
Low patient satisfaction with PONV control	15.7%	10.0%	0.313

PONV postoperative nausea and vomiting, *VAS* visual analog scale
[a]Simplified PONV impact scale [13]

Table 4 Severity of pain, frequency of rescue analgesic use, and cumulative morphine consumption

	Ondansetron	Palonosetron	*P* value
Severity of pain (VAS)[a]	4 (0/7)	5 (0/7)	0.377
Use of morphine	5.7%	8.6%	0.745
Cumulative morphine consumption (mg)[a]	0 (0/0)	0 (0/0)	0.501

VAS visual analog scale
[a]Presented as median (1st and 3rd quartile)

Few studies have focused on PONV in patients undergoing regional anesthesia with neuraxial opioids [5]. In a recent meta-analysis, 5HT-3 receptor antagonists (not including palonosetron) were shown to significantly reduce the incidence of PONV after caesarean section performed under spinal anesthesia with intrathecal morphine [19]. In the only study evaluating the efficacy of palonosetron after spinal anesthesia, palonosetron was associated with a lower incidence of PONV than ramosetron, another long-acting 5HT-3 receptor antagonist [10]. That study was performed in patients who underwent caesarean section without receiving neuraxial opioids; thus, the incidence of PONV and other pathophysiological considerations in that study may not be comparable to those of the current study.

Nausea and vomiting are well-known side effects of opioids that may have different central and peripheral components. The precise mechanisms of opioid-induced nausea and vomiting (OINV) are not entirely certain; however, known aspects include the activation of mu opioid receptors in the chemoreceptor trigger zone, direct stimulation of the vestibular apparatus, and peripheral action of opioids on the gastrointestinal tract [20]. The use of morphine in neuraxial anesthesia is related to a high incidence of PONV. Any hydrophilic substance (e.g., morphine), when injected into the subarachnoid space, tends to remain in the cerebrospinal fluid for a long period; during this period, it moves rostrally and reaches areas in the brainstem that induce nausea and vomiting [5].

It is likely that the addition of morphine in neuraxial anesthesia contributed to the high incidence of nausea and vomiting observed in this study. However, because several mechanisms and risk factors were involved (e.g., young age, female sex, a history of nonsmoking, and a history of gynecological surgery), it is difficult to clearly separate "pure" OINV from the broader definition of PONV.

The underlying pathophysiological mechanisms of PONV after neuraxial anesthesia include the use of hydrophilic opioids, arterial hypotension, increased sensory blockade, symptomatic liquoric hypotension, and gastrointestinal hyperactivity due to sympathetic blockade [5]. Serotonin receptor antagonists may only counteract some of these factors. Therefore, other strategies for PONV prevention must be used in some cases.

Dexamethasone is an effective drug for PONV prophylaxis, including in patients who receive neuraxial opioids [21]. The combination of dexamethasone and ondansetron has been shown to be particularly effective in patients at high risk of PONV [22]. Moreover, it has recently been reported that the combination of dexamethasone and palonosetron is more effective than palonosetron alone for reducing PONV after laparoscopic surgery [23].

Considering the high incidence of PONV in our study population, we believed it was ethically appropriate to use a combination therapy for PONV prevention rather than a single drug [1]. As patients in both groups received dexamethasone for this purpose, the overall incidence of PONV was probably diminished, which may have increased the chance of a type II error and reduced the detection power of this study. A similar limitation is applicable to secondary outcomes, such as the incidence of clinically significant PONV as determined by the simplified PONV impact scale. Notably, the incidences of clinically significant PONV were low in both groups.

The long-acting effect of palonosetron seems to be useful when a hydrophilic opioid, such as morphine, is administered intrathecally. However, despite the pharmacological benefits of palonosetron, the incidence of PONV remained high in the current study. Further studies are necessary to evaluate the role of palonosetron in the prevention of PONV in patients who undergo neuraxial anesthesia, particularly when a neuraxial opioid is used. It is also important to study the role of palonosetron in association with other PONV prophylaxis strategies.

Conclusion

In conclusion, palonosetron exhibited efficacy similar to that of ondansetron for reducing the overall incidence of PONV in patients who underwent TAH under spinal anesthesia with intrathecal morphine; however, palonosetron did reduce the incidence of late-onset vomiting better than ondansetron.

Abbreviations

OINV: Opioid-induced nausea and vomiting; PONV: Postoperative nausea and vomiting; TAH: Total abdominal hysterectomy; VAS: Visual analogue scale

Acknowledgements

None.

Authors' contributions

Study design: GOC, RLA, CNL, PRRO, NSPM. Data collection: GOC, GNJ, JCMFOJr, PRRO, CNL. Data analysis: GOC, RLA, MJM, LJSCA. Drafting paper: GOC, RLA, MJM, LJSCA, NSPM. The manuscript was reviewed and approved by all the authors.

Author details

[1]Department of Anesthesiology, São Rafael Hospital, D'Or Institute for Research and Education (IDOR), Salvador, Brazil. [2]Department of

Anesthesiology, Cardiopulmonar Hospital, Salvador, Brazil. [3]Department of Anesthesiology, São Paulo State University, Botucatu, Brazil. [4]Federal University of Bahia, Salvador, Brazil. [5]Department of Gynecology, São Rafael Hospital, D'Or Institute for Research and Education (IDOR), Salvador, Brazil. [6]Department of Anesthesiology, Santo Antonio Hospital, Salvador, Brazil.

References

1. Gan TJ, Diemunsch P, Habib AS, Kovac A, Kranke P, Meyer TA, Watcha M, Chung F, Angus S, Apfel CC, Bergese SD, Candiotti KA, Chan MT, Davis PJ, Hooper VD, Lagoo-Deenadayalan S, Myles P, Nezat G, Philip BK, Tramer MR. Society for Ambulatory Anesthesia. Consensus guidelines for the management of postoperative nausea and vomiting. Anesth Analg. 2014; 118:85–113.
2. Catro-Alves LJ, De Azevedo VL, De Freitas Braga TF, Goncalves AC, De Oliveira GS Jr. The effect of neuraxial versus general anesthesia techniques on postoperative quality of recovery and analgesia after abdominal hysterectomy: a prospective, randomized, controlled trial. Anesth Analg. 2011;113:1480–6.
3. Chinachoti T, Nilrat P, Samarnpiboonphol P. Nausea, vomiting and pruritus induced by intrathecal morphine. J Med Assoc Thail. 2013;96:589–94.
4. Apfel CC, Heidrich FM, Jukar-Rao S, Jalota L, Hornuss C, Whelan RP, Zhang K, Cakmakkaya OS. Evidence-based analysis of risk factors for postoperative nausea and vomiting. Br J Anaesth. 2012;109:742–53.
5. Borgeat A, Ekatodramis G, Schenker CA. Postoperative nausea and vomiting in regional anesthesia: a review. Anesthesiology. 2003;98:530–47.
6. Chandrakantan A, Glass PS. Multimodal therapies for postoperative nausea and vomiting, and pain. Br J Anaesth. 2011;107:i27–40.
7. Dominguez JE, Habib AS. Prophylaxis and treatment of the side-effects of neuraxial morphine analgesia following cesarean delivery. Curr Opin Anaesthesiol. 2013;26:288–95.
8. Kovac AL, Eberhart L, Kotarski J, Clerici G, Apfel C. A randomized, double-blind study to evaluate the efficacy and safety of three different doses of palonosetron versus placebo in preventing postoperative nausea and vomiting over a 72-hour period. Anesth Analg. 2008;107:439–44.
9. Candiotti KA, Kovac AL, Melson TI, Clerici G, Joo Gan T. A randomized, double-blind study to evaluate the efficacy and safety of three different doses of palonosetron versus placebo for preventing postoperative nausea and vomiting. Anesth Analg. 2008;107:445–51.
10. Chattopadhyay S, Goswami S. Palonosetron versus ramosetron prophylaxis for control ofpostoperative nausea and vomiting after cesarean delivery under spinal anesthesia. J Obstet Gynaecol India. 2015;65:28–33.
11. Xiong C, Liu G, Ma R, Xue J, Wu A. Efficacy of palonosetron for preventing postoperative nausea and vomiting: a systematic review and meta-analysis. Can J Anaesth. 2015;62:1268–78.
12. Singh PM, Borle A, Gouda D, Makkar JK, Arora MK, Trikha A, Sinha A, Goudra B. Efficacy of palonosetron in postoperative nausea and vomiting (PONV)-a meta-analysis. J Clin Anesth. 2016;34:459–82.
13. Myles PS, Wengritzky R. Simplified postoperative nausea and vomiting impact scale for audit and post-discharge review. Br J Anaesth. 2012;108:423–9.
14. Apfel CC, Roewer N, Korttila K. How to study postoperative nausea and vomiting. Acta Anaesthesiol Scand. 2002;46:921–8.
15. Park SK, Cho EJ. A randomized, double-blind trial of palonosetron compared with ondansetron in preventing postoperative nausea and vomiting after gynaecological laparoscopic surgery. J Int Med Res. 2011;39:399–407.
16. Moon YE, Joo J, Kim JE, Lee Y. Anti-emetic effect of ondansetron and palonosetron in thyroidectomy: a prospective, randomized, double-blind study. Br J Anaesth. 2012;108:417–22.
17. Kim SH, Hong JY, Kim WO, Kil HK, Karm MH, Hwang JH. Palonosetron has superior prophylactic antiemetic efficacy compared with ondansetron or ramosetron in high-risk patients undergoing laparoscopic surgery: a prospective, randomized, double-blinded study. Korean J Anesthesiol. 2013; 64:517–23.
18. Chun HR, Jeon IS, Park SY, Lee SJ, Kang SH, Kim SI. Efficacy of palonosetron for the prevention of postoperative nausea and vomiting: a randomized, double-blinded, placebo-controlled trial. Br J Anaesth. 2014;112:485–90.
19. George RB, Allen TK, Habib AS. Serotonin receptor antagonists for the prevention and treatment of pruritus, nausea, and vomiting in women undergoing cesarean delivery with intrathecal morphine: a systematic review and meta-analysis. Anesth Analg. 2009;109:174–82.
20. Smith HS, Laufer A. Opioid induced nausea and vomiting. Eur J Pharmacol. 2014;722:67–78.
21. Allen TK, Jones CA, Habib AS. Dexamethasone for the prophylaxis of postoperative nausea and vomiting associated with neuraxial morphine administration: a systematic review and meta-analysis. Anesth Analg. 2012; 114:813–22.
22. Apfel CC, Korttila K, Abdalla M, Kerger H, Turan A, Vedder I, Zernak C, Danner K, Jokela R, Pocock SJ, Trenkler S, Kredel M, Biedler A, Sessler DI, Roewer N, investigators IMPACT. A factorial trial of six interventions for the prevention of postoperative nausea and vomiting. N Engl J Med. 2004;350: 2441–51.
23. Bala I, Bharti N, Murugesan S, Gupta R. Comparison of palonosetron with palonosetron-dexamethasone combination for prevention of postoperative nausea and vomiting in patients undergoing laparoscopic cholecystectomy. Minerva Anestesiol. 2014;80:779–84.

The effects of epidural anaesthesia and analgesia on T lymphocytes differentiation markers and cytokines in patients after gastric cancer resection

Liping Wang[1†], Si Liang[2†], Hong Chen[1], Yang Xu[1] and Yu Wang[1*]

Abstract

Background: Epidural use can prevent peri-operative neuro-endocrine stress responses, mitigate pain after surgery, and reduce opioid use, which all lead to immunosuppression.

Methods: Forty patients with gastric cancer were ultimately enrolled into the study. Patients who received general anaesthesia (GA group, $n = 20$) or a combination of general anaesthesia and peri-operative epidural use (EGA group, $n = 20$) were given intravenous analgesia or epidural analgesia, respectively. We collected visual analogue scale (VAS) scores, length of hospital stay, the time of the first passage of flatus and incidence of postoperative nausea and vomiting (PONV). We also collected data on the cluster of differentiation markers $(CD)^{3+}$, CD^{4+}, CD^{8+}, CD^{4+}/CD^{8+}, interleukin (IL)-4, IL-6, and interferon (IFN)-γ the day before surgery as well as on postoperative days 1, 3, and 7.

Results: VAS scores and PONV in the GA group were higher than in the EGA group on postoperative day 3. CD^{3+}, CD^{4+}, and CD^{4+}/CD^{8+} T cells declined on postoperative day 3 and nearly recovered to baseline seven days after surgery in both groups. CD^{3+} T cells decreased more in the GA group than in the EGA group. IL-4, IL-6, and IFN-γ increased on postoperative day 3 and nearly recovered to baseline seven days after surgery in both groups. IL-4 and IL-6 increased more in the GA group than in the EGA group. IFN-γ increased more in the EGA group than in the GA group.

Conclusions: A combination of general anaesthesia and peri-operative epidural use can relieve postoperative pain and PONV. A combination of general anaesthesia and peri-operative epidural use decreases immunosuppression in gastric cancer resection.

Keywords: Epidural anaesthesia, General anaesthesia, Patient-controlled analgesia, Immune function, Cluster of differentiation, Cytokines

* Correspondence: littlepigdiudiu@163.com
†Liping Wang and Si Liang contributed equally to this work.
[1]Department of Anaesthesiology, Harbin Medical University Cancer Hospital, No. 150 Haping Rd., Nangang District, Harbin 150081, China

Background

The stress response induced by surgery can activate the immune regulation mechanism during a systemic inflammatory reaction [1–4]. There are many important contributors to the tumor microenvironment, such as cytokines, chemokines, inflammatory mediators, which exists in many stages of progression to metastasis [5–7]. Some clinical factors, such as general anaesthetics, postoperative pain, and opioid analgesia, have been recognized as immunosuppressive and have influenced the development of tumours [8–14]. In some studies, epidural anaesthesia (EA) was associated with improved overall survival in patients with gastric cancer; in other studies, EA did not improve overall survival [15–17]. EA may reduce cytokines and neuroendocrine stress immune stimulation, prevent nerve impulses, decrease excitability of the sympathetic adrenal medulla axis, reduce cortisol production, and improve the function of T lymphocytes [18, 19].

Among cytokines, interleukin (IL)-4, IL-6, and interferon (IFN)-γ play prominent roles in chronic inflammation, autoimmunity, infectious diseases and cancer, where they often act as diagnostic or prognostic indicators of disease activity and response to therapy [20, 21]. Therefore, we designed this study to explore the interaction between epidural use and the aforementioned cytokines in patients with gastric cancer.

Methods

Patient identification and exclusion

This study was a single-centre, randomized, observer-blinded study. The study procedures were approved by the Ethics Committee of The Harbin Medical University Cancer Hospital. This study was registered prospectively at http://www.chictr.org.cn/index.aspx on October 10, 2017 (Registered ChiCTR-INR-17012939). After the written consent was obtained from study participants, 50 American Society of Anesthesiologists (ASA) I-II patients aged 20–80 yr. who underwent radical resection of gastric cancer in our hospital were enrolled in this study between November 12, 2017, and December 15, 2017. Exclusion criteria were: (1) emergency operations, (2) laparoscopic procedures,(3) neoadjuvant treatment,(4) abnormally white blood cell count, (5) peri-operative transfusion, (6) severe heart, lung, liver, kidney, or endocrine diseases, After confirming understanding of the recruiter's description of the trial, all the patients signed informed consent forms. Anaesthesia and analgesia protocols were standardized as follows. Patients were randomly assigned to the general anaesthesia (GA) group or epidural anaesthesia (EGA) group by computer-generated codes on the beginning of the study.

Sample size calculation and masking method

The clear primary outcome of this study was inflammatory response, which was evaluated via the concentration of IL-6. Previously published studies on IL-6 suggested that its standard deviation (SD) in vivo is in the order of 7.6 pg/ml. Twenty patients were calculated based on detecting a reduction of 6.8 pg/ml deviation on α-value 0.05 and a power of 0.8. To compensate for potential dropouts, we enrolled Twenty-five patients.

The patients were randomly divided into two groups by computer-generated codes on the time of the study onset. Physicians who completed postoperative assessment and biological detection were blinded to the group assignments throughout the study period until follow-up was completed for final analysis.

Anaesthesia technique and grouping method

On arrival to the operating room, patients were monitored via electrocardiogram and blood pressure as well as pulse oximetry. Patients randomly assigned to the GA group underwent induction of balanced GA with 0.05 mg/kg midazolam (Enhua Pharmaceutical Co., Jiangsu, China), 0.2 μg/kg sufentanil (Renfu Pharmaceutical Co., Beijing, China), 1–1.5 mg/kg propofol (AstraZeneca Pharmaceutical Co., Shanghai, China), and 0.15 mg/kg cisatracurium (Hengrui Medicine Co., Jiangsu, China). Anaesthesia was maintained with propofol when the bispectral index (BIS) was 40–60, and intraoperative analgesia consisted of remifentanil (Enhua Pharmaceutical Co., Jiangsu, China). Oesophageal temperature was monitored and maintained above 36 °C. Patient-controlled intravenous analgesia (PCIA) with sufentanil (0.5 μg/ml) was available for 72–120 h. The PCIA protocol of the sufentanil group (S group) consisted of 0.5 μg/ml sufentanil (total 300 ml) with a background infusion rate of 4 ml h^{-1}, a bolus dose of 3 ml, and a lockout time of 15 min. Patients in the EGA group were given T_{8-10} epidural anaesthesia before general anaesthesia. An infusion of 0.5% ropivacaine (AstraZeneca Pharmaceutical Co., Shanghai, China) was administered during surgery, and the loading dose (0.5% ropivacaine, 5-7 ml) depended on the height and weight of the patient. GA was induced with 0.05 mg/kg midazolam, 0.2 μg/kg sufentanil, 1–1.5 mg/kg propofol, and 0.15 mg/kg cisatracurium, and anaesthesia was maintained with propofol when the bispectral index (BIS) was 40–60. Patient-controlled epidural analgesia (PCEA) with a combination of 0.2% ropivacaine and 0.5 μg/ml sufentanil was available for 72–120 h. Acute rescue analgesic medications could be used when the VAS score was more than 4 and a bolus of 100 mg tramadol, administered via intravenous injection, was required more than 3 times.

Indicator and data

A physician who was blinded to the group assignment assessed postoperative pain intensity using the visual analogue scale (VAS) on postoperative days 1, 2, and 3. The demographic data, cancer stage, degree of differentiation, duration of the operation, length of hospital stay, time of the first passage of flatus and incidence of postoperative nausea and vomiting (PONV) were recorded. A physician who was blinded to the group assignment collected data on cluster of differentiation markers $(CD)^{3+}$, CD^{4+}, CD^{8+}, and CD^{4+}/CD^{8+}, Interleukin (IL)-4, IL-6, and Interferon (IFN)-γ through peripheral blood (10 ml) on the day before surgery, day (d) 0, and on postoperative days 1, 3, and 7.CD^{3+}, CD^{4+}, CD^{8+} were measured by flow cytometric analysis. The plasma level of IL-4, IL-6, and Interferon IFN-γ were measured by enzyme-linked immunosorbent assay (ELISA). All samples were measured using three independent experiments.

Statistical approach

Statistical analysis was performed using SPSS version 22.0 for Windows (IBM Corp., USA). Normally distributed data were expressed as the means ± SDs. Categorical variables were described using frequencies and were analysed using the χ^2 test. Fisher's exact test was used for small sample sizes (expected frequencies < 5). We checked for normality of the data with the Shapiro Wilk test and used a one-way ANOVA between the two groups. The results with $P < 0.05$ were considered statistically significant.

Results

Patient characteristics

Between November 12, 2017, and December 15, 2017, fifty patients were screened for this study, and forty patients were ultimately included in this study. Five patients with metastases or peri-operative transfusions were excluded. Five patients had their analgesic regimen modified because of hypotension and severe nausea (Fig. 1). The two groups were similar with respect to age, height, weight, gender, ASA grade, cancer stage and degree of differentiation, duration of surgery, surgical procedure and surgical manner between the two groups (Table 1).

Association between epidural use and postoperative variables

The VAS scores in the GA group were higher than in the EGA group on postoperative day 3, and the incidence of PONV in the EGA group was lower ($P < 0.05$, Table 2). There were no differences in days of analgesia, the time of the first passage of flatus, and length of hospital stay. CD^{3+}, CD^{4+}, and CD^{4+}/CD^{8+} T cells declined on postoperative day 3 ($P < 0.05$) and nearly recovered to baseline seven days after surgery in both groups. CD^{3+} T cells decreased more in the GA group than in the EGA group ($P < 0.05$, Table 3). IL-4, IL-6, and IFN-γ increased on postoperative day 3 ($P < 0.05$; Figs. 2, 3, and 4) and nearly recovered to baseline seven days after surgery in both groups. IL-4 and IL-6 increased more in the GA group than in the EGA group ($P < 0.05$, Figs. 2 and 3). IFN-γ increased more in the EGA group than in the GA group ($P < 0.05$, Fig. 4).

Discussion

In our study, we found a beneficial effect of epidural use. The VAS scores in the GA group were higher than those in the EGA group on postoperative day three. The incidence

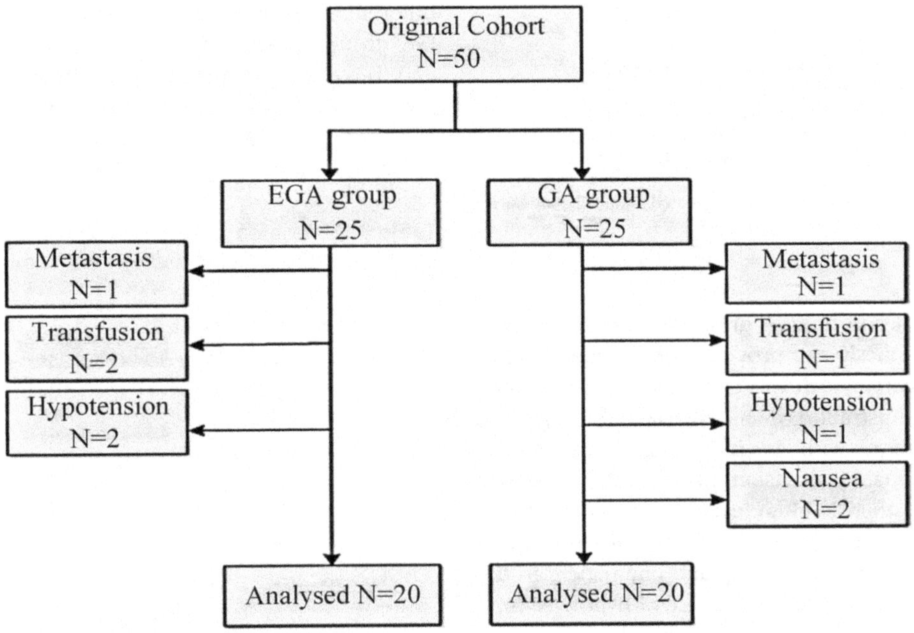

Fig. 1 Patient identification and exclusion

Table 1 Baseline and surgical characteristics of general anesthesia group and epidural combined general anesthesia group

Characteristics	GA group (*n* = 20)	EGA group (n = 20)	*P* value
Age (year)	59.3 ± 6.8	59.7 ± 8.5	0.870
Height (cm)	164.0 ± 6.1	164.5 ± 8.7	0.832
Weight (kg)	66.5 ± 8.4	64.3 ± 7.7	0.394
Gender (male)	11 (55%)	10 (50%)	0.752
ASA grade			
I	2 (10%)	2 (10%)	1.000
II	16 (80%)	17 (85%)	
III	2 (10%)	1 (5%)	
Cancer stage			
I	3 (15%)	4 (20%)	0.925
II	2 (10%)	2 (10%)	
III	12 (60%)	10 (50%)	
Cancer stageIV	3 (15%)	4 (20%)	
Degree of differentiation			
1	7 (35%)	5 (25%)	0.915
2	10 (50%)	11 (55%)	
3	2 (10%)	2 (10%)	
4	1 (5%)	2 (10%)	
Duration of surgery (h)	2.25 (2.00,3.75)	2.25 (2.00,3.50)	0.577
Surgical procedure			
open	20 (100%)	20 (100%)	1.000
minimal invasive	0 (0%)	0 (0%)	
Surgical manner			
total	20 (100%)	20 (100%)	1.000
partial	0 (0%)	0 (0%)	

GA = general anesthesia group
EGA = epidural anesthesia combined with general anesthesia group
ASA = American Society of Anesthesiologists
Cancer stages: I grade-T1, N0, M0/T2, N0, M0/T1, N1, M0; II grade-T3, N0, M0/T4a, N1, M0/T3, N1, M0/T2, N2, M0/T1, N3, M0; III grade-T2, N3, M0/T3, N2, M0/T3, N3, M0/T4a, N2, M0/T4a, N3, M0/ any T4b, any N, M0; IV grade, any T, any N, M1
Degrees of differentiation: Degree1, poorly differentiated; Degree2, moderately differentiated; Degree3, well differentiated; Degree 4, other/unknown differentiated

of PONV was higher in the GA group. It has been proven that epidural anaesthesia can provide better analgesia after gastric cancer surgery, which was consistent with our study [22]. Epidural administration of anaesthesia and analgesia is considered a technique with risk of complications, such as neuraxial haematoma, hypotension, pruritus; the subjective experience of anaesthetists often leads to the failure of epidural anaesthesia and analgesia [23, 24]. In our study, there were two patients in the EGA group and one patient in the GA group who could not use EA because of hypotension.

Many studies have reported that opioids impair the peri-operative immune system and increase vascular

Table 2 The VAS scores of patients in the postoperative days 1, 2, 3 between general anesthesia group and epidural combined general anesthesia group

Characteristics	GA group (n = 20)	EGA group (n = 20)	*P* value
VAS scores			
POD1	3 (2,5)	2 (1,4)	0.004*
POD2	2 (1,4)	1 (0,3)	0.003*
POD3	1 (0,3)	0 (0,2)	0.003*
Days of analgesia	3 (3,5)	3 (3,5)	0.527
Days of flatus time	3 (3,4)	3 (2,4)	0.764
Nausea and vomiting (%)	8(40%)	1 (5%)	0.020*
Length of stay	11 (9,12)	11 (9,12)	0.795

VAS=Visual analogue scale (VAS) scores
POD = Postoperative day
*: Compare between two groups, $P < 0.05$

permeability, and the use of epidural anaesthesia may prevent these peri-operative immunosuppressive changes during major surgery because it can decrease neuroendocrine stress responses [18, 25–28]. Immune surveillance is the primary indicator for stopping the metastasis of tumours, and immunosuppression may destroy the defensive barrier [29]. Clinical events that may lead to immunosuppressive changes facilitated by surgery include injury, pain, and use of anaesthetic medications [30–32]. CD^{3+} T cells, CD^{4+} T cells, and CD^{8+} T cells are the main cells which take part in antitumour immunity [33]. The ratio of CD^{4+}/CD^{8+} cells decreases as the serum cortisol levels increase [34, 35]. In our study, CD^{3+}, CD^{4+}, and CD^{4+}/CD^{8+} T cells were inhibited and had a negative trend. All patients' CD^{3+} and CD^{4+} T cells decreased to different degrees on the first postoperative day, but in the GA group, patients' CD^{3+} T cells significantly decreased and recovered to preoperative levels until the seventh postoperative day. The change in CD^{8+} T cells was not statistically significant. These results are consistent with some prior studies [36, 37],they described a lymphocyte

Table 3 Comparison of T lymphocyte subsets of patients in general anesthesia group and epidural combined general anesthesia group

Characteristics	Group	d0	d1	d3	d7
$CD3^+$ (%)	GA	54.3 ± 3.5	42.5 ± 2.3#	44.6 ± 3.2#	51.8 ± 6.7
	EGA	55.6 ± 4.1	46.1 ± 2.9#*	48.1 ± 2.2#*	51.2 ± 6.9
$CD4^+$ (%)	GA	32.4 ± 4.3	21.5 ± 3.4#	23.2 ± 1.6#	31.7 ± 2.8
	EGA	34.5 ± 3.5	23.4 ± 3.5#	24.5 ± 2.1#	33.0 ± 2.0
$CD8^+$ (%)	GA	21.1 ± 1.8	20.7 ± 1.8	21.0 ± 1.9	20.9 ± 1.3
	EGA	21.5 ± 1.2	21.2 ± 1.1	22.9 ± 2.0	21.3 ± 1.5
$CD4^+/CD8^+$	GA	1.5 ± 0.5	1.0 ± 0.2#	1.0 ± 0.1#	1.5 ± 0.2
	EGA	1.6 ± 0.5	1.2 ± 0.2#	1.2 ± 0.3#	1.5 ± 0.1

CD = Clusters of Differentiation
#: Compare to d0 $P < 0.05$, *:Compare between two groups, $P < 0.05$

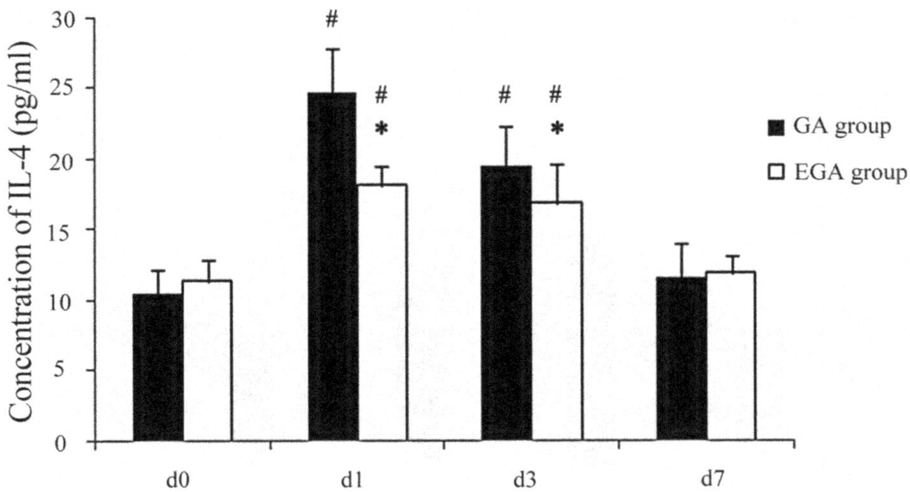

Fig. 2 Comparison of IL-4 between the general anaesthesia group and epidural combined with general anaesthesia group on day (d) 0, the day before surgery, and on postoperative days 1, 3, and 7

depressing factor that was present in the serum of patients in the GA group but was absent in the serum of patients in the EGA group.

Many cytokines can modulate the immune system. Pro-inflammatory cytokines may favour tumour progression. Activated biological cascades lead to immunosuppression, which affects the immune response and decreases IL-4 and IFN-γ [38, 39]. As a pro-inflammatory factor, IL-4 stimulates the proliferation of B cells and participates in the differentiation of Th2 cells. The combination of the cytokine IL-6 with prostaglandin 2 can reduce the production of the immune factor IL-2 by Th1 cells and affect the activation of NK cells [40]. IL-6 has a major influence on the proliferation, survival and metastatic properties of cancerous cells, and studies using preclinical mouse models indicate that treatments targeting IL-6 or its receptor display therapeutic efficacy as anticancer agents [20].In our study, the pro-inflammatory cytokines IL-4 and IL-6 increased more in the GA group than in the EGA group, which may indicate that immune function was less suppressed in the EGA group. IFN-γ can kill tumour cells directly and transform Th0 cells into Th1 cells, which play a large role in the activation of NK cells and T cells. The level of IFN-γ expression embodies the memory ability of this antitumour cytokine [41, 42]. In our study, IFN-γ increased more in the EGA group than

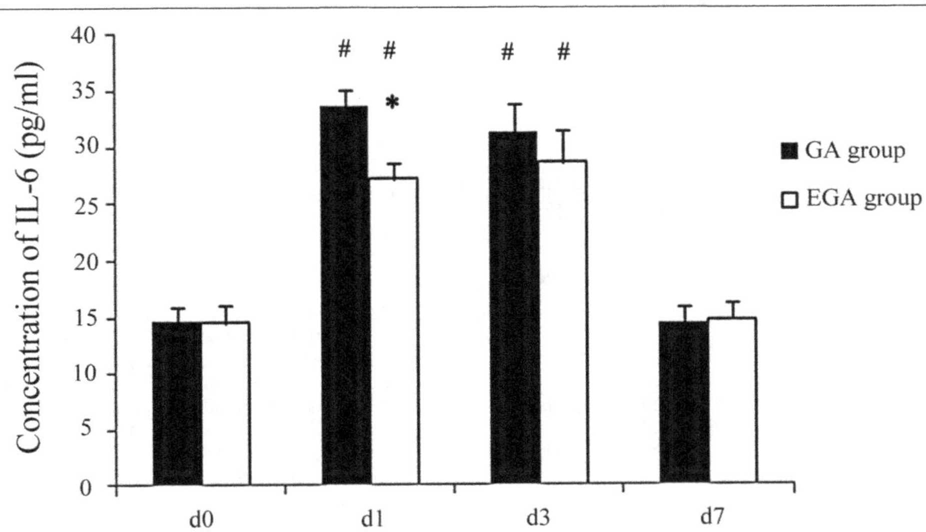

Fig. 3 Comparison of IL-6 between the general anaesthesia group and epidural combined with general anaesthesia group on day (d) 0, the day before surgery, and on postoperative days 1, 3, and 7

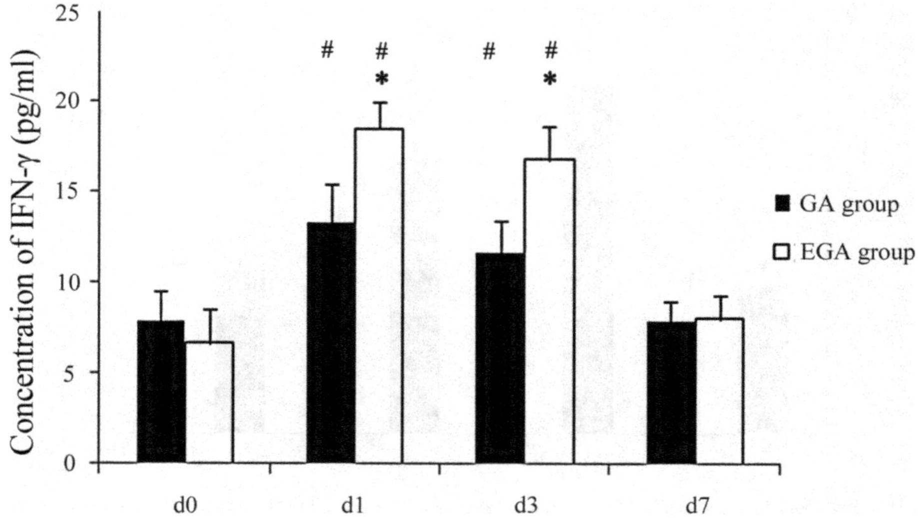

Fig. 4 Comparison of IFN-γ between the general anaesthesia group and epidural combined with general anaesthesia group on day (d) 0, the day before surgery, and postoperative days 1, 3, and 7

in the GA group, which may indicate that immune function was less suppressed in the EGA group. Therefore, in our study, EA was able to relieve postoperative pain and PONV, was able to decrease immunosuppression, and may have reduced inflammatory-associated metastasis in gastric cancer.

There were a few limitations in our study. First, we only measured some T cell subsets and some important immune factors. The immune system is a complex system. There are many immune cells, such as NK cells, and other immune factors, such as IL-2 and IL-12, which may be investigated in the future because these antitumourigenic cytokines were increased by EA. Second, these patients' long-term outcomes, such as long-term survival, recurrence rates and metastasis rates, could not be obtained at present. We will evaluate these results in 3 to 5 years.

Conclusions

A combination of general anaesthesia and peri-operative epidural use can relieve postoperative pain and PONV. A combination of general anaesthesia and peri-operative epidural use decreases immunosuppression in gastric cancer resection.

Abbreviations

(NK) cell: Natural killer cell; ASA: American Society of Anesthesiologists; BIS: Bispectral index; EGA: Epidural general anaesthesia; GA: General anaesthesia; IFN: Interferon; IL: Interleukin; PCEA: Patient-controlled epidural analgesia; PCIA: Patient-controlled intravenous analgesia; PONV: Postoperative nausea and vomiting; VAS: Visual analogue scale

Acknowledgements

Not applicable.

Authors' contributions

Y.W. and L.W. contributed to the study conception and the designing and drafting of the manuscript. L.W., S.L., C.H. and Y.X. contributed to acquisition and interpretation of the data. H.C. and L.W. were responsible for the revision of important intellectual content and final approval of the version to be published. All authors read and approved the final manuscript.

Author details

[1]Department of Anaesthesiology, Harbin Medical University Cancer Hospital, No. 150 Haping Rd., Nangang District, Harbin 150081, China. [2]Department of Anaesthesiology, Affiliated Hospital of HeBei University, Baoding, China.

References

1. Cassinello F, Prieto I, del OM, Rivas S, Strichartz GR. Cancer surgery: how may anesthesia influence outcome. J Clin Anesth. 2015;27(3):262–72.
2. Shakhar G, Ben-Eliyahu S. Potential prophylactic measures against postoperative immunosuppression: could they reduce recurrence rates in oncological patients. Ann Surg Oncol. 2003;10(8):972–92.
3. Xu YJ, Li SY, Cheng Q, et al. Effects of anaesthesia on proliferation, invasion and apoptosis of LoVo colon cancer cells in vitro. Anaesthesia. 2016;71(2):147–54.
4. O'Dwyer MJ, Owen HC, Torrance HD. The perioperative immune response. Curr Opin Crit Care. 2015;21(4):336–42.
5. Luo JL, Maeda S, Hsu LC, Yagita H, Karin M. Inhibition of NF-kappaB in cancer cells converts inflammation- induced tumor growth mediated by TNFalpha to TRAIL-mediated tumor regression. Cancer Cell. 2004;6(3):297–305.
6. Tan W, Zhang W, Strasner A, et al. Tumour-infiltrating regulatory T cells stimulate mammary cancer metastasis through RANKL-RANK signalling. Nature. 2011;470(7335):548–53.
7. Hou M, Zhou NB, Li H, et al. Morphine and ketamine inhibit immune function of gastric cancer patients by increasing percentage of CD4(+)CD25(+)Foxp3(+) regulatory T cells in vitro. J Surg Res. 2016;203(2):306–12.
8. Oka M, Hazama S, Suzuki M, et al. Depression of cytotoxicity of nonparenchymal cells in the liver after surgery. Surgery. 1994;116(5):877–82.
9. Müller-Edenborn B, Frick R, Piegeler T, et al. Volatile anaesthetics reduce neutrophil inflammatory response by interfering with CXC receptor-2 signalling. Br J Anaesth. 2015;114(1):143–9.
10. Wigmore TJ, Mohammed K, Jhanji S. Long-term survival for patients undergoing volatile versus IV anesthesia for Cancer surgery: a retrospective analysis. Anesthesiology. 2016;124(1):69–79.
11. Cata JP, Chavez-MacGregor M, Valero V, et al. The impact of paravertebral block analgesia on breast Cancer survival after surgery. Reg Anesth Pain Med. 2016;41(6):696–703.
12. Yi W, Li D, Guo Y, Zhang Y, Huang B, Li X. Sevoflurane inhibits the migration

and invasion of glioma cells by upregulating microRNA-637. Int J Mol Med. 2016;38(6):1857–63.

13. Connolly C, Buggy DJ. Opioids and tumour metastasis: does the choice of the anesthetic-analgesic technique influence outcome after cancer surgery. Curr Opin Anaesthesiol. 2016;29(4):468–74.
14. Kim R. Anesthetic technique and cancer recurrence in oncologic surgery: unraveling the puzzle. Cancer Metastasis Rev. 2016.
15. Hiller JG, Hacking MB, Link EK, Wessels KL, Riedel BJ. Perioperative epidural analgesia reduces cancer recurrence after gastro-oesophageal surgery. Acta Anaesthesiol Scand. 2014;58(3):281–90.
16. Cummings KC, Patel M, Htoo PT, Bakaki PM, Cummings LC, Koroukian S. A comparison of the effects of epidural analgesia versus traditional pain management on outcomes after gastric cancer resection: a population-based study. Reg Anesth Pain Med. 2014;39(3):200–7.
17. Pérez-González O, Cuéllar-Guzmán LF, Navarrete-Pacheco M, Ortiz-Martínez JJ, Williams WH, Cata JP. Impact of regional anesthesia on gastroesophageal Cancer surgery outcomes: a systematic review of the literature. Anesth Analg. 2018;127(3):753–8.
18. Ben-David B. Anaesthesia in Cancer surgery: can it affect Cancer survival. Curr Clin Pharmacol. 2016;11(1):4–20.
19. Byrne K, Levins KJ, Buggy DJ. Can anesthetic-analgesic technique during primary cancer surgery affect recurrence or metastasis. Can J Anaesth. 2016; 63(2):184–92.
20. Jones SA, Jenkins BJ. Recent insights into targeting the IL-6 cytokine family in inflammatory diseases and cancer. Nat Rev Immunol. 2018;18(12):773–89.
21. Cui M, Gong C, Jiang B, et al. Evaluation of immune responses of gastric cancer patients treated by laparoscopic and open gastrectomy. Med Oncol. 2015, 32(11):253.
22. Yanagimoto Y, Takiguchi S, Miyazaki Y, et al. Comparison of pain management after laparoscopic distal gastrectomy with and without epidural analgesia. Surg Today. 2016;46(2):229–34.
23. Salicath JH, Yeoh EC, Bennett MH. Epidural analgesia versus patient-controlled intravenous analgesia for pain following intra-abdominal surgery in adults. Cochrane Database Syst Rev. 2018;(8):CD010434.
24. Wang L, Li X, Chen H, Liang J, Wang Y. Effect of patient-controlled epidural analgesia versus patient-controlled intravenous analgesia on postoperative pain management and short-term outcomes after gastric cancer resection: a retrospective analysis of 3,042 consecutive patients between 2010 and 2015. J Pain Res. 2018;11:1743–9.
25. Hole A, Terjesen T, Breivik H. Epidural versus general anaesthesia for total hip arthroplasty in elderly patients. Acta Anaesthesiol Scand. 1980;24(4):279–87.
26. Rem J, Brandt MR, Kehlet H. Prevention of postoperative lymphopenia and granulocytosis by epidural analgesia. Lancet. 1980;1(8163):283–4.
27. Neeman E, Ben-Eliyahu S. Surgery and stress promote cancer metastasis: new outlooks on perioperative mediating mechanisms and immune involvement. Brain Behav Immun. 2013, 30 Suppl:S32–40.
28. Ahlers O, Nachtigall I, Lenze J, et al. Intraoperative thoracic epidural anaesthesia attenuates stress-induced immunosuppression in patients undergoing major abdominal surgery. Br J Anaesth. 2008;101(6):781–7.
29. Melamed R, Rosenne E, Shakhar K, Schwartz Y, Abudarham N, Ben-Eliyahu S. Marginating pulmonary-NK activity and resistance to experimental tumor metastasis: suppression by surgery and the prophylactic use of a beta-adrenergic antagonist and a prostaglandin synthesis inhibitor. Brain Behav Immun. 2005;19(2):114–26.
30. Sekandarzad MW, van Zundert AA, Lirk PB, Doornebal CW, Hollmann MW. Perioperative anesthesia care and tumor progression. Anesth Analg. 2016.
31. Buckley A, McQuaid S, Johnson P, Buggy DJ. Effect of anaesthetic technique on the natural killer cell anti-tumour activity of serum from women undergoing breast cancer surgery: a pilot study. Br J Anaesth. 2014, 113(Suppl 1):i56–62.
32. Xu YJ, Chen WK, Zhu Y, Wang SL, Miao CH. Effect of thoracic epidural anaesthesia on serum vascular endothelial growth factor C and cytokines in patients undergoing anaesthesia and surgery for colon cancer. Br J Anaesth. 2014, 113(Suppl 1):i49–55.
33. Gasparini G, Longo R, Sarmiento R, Morabito A. Inhibitors of cyclo-oxygenase 2: a new class of anticancer agents. Lancet Oncol. 2003;4(10):605–15.
34. Hosokawa T. Effect of anesthesia and surgery on cell-mediated immunity--the application of two color analysis to classification of functional lymphocyte subpopulation. Masui. 1987;36(6):956–61.
35. Hosokawa T, Hori Y, Ohtsuka T, Nakagawa H, Miyazaki M. Effect of anesthesia and surgery on immunity in patients with benign and malignant diseases. Masui. 1989;38(3):343–9.
36. Hashimoto T, Hashimoto S, Hori Y, Nakagawa H, Hosokawa T. Epidural anaesthesia blocks changes in peripheral lymphocytes subpopulation during gastrectomy for stomach cancer. Acta Anaesthesiol Scand. 1995;39(3):294–8.
37. Hole A, Unsgaard G. The effect of epidural and general anaesthesia on lymphocyte functions during and after major orthopaedic surgery. Acta Anaesthesiol Scand. 1983;27(2):135–41.
38. Page GG, Blakely WP, Ben-Eliyahu S. Evidence that postoperative pain is a mediator of the tumor-promoting effects of surgery in rats. Pain. 2001;90(1–2):191–9.
39. Greenfeld K, Avraham R, Benish M, et al. Immune suppression while awaiting surgery and following it: dissociations between plasma cytokine levels, their induced production, and NK cell cytotoxicity. Brain Behav Immun. 2007;21(4):503–13.
40. Goldfarb Y, Ben-Eliyahu S. Surgery as a risk factor for breast cancer recurrence and metastasis: mediating mechanisms and clinical prophylactic approaches. Breast Dis. 2006;26:99–114.
41. Sasada T, Kimura M, Yoshida Y, Kanai M, Takabayashi A. CD4+CD25+ regulatory T cells in patients with gastrointestinal malignancies: possible involvement of regulatory T cells in disease progression. Cancer. 2003;98(5):1089–99.
42. Liu S, Carpenter RL, Neal JM. Epidural anesthesia and analgesia. Their role in postoperative outcome. Anesthesiology. 1995;82(6):1474–506.

Permissions

All chapters in this book were first published by BioMed Central; hereby published with permission under the Creative Commons Attribution License or equivalent. Every chapter published in this book has been scrutinized by our experts. Their significance has been extensively debated. The topics covered herein carry significant findings which will fuel the growth of the discipline. They may even be implemented as practical applications or may be referred to as a beginning point for another development.

The contributors of this book come from diverse backgrounds, making this book a truly international effort. This book will bring forth new frontiers with its revolutionizing research information and detailed analysis of the nascent developments around the world.

We would like to thank all the contributing authors for lending their expertise to make the book truly unique. They have played a crucial role in the development of this book. Without their invaluable contributions this book wouldn't have been possible. They have made vital efforts to compile up to date information on the varied aspects of this subject to make this book a valuable addition to the collection of many professionals and students.

This book was conceptualized with the vision of imparting up-to-date information and advanced data in this field. To ensure the same, a matchless editorial board was set up. Every individual on the board went through rigorous rounds of assessment to prove their worth. After which they invested a large part of their time researching and compiling the most relevant data for our readers.

The editorial board has been involved in producing this book since its inception. They have spent rigorous hours researching and exploring the diverse topics which have resulted in the successful publishing of this book. They have passed on their knowledge of decades through this book. To expedite this challenging task, the publisher supported the team at every step. A small team of assistant editors was also appointed to further simplify the editing procedure and attain best results for the readers.

Apart from the editorial board, the designing team has also invested a significant amount of their time in understanding the subject and creating the most relevant covers. They scrutinized every image to scout for the most suitable representation of the subject and create an appropriate cover for the book.

The publishing team has been an ardent support to the editorial, designing and production team. Their endless efforts to recruit the best for this project, has resulted in the accomplishment of this book. They are a veteran in the field of academics and their pool of knowledge is as vast as their experience in printing. Their expertise and guidance has proved useful at every step. Their uncompromising quality standards have made this book an exceptional effort. Their encouragement from time to time has been an inspiration for everyone.

The publisher and the editorial board hope that this book will prove to be a valuable piece of knowledge for researchers, students, practitioners and scholars across the globe.

List of Contributors

Wolfgang Baar, Ulrich Goebel, Hartmut Buerkle, Kai Kaufmann and Sebastian Heinrich
Department of Anesthesiology and Critical Care, Medical Center, Faculty of Medicine, University of Freiburg, Hugstetter Strasse 55, 79106 Freiburg, Germany

Bernd Jaenigen
Department of General and Visceral Surgery, Medical Center, Faculty of Medicine, University of Freiburg, Hugstetter Strasse 55, 79106 Freiburg, Germany

Thomas Rössel, Christopher Uhlig, Thea Koch, Torsten Richter and Peter Markus Spieth
Department of Anaesthesiology and Critical Care Medicine, University Hospital Carl Gustav Carus Dresden, Technische Universität Dresden, Fetscherstr. 74, 01307 Dresden, Germany

Jörg Pietsch
Institute of Legal Medicine, Technische Universität Dresden, Dresden, Germany

Stefan Ludwig
Department of Visceral, Thoracic and Vascular Surgery, University Hospital Carl Gustav Carus, Technische Universität Dresden, Dresden, Germany

Stephan Kersting
Department of Visceral, Thoracic and Vascular Surgery, University Hospital Carl Gustav Carus, Technische Universität Dresden, Dresden, Germany
Department of General Surgery, University Hospital of Friedrich-Alexander-University, Erlangen, Germany

Pasquale Sansone, Luca Gregorio Giaccari, Caterina Aurilio, Francesco Coppolino, Maria Beatrice Passavanti, Vincenzo Pota and Maria Caterina Pace
Department of Woman, Child and General and Specialized Surgery, University of Campania "Luigi Vanvitelli", Piazza Luigi Miraglia, 2, Naples, Italy

Mario Faenza, Pasquale Di Costanzo and Sara Izzo
Multidisciplinary Department of Medical Surgical and Dental Sciences - Plastic Surgery Unit, University of Campania "Luigi Vanvitelli", Naples, Italy

Yanshuang Wang and Mingjun Xu
Department of Anesthesiology, Beijing Obstetrics and Gynecology Hospital, Capital Medical University, Beijing 100029, China

Jinguo Wang and Junyan Liu
Department of Urology, The First Hospital of Jilin University, No.1 Xinmin Street, Changchun, Jilin 130021, China

Zaitang Wang
Department of Taxation, School of Public Economics and Administration of Shanghai University of Finance and Economics, NO.777, Guoding Road, Yangpu District, Shanghai 200433, China

Na Wang
Department of Anesthesiology, The First Hospital of Jilin University, No.1 Xinmin Street, Changchun, Jilin 130021, China

Bo Qu, Luying Chen, Yuling Zhang and Mengting Jiang
Guangzhou University of Chinese Medicine, Guangzhou 510405, Guangdong, China

Caineng Wu, Wuhua Ma and Yuhui Li
Department of Anesthesiology, The First Affiliated Hospital of Guangzhou University of Chinese Medicine, Guangzhou 510405, Guangdong, China

Andrés Felipe Gil Blanco, Pascal Laferrière-Langlois, Frédérick D'Aragon, Yanick Sansoucy and Pablo Echave
Department of Anesthesiology, Medicine and Health Sciences Faculty, Centre Hospitalier Universitaire de Sherbrooke (CHUS), 3001, 12e Avenue Nord, Sherbrooke, QC J1H 5N4, Canada

David Jessop and Natalie Albert
Department of Anesthesiology, Medicine and Health Sciences Faculty, Centre Hospitalier Universitaire de Laval (CHUL), 2705 boul Laurier, Quebec G1V 4G2, QC, Canada

Pascal Tétreault
Department of Biomedical Engineering, Faculty of medicine and Dentistry, University of Alberta, 1098 Research Transition Facility, Edmonton T6G 2V2, AB, Canada

Xiao-xiao Li, Xue-li Lv and Xing-he Wang
Jiangsu Province Key Laboratory of Anesthesiology, Xuzhou Medical University, Xuzhou, Jiangsu, China

Yu-mei Li
Feng Xian People's Hospital of Jiangsu Province, Xuzhou, Jiangsu, China

Su Liu
Jiangsu Province Key Laboratory of Anesthesiology, Xuzhou Medical University, Xuzhou, Jiangsu, China
Department of Anesthesiology, the Affiliated Hospital of Xuzhou Medical University, 99 Huaihai West Road, Xuzhou 221000, Jiangsu, China

Heba Omar, Amany Hassan, Passaint Hassan, Ahmed Elshall, Dalia Khaled, Maha Mostafa, Pierre Zarif Tawadros, Mona Hossam Eldin, Mai Wedad and Bassant Mohamed Abdelhamid
Anesthesia Department, Faculty of Medicine, Cairo University, Cairo, Egypt

Wessam Adel Aboella
El Sahel Teaching Hospital, Cairo, Egypt

Mohammed Mahmoud Hassan
Anesthesia Department, National Cancer Institute, Cairo University, Cairo, Egypt

J. U. Han, B. G. Kim, C. Yang, W. H. Choi, J. Jeong, K. J. Lee and H. Kim
Department of Anesthesiology and Pain Medicine, Inha University College of Medicine, 27, Inhang-ro, Jung-gu, Incheon, Republic of Korea

Bruno Antonio Zanfini, Salvatore De Martino, Luciano Frassanito, Stefano Catarci, Francesco Vitale di Maio, Pietro Paolo Giuri, Gian Luigi Gonnella and Gaetano Draisci
Fondazione Policlinico Universitario Agostino Gemelli IRCCS, Università Cattolica del Sacro Cuore, Scienze dell'Emergenza, Anestesiologiche e della Rianimazione, Largo A. Gemelli 8, 00168 Rome, Italy

Daniel Hägi-Pedersen and Kasper Højgaard Thybo
Department of Anesthesiology, Naestved Hospital, Naestved, Denmark

Frederik Vilhelmsen and Mariam Nersesjan
Department of Anesthesiology, Naestved Hospital, Naestved, Denmark
CAR, Department of Anesthesiology, Centre of Anaesthesiological Research-Zealand University Hospital, Koege, Denmark

Jakob Hessel Andersen, Jakob Klim Danker and Ole Mathiesen
CAR, Department of Anesthesiology, Centre of Anaesthesiological Research-Zealand University Hospital, Koege, Denmark

Leif Broeng
Department of Orthopedics, Zealand University Hospital, Koege, Denmark

Eun Hee Chun
Department of Anesthesiology and Pain Medicine, Kangnam Sacred Heart Hospital, Hallym University College of Medicine, Seoul, Republic of Korea

Sooyoung Cho, Jae Hee Woo and Youn Jin Kim
Department of Anesthesiology and Pain Medicine, College of Medicine, Ewha Womans University, 25 Magokdong-ro 2-gil, Gangseo-gu, Seoul, Republic of Korea

Antonio Moraitis and Jakob Walldén
Department of Surgical and Perioperative Sciences, Anaesthesiology and Intensive Care Medicine (Sundsvall), Umeå University, Sundsvall, Sweden

Magnus Hultin
Department of Surgical and Perioperative Sciences, Anaesthesiology and Intensive Care Medicine (Umeå), Umeå University, Umeå, Sweden

Roser Vives and Caridad Pontes
Departament de Farmacologia, de Terapèutica i de Toxicologia, UAB, Clinical Pharmacology Unit, Parc Taulí Hospital Universitari, Institut d'Investigació i Innovació Parc Taulí I3PT, Universitat Autònoma de Barcelona, Parc Taulí 1, 08028 Sabadell (Barcelona), Spain

Diana Fernandez-Galinski, Francisca Gordo, Alberto Izquierdo and Carmen Colilles
Anesthesiology Department, Parc Taulí Hospital Universitari, Institut d'Investigació i Innovació Parc Taulí I3PT, Universitat Autònoma de Barcelona, Parc Taulí 1, 08028 Sabadell (Barcelona), Spain

Joan C. Oliva
Statistics Unit, Parc Taulí Hospital Universitari, Institut d'Investigació i Innovació Parc Taulí I3PT, Universitat Autònoma de Barcelona, Parc Taulí 1, 08028 Sabadell (Barcelona), Spain

Irwin Gratz, Magdy Takla, Brian McEniry and Edward Deal
Cooper University Hospital, 1 Cooper Plaza, Camden, NJ 08103, USA

Martin Baruch
Caretaker Medical, Charlottesville, VA, USA

Julia Seaman
Quahog Research Group, Oakland, CA, USA

Isabel Allen
University of California - San Francisco, San Francisco, CA, USA

Young Sung Kim, Hyo Sung Kim, Hyerim Jeong, Chung Hun Lee, Mi Kyoung Lee and Sang Sik Choi
Department of Anesthesiology and Pain Medicine, Korea University Guro Hospital, 148 Gurodong-ro, Guro-gu, Seoul 08308, South Korea

Yamini Subramani, Mahesh Nagappa, Yun Fei Zhu and Sudha (Indu) Singh
Department of Anesthesia and Perioperative Medicine, Schulich School of Medicine, & Dentistry, Western University, London Health Sciences Centre- University Hospital, (LHSC-UH), London, Ontario, Canada

Lee-Anne Fochesato, Moaz Bin Yunus Chohan and Kevin Armstrong
Department of Anesthesia and Perioperative Medicine, London Health Sciences Centre and St. Joseph's Health Care, Western University, London, Ontario, Canada

Kamal Kumar
Department of Anesthesia and Perioperative Medicine, Schulich School of Medicine, & Dentistry, Western University, London Health Sciences Centre- Victoria Hospital, (LHSC-VH) , London, Ontario, Canada

Dan Huang, Linjie Zhu, Jie Chen and Jie Zhou
Department of Anesthesiology, Renji Hospital, School of Medicine, Shanghai Jiaotong University, Shanghai 200127, China

George L.Tewfik, Adam N.Work, Steven M.Shulman and Patrick Discepola
Department of Anesthesiology, Rutgers, New Jersey Medical School, 185 South Orange Ave., Newark, NJ 07103, USA

Alessandro Svelato and Antonio Ragusa
Department of Obstetrics and Gynecology, Massa Carrara General Hospital, Via Enrico Mattei, 54100 Massa Carrara, Italy

Alberto Rutili and Caterina Bertelloni
Department of Anaesthesia, Massa Carrara General Hospital, Massa Carrara, Italy

Domenico Foti
Department of Neurosurgery, S. Chiara Hospital, Pisa, Italy

Angela Capizzi
Department of Obstetrics and Gynecology, Imperia General Hospital, Imperia, Italy

Hoda Shokri
Assistant Professor of Anaesthesiology, Ain Shams University, Cairo, Egypt

Amr A. Kasem
Lecturer of Anaesthesiology, Ain Shams University, Cairo, Egypt

Wei Bing Wang, Ai Jiao Sun, Hong Ping Yu, Jing Chun Dong and Huang Xu
Department of Anesthesiology, The Affiliated AnQing Hospitals of Anhui Medical University, 352th, Renming Road, AnQing 246003, AnHui province, China

Ting-ting Ni
Department of Anesthesiology, NO.7 Hospital of Ningbo, Ningbo, Zhejiang Province, China

Zhen-feng Zhou
Department of Anesthesiology, People's Hospital of Zhejiang Provincial (People's Hospital of Hangzhou Medicine College), Hangzhou, Zhejiang Province, China

Bo He
Department of Gynecology, NO.7Hospital of Ningbo, Ningbo, Zhejiang Province, China

Qing-he Zhou
Department of Anesthesiology, The Affiliated Hospital of Jiaxing University, Jiaxing, Zhejiang Province, China

João Carlos Macêdo Fernandes de Oliveira Junior
Department of Anesthesiology, São Rafael Hospital, D'Or Institute for Research and Education (IDOR), Salvador, Brazil

Guilherme Oliveira Campos
Department of Anesthesiology, São Rafael Hospital, D'Or Institute for Research and Education (IDOR), Salvador, Brazil
Department of Anesthesiology, Cardiopulmonar Hospital, Salvador, Brazil

Marcelo de Jesus Martins and Norma Sueli Pinheiro Módolo
Department of Anesthesiology, São Paulo State University, Botucatu, Brazil

Gabriel Nascimento Jesus and Rodrigo Leal Alves
Department of Anesthesiology, São Rafael Hospital, D'Or Institute for Research and Education (IDOR), Salvador, Brazil
Federal University of Bahia, Salvador, Brazil

Paulo Roberto Rios de Oliveira and Caio Nogueira Lessa
Department of Gynecology, São Rafael Hospital, D'Or Institute for Research and Education (IDOR), Salvador, Brazil

Lucas Jorge Santana de Castro Alves
Department of Anesthesiology, Santo Antonio Hospital, Salvador, Brazil

Liping Wang, Hong Chen, Yang Xu and Yu Wang
Department of Anaesthesiology, Harbin Medical University Cancer Hospital, No. 150 Haping Rd., Nangang District, Harbin 150081, China

Si Liang
Department of Anaesthesiology, Affiliated Hospital of HeBei University, Baoding, China

Index

www.ingramcontent.com/pod-product-compliance
Lightning Source LLC
LaVergne TN
LVHW060514210926
848485LV00005B/1079